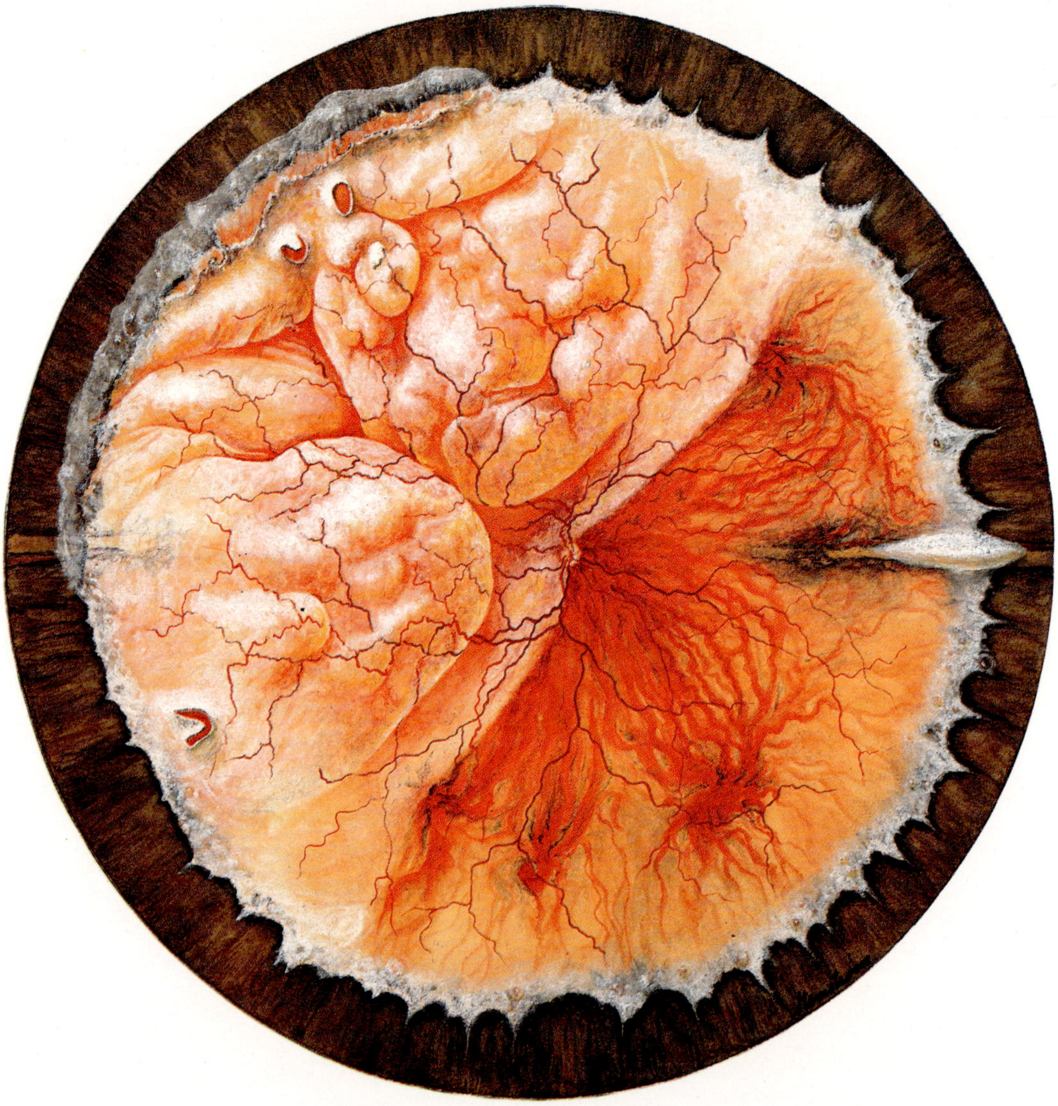

atlas of the PERIPHERAL RETINA

Frank C. Bell, M.D.
Chief of Ophthalmology, St. Joseph's Hospital, Atlanta, Georgia
Clinical Assistant Professor of Ophthalmology
Emory University School of Medicine, Atlanta, Georgia

William J. Stenstrom, M.Ed.
Professor of Medical Illustration
Medical College of Georgia, Augusta, Georgia

W.B. SAUNDERS COMPANY 1983
Philadelphia London Toronto Mexico City Rio de Janeiro Sydney Tokyo

W. B. Saunders Company: West Washington Square
Philadelphia, PA 19105

1 St. Anne's Road
Eastbourne, East Sussex BN21 3UN, England

1 Goldthorne Avenue
Toronto, Ontario M8Z 5T9, Canada

Apartado 26370—Cedro 512
Mexico 4, D.F., Mexico

Rua Coronel Cabrita, 8
Sao Cristovao Caixa Postal 21176
Rio de Janeiro, Brazil

9 Waltham Street
Artarmon, N.S.W. 2064, Australia

Ichibancho, Central Bldg., 22-1 Ichibancho
Chiyoda-Ku, Tokyo 102, Japan

Library of Congress Cataloging in Publication Data

Bell, Frank C.

Atlas of the peripheral retina.

1. Retina—Diseases—Atlases. I. Stenstrom, William J. II. Title. [DNLM: 1. Retinal diseases—Atlases. 2. Retina—Atlases. WW 17 B433a]

RE551.B43 1983 617.7'3075 82-24063

ISBN 0-7216-1669-0

Atlas of the Peripheral Retina ISBN 0-7216-1669-0

Last digit is the print number: 9 8 7 6 5 4 3 2 1

To
Kathy
and
Bobbie

PREFACE

Our purpose in publishing this atlas is to present the clinical appearances found in the peripheral retina in an interesting and educational manner. This is a book for the practitioner; a book to aid in the diagnosis of confusing cases. It is not meant as an exhaustive treatise on the pathology or treatment of peripheral fundus lesions. The references included are intended to be pertinent, not exhaustive.

We have chosen the artist's color illustrations as the best means to present the lesions of the peripheral fundus. The artist has the advantage of being able to synthesize many features of a disease process into a single picture, in a manner photographs alone cannot do.

It is our hope that this book will aid the student as well as the experienced practitioner in making the correct diagnosis of peripheral fundus disease.

FRANK C. BELL
WILLIAM J. STENSTROM

CONTENTS

Chapter One

BASIC ANATOMY, ORIENTATION, AND MAJOR LANDMARKS

BASIC ANATOMY

The retina of the eye performs the miraculous function of changing light energy into images that we can perceive. The retina normally lines the inside of the eye, as shown in Figure 1–1. The cornea and lens are optical components of the eye that form an image on the retina, while the iris controls the amount of light

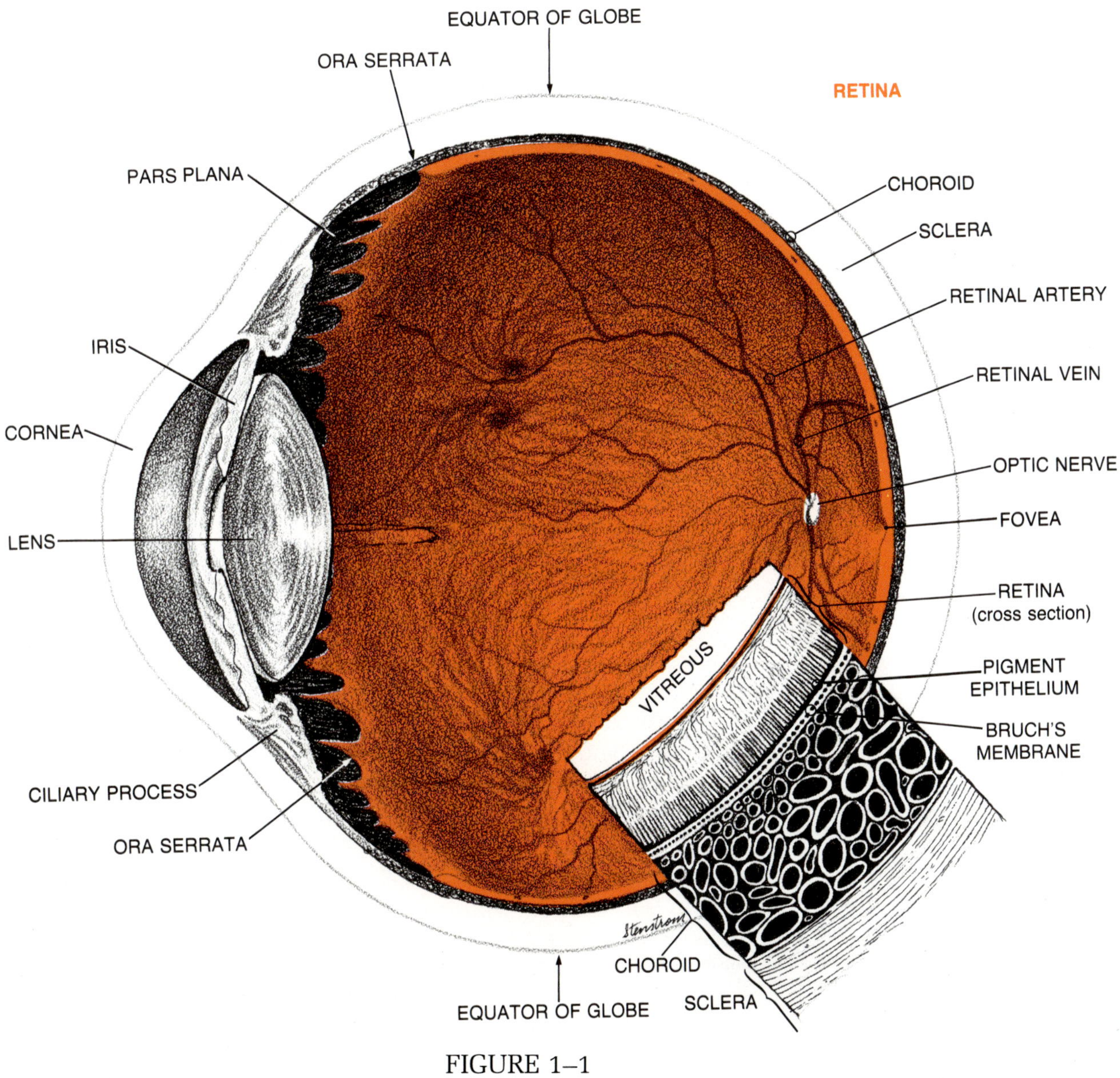

FIGURE 1–1

entering the eye. The pigment epithelium, Bruch's membrane, and choroid lie adjacent to the retina and perform nutritive and regenerative functions. The vitreous, a clear gel, fills the central cavity of the eye, while the sclera functions as a rigid outer wall of the eye.

The optic nerve is composed of neurons that originate in the retina and exit from the eye to the brain. The retinal arteries and veins emerge from the optic nerve and provide much of the blood supply for the retina. The arteries divide into many branches and become smaller and smaller until they become a capillary network too small to see with the opththalmoscope. The capillaries then coalesce into small venules and finally into the retinal veins. At the optic nerve, the retinal arteries and veins can be distinguished by their color and size. The arteries are brighter red and smaller in diameter; the veins are darker red and larger in size.

The macula is the specialized portion of the retina on which the cornea and lens focus the optical image. The macula is more darkly pigmented than the remainder of the retina. In the direct center of the macula is the fovea, a pinpoint area devoid of blood vessels. The fovea has the sharpest visual acuity of any part of the retina.

In the periphery, the equator represents the greatest circumference of the retina. At the edge of the retina is the ora serrata, the boundary between the seeing retina and the nonseeing pars plana.

Marchesani O, Sautter H: Atlas of the Ocular Fundus, New York, Hafner Publishing Co, 1959 (Translated by A Phillipp)

Michaelson IC: Textbook of the Fundus of the Eye. 3rd ed, Baltimore, Williams & Wilkins, 1981

Polyak SL: The Retina. Chicago, University of Chicago Press, 1941

Straatsma DR, Hall MV, Allen RA, Crescitelli F: The Retina. Los Angeles, University of California Press, 1969

Thiel R: Atlas of Diseases of the Eye, Vol II, Amsterdam, Elsevier Publishing Co, 1963 (Translated by D Guerry, W J Geeraets, and H Wiesinger)

Wolff E: Anatomy of the Eye and Orbit. 7th ed,. Philadelphia, W B Saunders Co, 1977 (Revised by R Warwick)

ORIENTATION

The retina is the innermost layer of the spherical eye. From the science of cartography (map making), it is known that spherical surfaces cannot be represented on flat surfaces without distortion. In drawings and paintings of the retina, however, the retina is represented as a flat surface with the understanding that certain distortions are present. Figure 1–2 shows the retina portrayed on a flat surface, the standard fundus drawing chart. The accepted distortions include the fact that the disc and macula are relatively minified, while the peripheral retina, the equator, and ora serrata are relatively magnified. Also, the ora serrata is represented as larger in circumference than the equator, while in reality the equator is larger.

In the center of the diagram, the optic nerve is represented by a small circle, while the fovea, the area of sharpest vision, is

Close inspection of the ora serrata reveals that it is not entirely straight but composed of a series of gentle, crescent-shaped indentations. These crescent-shaped scallops of the ora serrata are called ora bays. Ora bays are much more prominent in the nasal ora serrata than in the temporal ora. Between each ora bay is an anteriorly directed finger of retina called an ora serrata tooth, or dentate process, that extends out onto the pars plana. Further anteriorly, the posterior portion of the ciliary processes can be observed with the usual examining method of indirect ophthalmoscopy and scleral depression.

In many eyes, there can be observed a transition between the more deeply crescentic nasal ora serrata and the relatively straighter temporal ora serrata. This transition occurs superiorly and inferiorly, but not at exactly the 12 o'clock and 6 o'clock meridians. The transition is usually slightly temporal to the 12 o'clock meridian superiorly and nasal to the 6 o'clock meridian inferiorly (Fig. 1–12). This change, from the more scalloped nasal ora to the less scalloped temporal ora, is called the anatomical vertical meridian. This transition marks the watershed between the drainage fields of the nasal and temporal vortex vein collection systems.

Foos R Y: Vitreoretinal juncture, topographical variations. Invest Ophthalmol *11*:801–808, 1972

Okun E: Gross and microscopic pathology in autopsy eyes. I. Introduction and long posterior ciliary nerves. Am J Ophathalmol *50*:424–429, 1960

Rutnin U: Fundus appearance in normal eyes. I. The choroid. Am J Ophthalmol *64*:821–839, 1967

Salzman M: The Anatomy and Histology of the Human Eyeball in the Normal State: Its Development and Senescence. Chicago, 1912, University of Chicago Press (Translated by E U L Brown)

Straatsma BR, Landers MB, Kreiger AE: The ora serrata in the adult human eye. Arch Ophthalmol *80*:3–20, 1968

Tasman W, Shields JA: Disorders of the Peripheral Fundus. Hagerstown, Maryland, Harper & Row Publishers, 1980

Thiel HL: Bietrage zur Anatomie der Ora serrata. Ber Deutsch Ophth Ges *58*:249–256, 1953

Thiel HL: Zur topographischen and histologischen Situation der Ora serrata. Grafe Arch Ophthal *156*:590–629, 1955

Chapter Two

PERIPHERAL RETINAL APPEARANCES AND DEGENERATIONS

CYSTOID DEGENERATION

Cystoid degeneration of the retina is characterized by small bubbles or vacuoles in the peripheral retina near the ora serrata. These small cysts occur in the outer plexiform and inner nuclear layers of the retina. Cystoid degeneration is of universal occurrence, having been found in virtually all eyes, including those of premature infants and octogenarians. The cysts increase in number with advancing age, rarely becoming numerous before the age of eight and becoming widespread only after the fourth decade. Males and females are equally affected, and the eyes of a given patient are usually bilaterally symmetrical. There usually is more cystoid degeneration in the temporal retina than in the nasal area, and the degeneration occurs more superiorly than inferiorly. In the nasal retina, cysts may occur in the dentate processes and in clumps at the base of a dentate process. In the temporal retina, the cysts are aligned parallel to the ora serrata, with the more recently formed cysts developing posteriorly to the established cysts. Multiple rows of cystoid degeneration give the peripheral margin of the retina a thickened, white appearance.

The inner wall of a single cyst may be absent, giving the appearance of a retinal hole. Usually this is a pseudo-hole, since the outer wall of the cyst is intact. Most observers believe that retinal detachment seldom, if ever, is caused by a retinal hole in cystoid degeneration. There is also no known relationship between cystoid degeneration and any systemic disease.

A second type of cystoid degeneration, called reticular cystoid degeneration, has been seen in eyes of cadavers. Reticular cystoid degeneration occurs posterior to regular cystoid degeneration, and differs histologically from the regular cystoid.

Foos RY, Feman SS: Reticular cystoid degeneration of the peripheral retina. Am J Ophthalmol 69:392–403, 1970

Gottinger W: Rasterelektronen mikroskopische Befunde bei peripheren cystoiden Degenerationen. Deutsch Ophthal Ges 74:147–149, 1967

O'Malley PF, Allen RA: Peripheral cystoid degeneration of the retina. Arch Ophthalmol 77:769–776, 1967

Rutnin U, Schepens CL: Fundus appearance in normal eyes III. Peripheral degenerations. Am J Ophthalmol 64:1040–1062, 1967

Teng CC, Katzin HM: An anatomic study of the peripheral retina II. Peripheral cystoid degeneration of the retina, formation of cysts and holes. Am J Ophthalmol 36:29–49, 1953

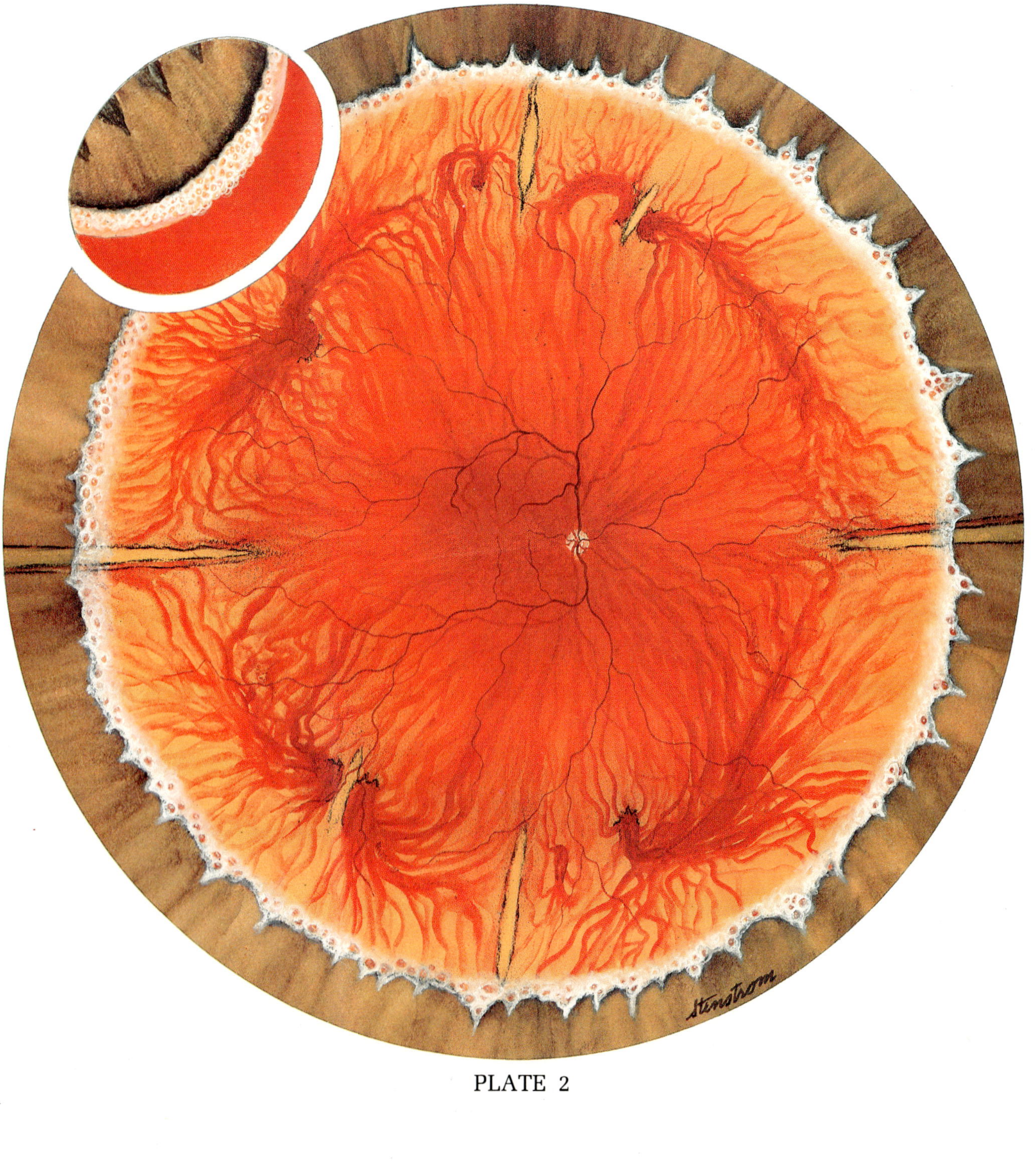

PLATE 2

IRREGULAR ORA BAYS AND TEETH

Normal anatomic variations of ora bays and teeth are frequently confused with pathological structures. In this composite illustration, several interesting variations of the ora structures are visualized as they are seen with indirect ophthalmoscopy and scleral depression.

In the 1:30 o'clock meridian is one of the most interesting of these variations, a bridging dentate process. This large, white dentate process extends from just behind the ora serrata to the mid pars plana. It is entirely elevated into the vitreous base, touching the retina and pars plana only at its ends. Extensive cystoid changes are frequently present in these bridging dentate processes.

In the 3 o'clock meridian a large ora bay extends posterior to the normal curve of the ora serrata. A similar large ora bay is present in the 9 o'clock meridian that is almost completely enclosed. These partially or completely enclosed posteriorly extending ora bays should not be considered as open retinal holes, as they are completely covered by ciliary epithelium from the pars plana. It is not unusual for a partial thickness retinal erosion to be present immediately posterior to a large posteriorly extending ora bay, and if a posterior vitreous detachment occurs, a full thickness retinal hole may be torn in the retina at the time of vitreous detachment.

In the 4:30 o'clock meridian two adjacent dentate processes curve toward one another, almost completely enclosing a portion of the pars plana. A smaller, completely enclosed area of pars plana is shown in the 7 o'clock meridian, immediately behind a dentate process. Neither partially nor completely enclosed areas of the pars plana should be confused with retinal holes.

In the 10:30 o'clock meridian a giant dentate process is seen as a broad expanse extending far peripherally. Frequently there is extensive cystoid degeneration in such giant dentate processes. Usually such giant processes are meridionally aligned with a ciliary process, producing a structure known as a meridional complex. Retinal erosion may be present immediately behind a meridional complex, sometimes developing into a full thickness retinal hole.

Rutnin U, Schepens CL: Fundus appearance in normal eyes II. The standard peripheral fundus and developmental variations. Am J Ophthalmol *64*:840–852, 1967

Spencer LM, Foos RY, Straatsma BR: Meridional folds and meridional complexes of the peripheral retina. Trans Am Acad Ophthalmol Otolaryngol *73*:204–221, 1969

Spencer LM, Foos RY, Straatsma BR: Enclosed bays of the ora serrata. Arch Ophthalmol *83*:421–425, 1970

Straatsma BR, Landers MB, Kreiger AE: The ora serrata in the adult human eye. Arch Ophthalmol *80*:3–20, 1968

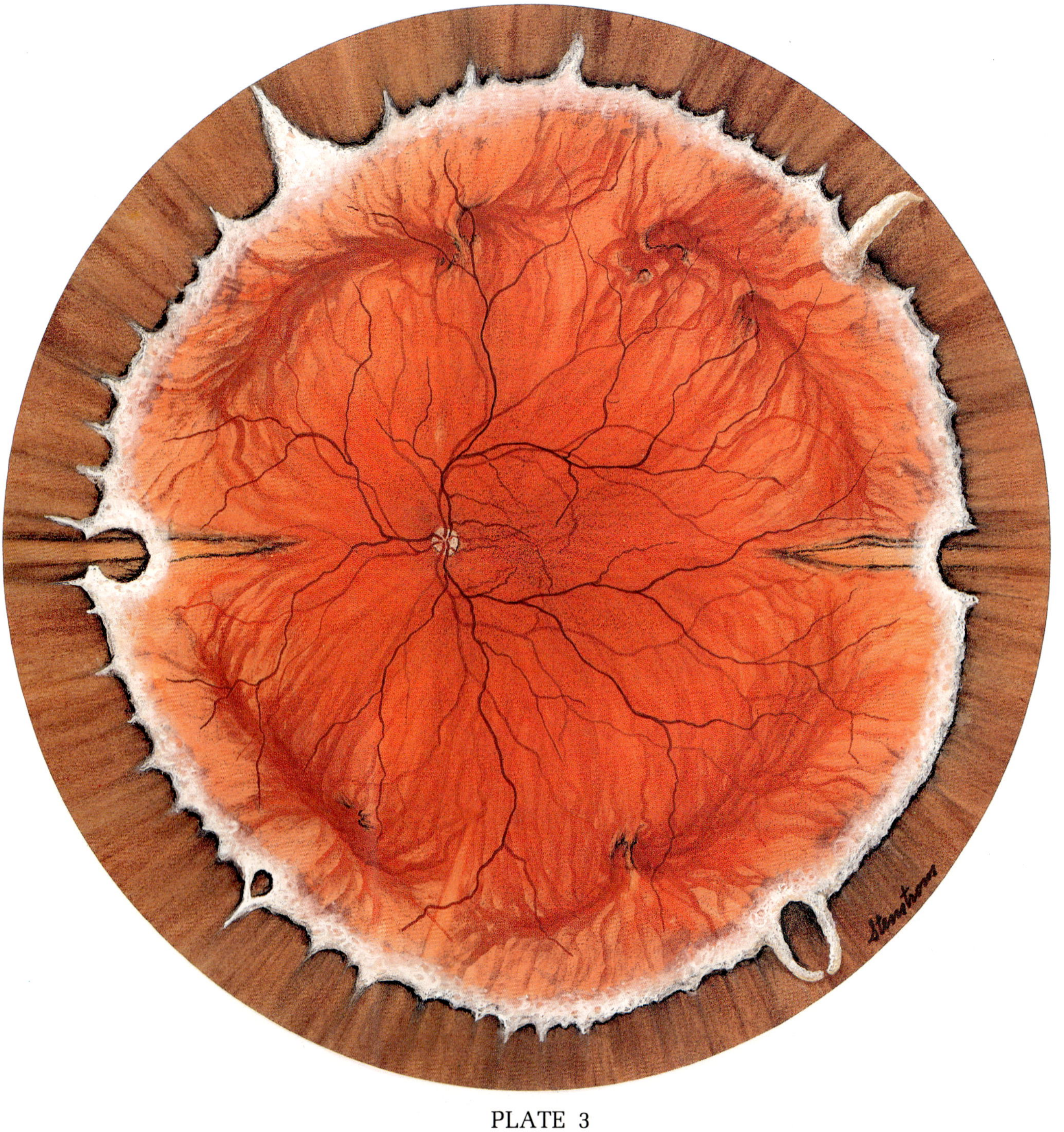

PLATE 3

GRANULAR TAGS AND ORA PEARLS

Typical granular tags are shown in the illustration on the left. These discrete white to gray irregular clumps on the retinal surface are called granular tags, patches, globules, or cystic retinal tufts, depending on their size and configuration. These tags are elevated and have a granular-appearing surface. Most are located immediately posterior to the ora serrata and are more common nasally than temporally. Granular tags are very common, being observed in approximately 38 percent of patients. Histologic study shows small masses of cells similar to the nonpigmented epithelium that covers the pars plana. Frequently, granular tags are surrounded by cystic degeneration of the retina. It is believed that granular tags are congenital in origin.

Granular tags may separate from the retina either spontaneously or with the development of a posterior vitreous detachment. With spontaneous separation, the elevated tag is seen floating freely in the vitreous base unattached to the retina. It has been demonstrated microscopically that tiny fibrils may extend from the granular tag tissue into the vitreous, producing a firm vitreous adhesion. With posterior vitreous detachment the granular tag may be avulsed from the retinal surface, producing either a partial or full thickness retinal hole. A small percentage of retinal detachments are believed to be produced by this mechanism.

Ora serrata pearls appear exactly as the name implies. They are white, glistening round structures present on the pars plana or on the peripheral retina adjacent to the ora serrata. They are relatively common, occurring in approximately 20 percent of all eyes. The darkly colored pearls are believed to receive their pigmentation from the adjacent pigment epithelium. Most pearls, however, are white and appear calcified. Histologically they stain as an acid carbohydrate, staining positively with the periodic acid-Schiff reaction. Despite their distinctive appearance, ora serrata pearls have no pathologic significance.

Byer NE: Cystic retinal tufts and their relationship to retinal detachment. Arch Ophthalmol *99*:1788–1790, 1981

Foos RY: Vitreous base, retinal tufts, and retinal tears: Pathogenic relationships. *In* Pruett RC, Regan CDJ (eds): Retina Congress. New York, Appleton-Century-Crofts, 1972, pp 259–279

Foos RY, Allen RA: Retinal tears and lesser lesions of the peripheral retina in autopsy eyes. Am J Ophthalmol *64*:643–655, 1967

Lonn LI, Smith TR: Ora serrata pearls. Arch Ophthalmol *77*:809–813, 1967

Okun E: Gross and microscopic pathology in autopsy eyes III. Retinal breaks without detachment. Am J Ophthalmol *51*:369–391, 1961

Rutnin U, Schepens CL: Fundus appearance in normal eyes II. The standard peripheral fundus and developmental variations. Am J Ophthalmol *64*:840–854, 1967

Rutnin U, Schepens CL: Fundus appearance in normal eyes IV. Retinal breaks and other findings. Am J Ophthalmol *64*:1063–1078, 1967

Teng CC, Katzin HM: An anatomic study of the periphery of the retina I. Nonpigmented epithelial cell proliferation and hole formation. Am J Ophthalmol *34*:1237–1248, 1951

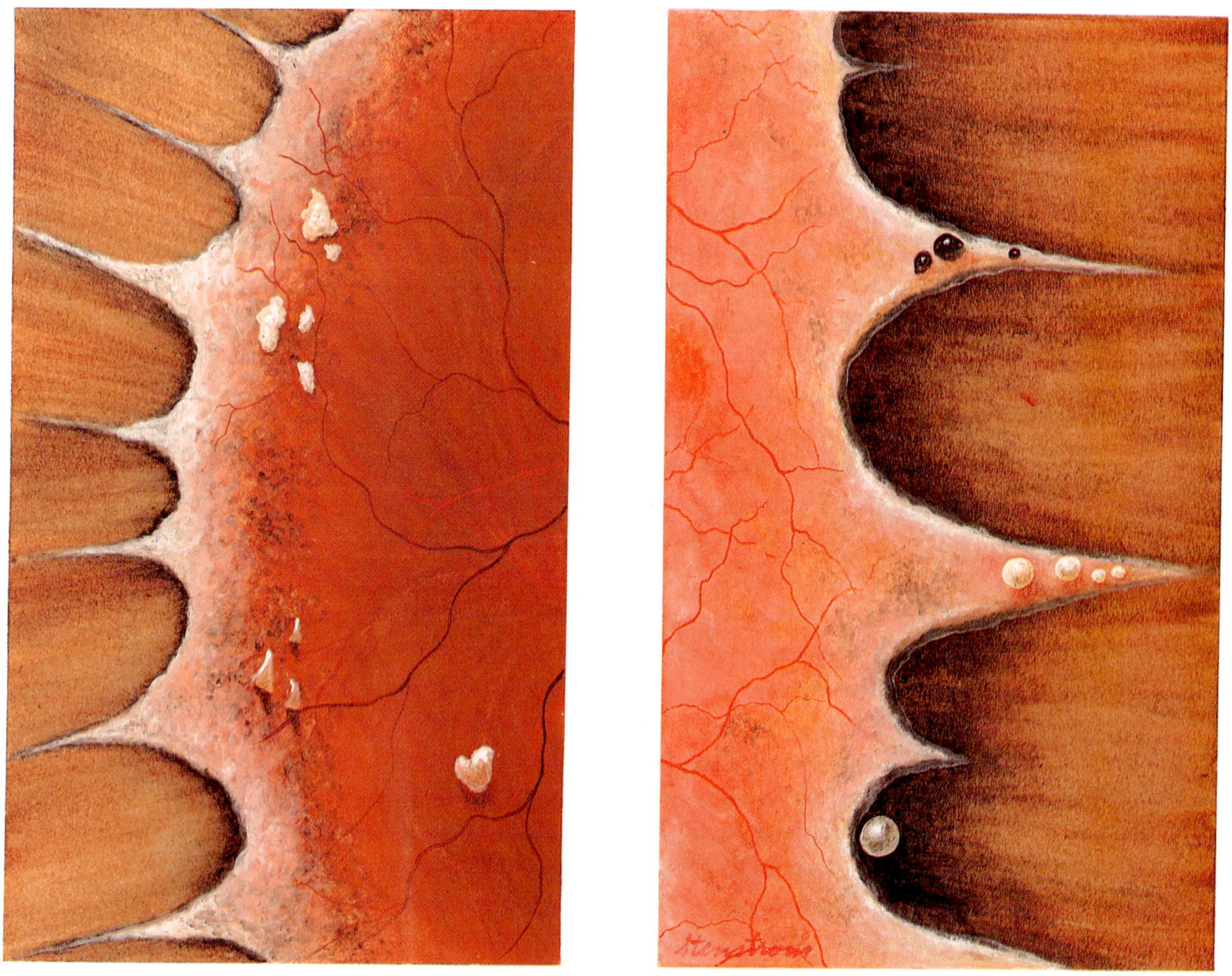

PLATE 4

MERIDIONAL FOLDS

Meridional folds are radially oriented gatherings or folds of retinal tissue oriented perpendicularly to the ora serrata. They are whiter than surrounding normal retina and are slightly elevated, with irregular cystoid degeneration present in the fold. Meridional folds are present in 20 percent of normal eyes, usually in the superior nasal quadrant, although they may be present in any meridian. Meridional folds are thought to be of congenital origin and to occur in an equal incidence in all age groups. There is no racial predilection, but for unknown reasons meridional folds are more common in males than females.

In the composite illustration, a meridional fold is shown in the 2 o'clock meridian extending from the ora serrata posteriorly almost to the equator. A normal retinal vessel courses over the fold. The meridional fold shown in the 5 o'clock meridian demonstrates a small retinal break in the posterior aspect of the fold. Such holes may produce a retinal detachment, particularly when they occur in a fold located in the temporal quadrants. Meridional folds may be aligned with either ora bays or dentate processes. The 8 o'clock meridional fold is located in the center of a prominent ora bay, a relationship noted in 19 percent of meridional folds. More commonly, a meridional fold is radially aligned with a dentate process, as shown in the 11 o'clock meridian. This relationship occurs in 81 percent of meridional folds. In addition to granular tags, peripheral retinal excavation, a partial thickness erosion of the retina, or retinal pigmentation may occur at the posterior extent of meridional folds.

Radial alignment of a dentate process and a ciliary process in the same meridian is called a meridional complex. Frequently, the dentate process is enlarged and contains a meridional fold. When such a meridional complex is observed, peripheral retinal excavation is particularly common posterior to the meridional fold.

Eisner G: Zur spaltlampenmikroskopischer Ora serrata und Pars plana Corporis ciliaris. Albrecht von Graefes Arch Klin Ophthalmol *177*:232–247, 1969

Rutnin U, Schepens CL: Fundus appearance in normal eyes II. The standard peripheral fundus and developmental variations. Am J Ophthalmol *64*:840–852, 1967

Spencer LM, Foos RY, Straatsma BR: Meridional folds and meridional complexes of the peripheral retina. Trans Am Acad Ophthalmol Otolaryngol *73*:204–221, 1969

Spencer LM, Foos RY, Straatsma BR: Meridional folds, meridional complexes, and associated abnormalities of the peripheral retina. Am J Ophthalmol *70*:697–714, 1970

Straatsma BR, Landers MB, Kreiger AE: The ora serrata in the adult human eye. Arch Ophthalmol *80*:3–20, 1968

Teng CC, Katzin HM: An anatomic study of the retina. Part I. Nonpigmented epithelial cell proliferation and hole formation. Am J Ophthalmol *34*:1237–1240, 1951

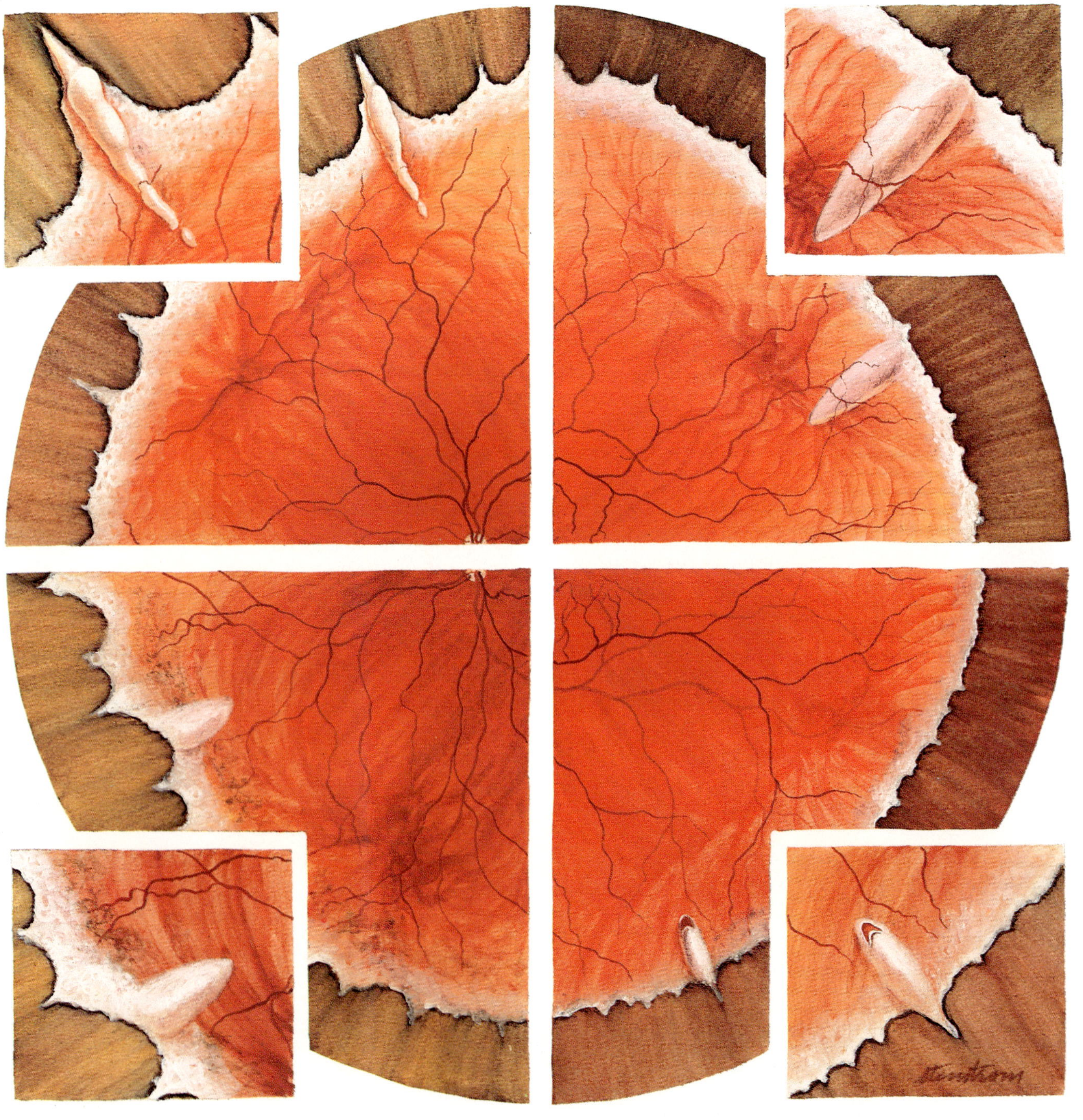

PLATE 5

WHITE WITH PRESSURE

White with pressure is a distinctive milky white or opalescent appearance of the peripheral retina that is observed in many normal eyes when examined with scleral depression. Without scleral depression the peripheral retina appears normal. When the depressor is applied, the peripheral retina between the ora serrata and equator appears to turn white and give the appearance of watered silk or moiré. The posterior margin is generally irregular and sharply demarcated from the posterior, normal-appearing retina. In the illustration, the retina is shown as it would be if the entire ora serrata were depressed.

White with pressure is common, being observed in approximately 32 percent of eyes examined with scleral depression. All quadrants may be involved, with the inferior nasal quadrant least likely to be affected. There is an equal incidence in males and females but there is an increase in incidence with age. White with pressure is particularly common in fundi that are heavily pigmented.

White with pressure is a benign condition and is not associated with peripheral retinal breaks. It is frequently observed around the margins of lattice degeneration and at the margins of cystoid degeneration and retinoschisis. The underlying choroidal markings are visible through the retina, but less so than in normal retina. White with pressure must be carefully distinguished from a peripheral subclinical retinal detachment.

Grignolo A: Ophthalmoscopy and other methods of examination. *In* Schepens CL, Regan CDJ (eds): Controversial Aspects of the Management of Retinal Detachment. Boston, Little Brown & Company, 1965, pp 2–28

Rutnin U, Schepens CL: Fundus appearance in normal eyes IV. Retinal breaks and other findings. Am J Ophthalmol 64:1063–1078, 1967

Schepens CL: Subclinical retinal detachments. Arch Ophthalmol 47:593–608, 1952

Watzke RC: The ophthalmic sign white with pressure. A clinicopathologic correlation. Arch Ophthalmol 66:812–823, 1961

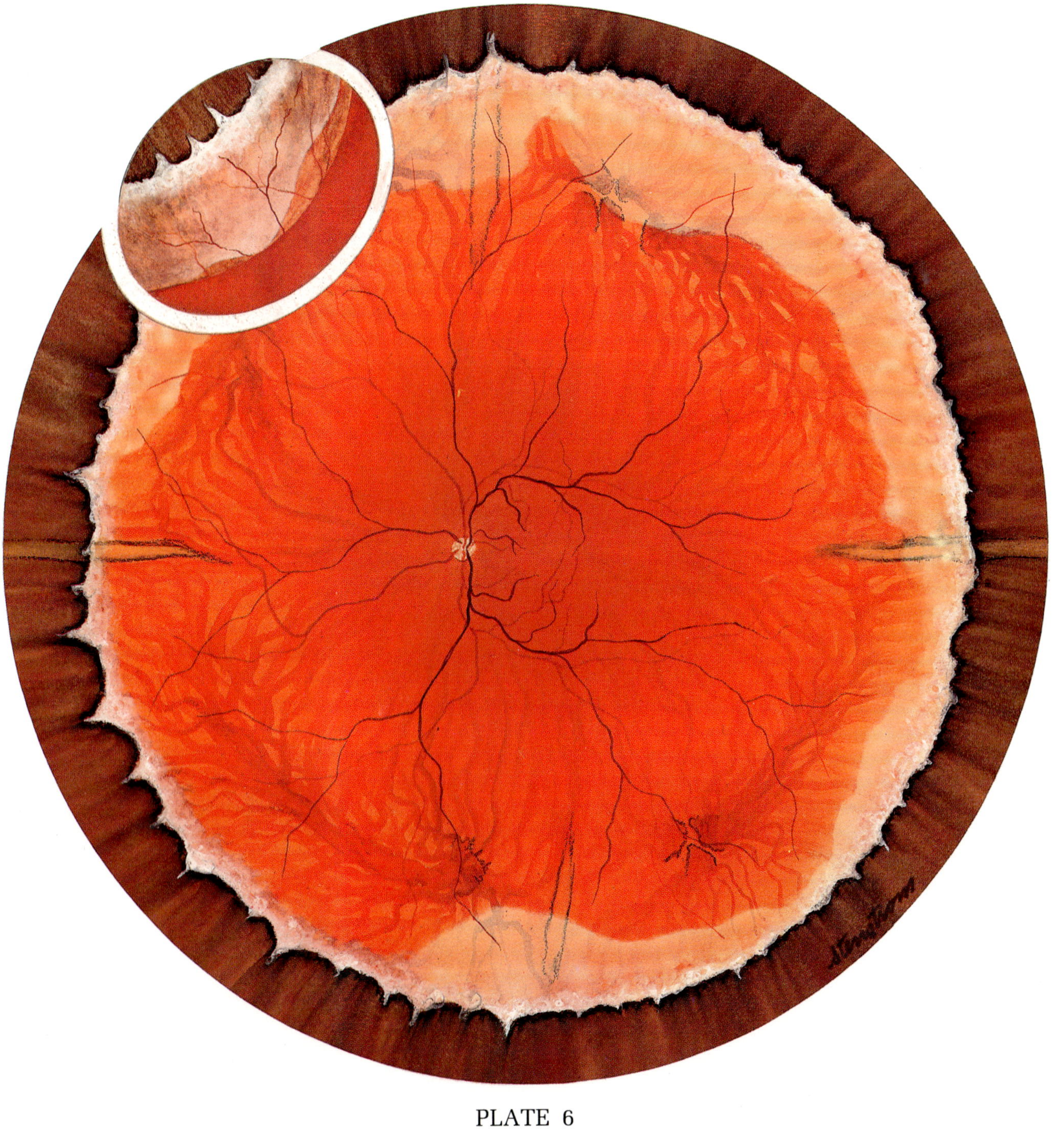

PLATE 6

WHITE WITHOUT PRESSURE

White without pressure is a distinctive white appearance of the peripheral retina that is visible without scleral depression. The retina appears whiter than in white with pressure, and the choroidal markings are almost obscured. The retinal vessels stand out in dramatic fashion but are entirely normal. If scleral depression is used, the whiteness of the peripheral retina is further accentuated. White without pressure generally occurs between the ora serrata and the equator, although it may extend posterior to the equator toward the optic nerve. Islands of normal retina may be incorporated in affected areas, and these islands should not be confused with retinal holes. The margins of white without pressure are very sharply demarcated from normal retina and may assume almost any configuration.

The cause of white without pressure is not precisely known, but the condition is generally assumed to be a manifestation of peripheral vitreous traction. There is, however, no necessary correlation with peripheral retinal holes. The dramatic appearance of white without pressure frequently causes confusion with subclinical retinal detachment and retinoschisis, but careful examination with scleral depression will reveal that the retina is in contact with the pigment epithelium and is not elevated.

Goldbaum MH, Joondeph H, Huamonte FU et al: White with pressure or white without pressure lesions. *In* Peyman GA, Sanders DR, Goldberg MF: Principles and Practice of Ophthalmology. Philadelphia, W. B. Saunders, 1980, pp 1027–1028

Karlin DB, Curtin BJ: Axial length measurements and peripheral fundus changes in the myopic eye. *In* Pruett RC, Regan CDJ (eds): Retina Congress. New York, Appleton-Century-Crofts, 1972, pp 629–642

Nagpal KC, Huamonte FU, Constantaras A, et al: Migratory white without pressure retinal lesions. Arch Ophthalmol *94*:576–579, 1976

Rutnin U, Schepens CL: Fundus appearance in normal eyes IV. Retinal breaks and other findings. Am J Ophthalmol *64*:1063–1078, 1967

Schepens CL: Subclinical retinal detachments. Arch Ophthalmol *47*:593–608, 1952

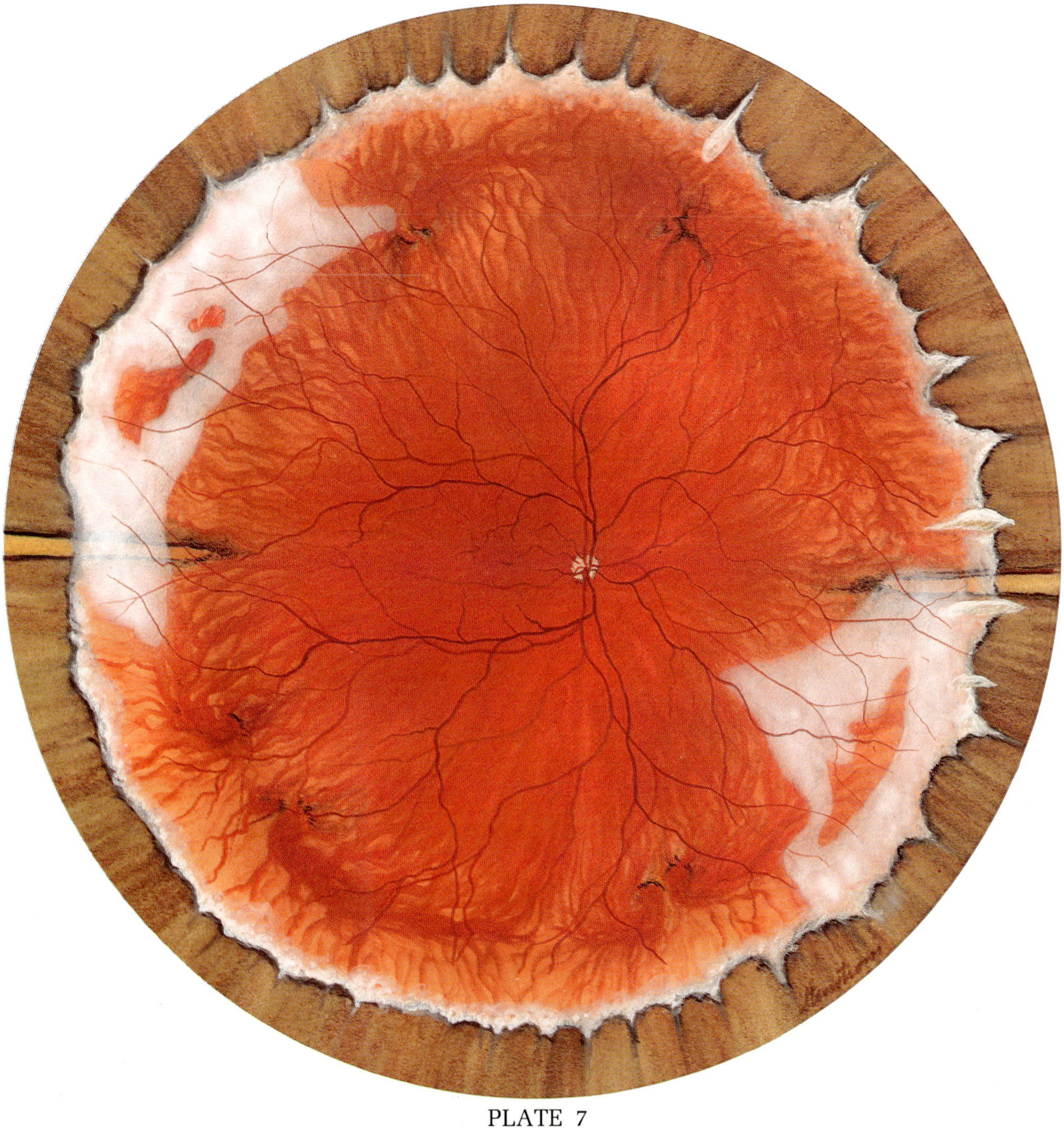

PLATE 7

PAVING STONE DEGENERATION

Paving stone degeneration has a dramatic appearance, revealing multiple rounded punched out areas of choroidal and retinal atrophy. These lesions are one to several disc diameters in size and are located in the far periphery of the retina between the equator and ora serrata. There is a definite predilection for the inferior nasal and temporal quadrants. The affected areas are yellow-white in color due to the sclera being partly visible through the atrophic choroid. Large choroidal vessels are seen running through the base of the lesion. The lesions are completely flat and have discrete margins which may have pigmented edges. Multiple round lesions may become confluent, producing a belt of choroidal atrophy in the peripheral retina.

Paving stone degeneration occurs in both sexes and becomes increasingly common with increasing age. Frequently it is bilateral. This relatively common degeneration is generally benign and should not be interpreted as multiple retinal holes.

O'Malley PF, Allen RA, Straatsma BR, O'Malley CC: Paving stone degeneration of the retina. Arch Ophthalmol 73:169–182, 1965

Schepens CL: Cobblestone degeneration of the retina. *In* Kimura SJ and Cagill WM (eds): Retinal Diseases. Philadelphia, Lea & Febiger, 1966, pp 195–203

Straatsma BR, Allen RA, O'Malley P, et al: Pathologic and clinical manifestations of paving stone degeneration of the retina. *In* McPherson A (ed): New and Controversial Aspects of Retinal Detachment. New York, Harper & Row, 1968, pp 76–99

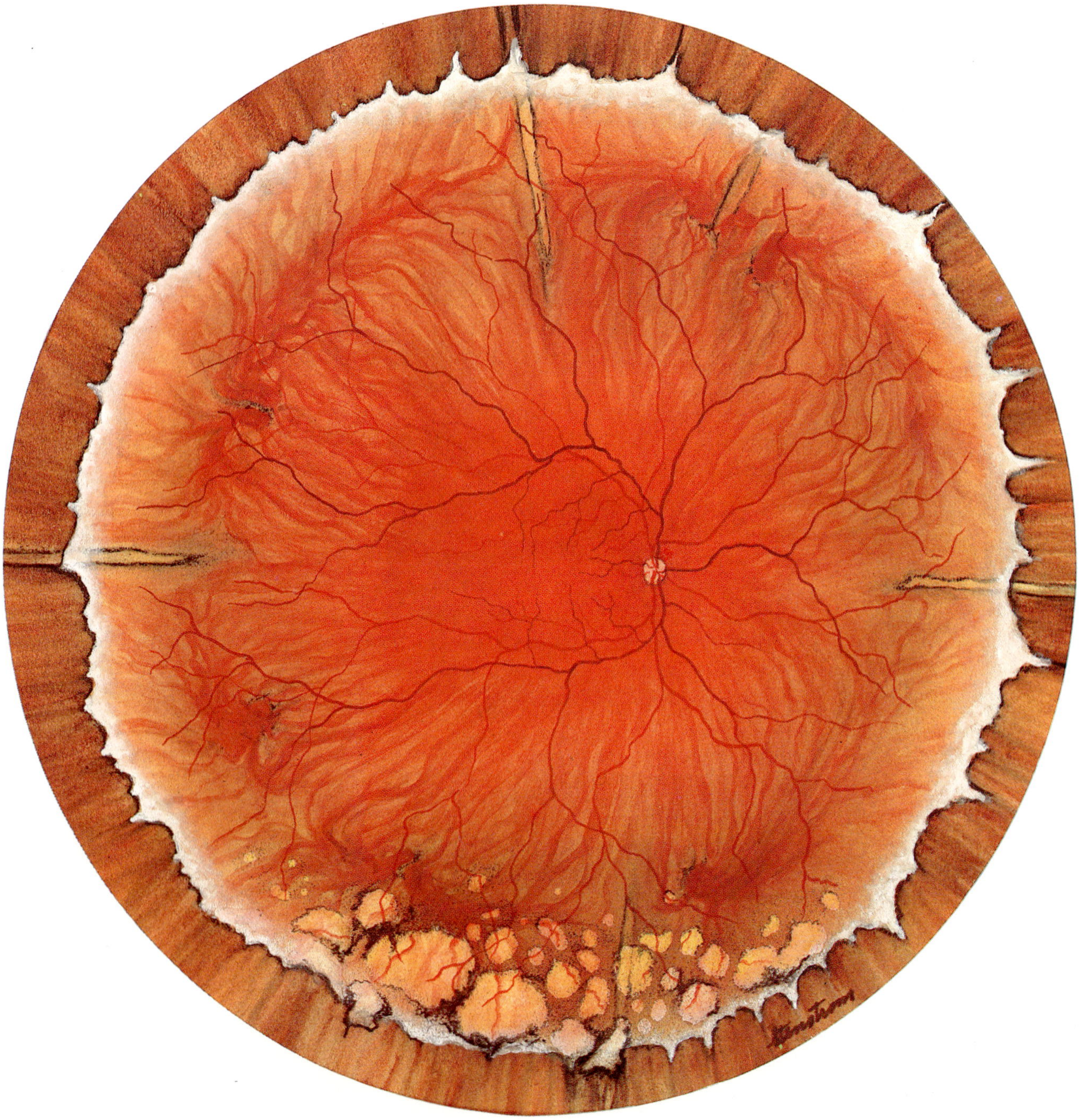

PLATE 8

PARS PLANA CYSTS

Pars plana cysts are clear bullous elevations of the nonpigmented ciliary epithelium of the pars plana. They resemble blisters on the pars plana. These cysts are usually more prominent temporally underneath the vitreous base. They are best viewed in profile by scleral depression. The surface is usually quite smooth, but sometimes gray tissue may occur on the cyst surface. The cyst content is usually clear and has been found to contain hyaluronic acid. In patients with abnormal serum proteins, such as in multiple myeloma, the cysts may contain abnormal protein, giving them a turbid appearance.

Cysts of the pars plana are usually found in adults, with 24 percent of patients over 40 and 34 percent of patients over 70 having at least one pars plana cyst. They are bilateral in about one third of cases and there is no sex predilection. Pars plana cysts are not associated with serious eye complications.

Allen RA, Miller DH, Straatsma BR: Cysts of the posterior ciliary body (pars plana). Arch Ophthalmol *66*:302–313, 1961

Grignolo A, Schepens CL, Heath P: Cysts of the pars plana ciliaris. Arch Ophthalmol *58*:530–545, 1957

Johnson BL, Storey JD: Proteinaceous cysts of the ciliary epithelium. I. Their clear nature and immunoelectrophoretic analysis in a case of multiple myeloma. II. Their occurrence in nonmyelomatous hypergammaglobulinemic conditions. Arch Ophthalmol *84*:166–175, 1970

Okun E: Gross and microscopic pathology in autopsy eyes IV. Pars plana cysts. Am J Ophthalmol *51*:1221–1228, 1961

Ruiz RS: Giant cysts of the pars plana. Am J Ophthalmol *72*:481–482, 1971

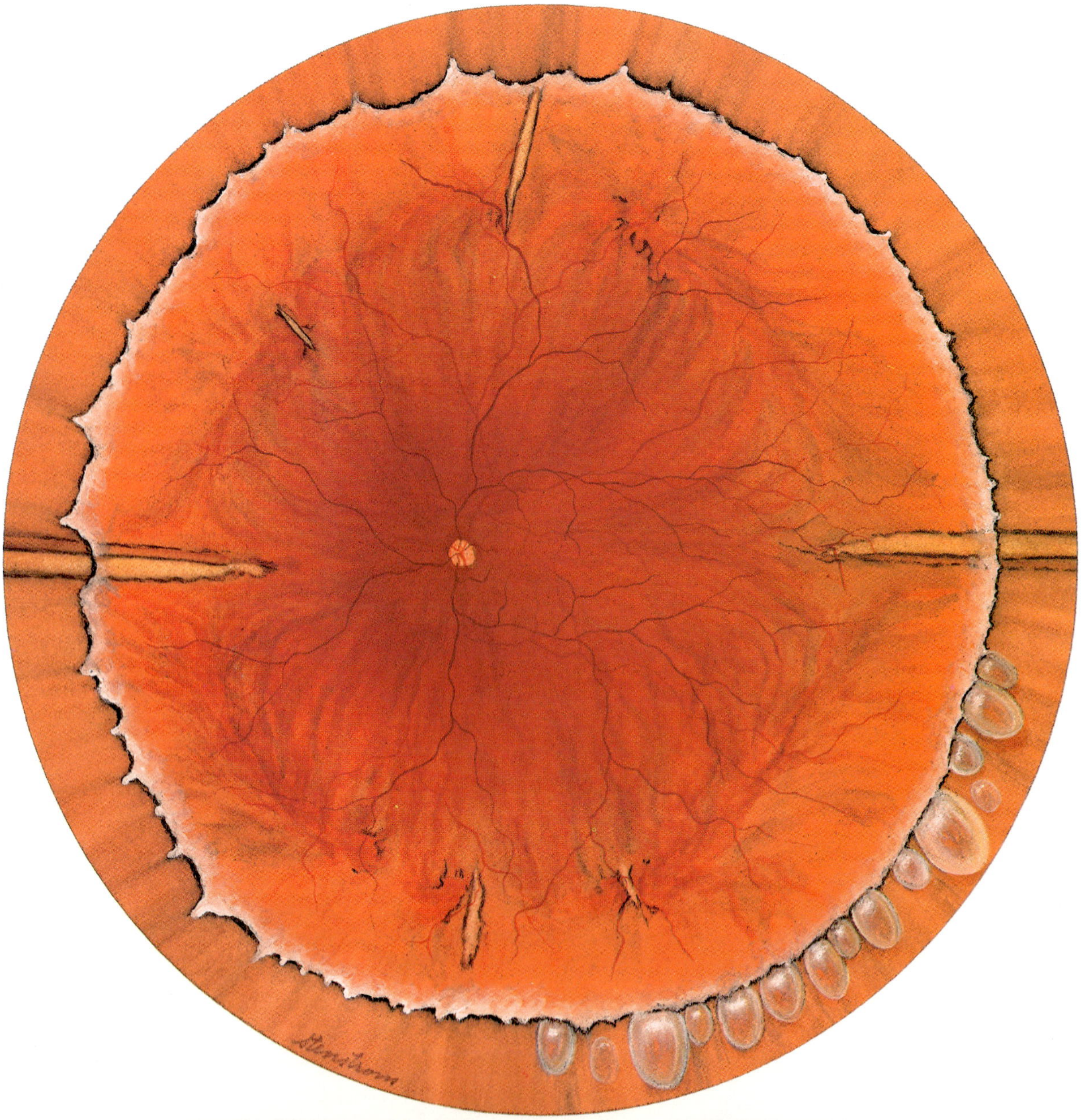

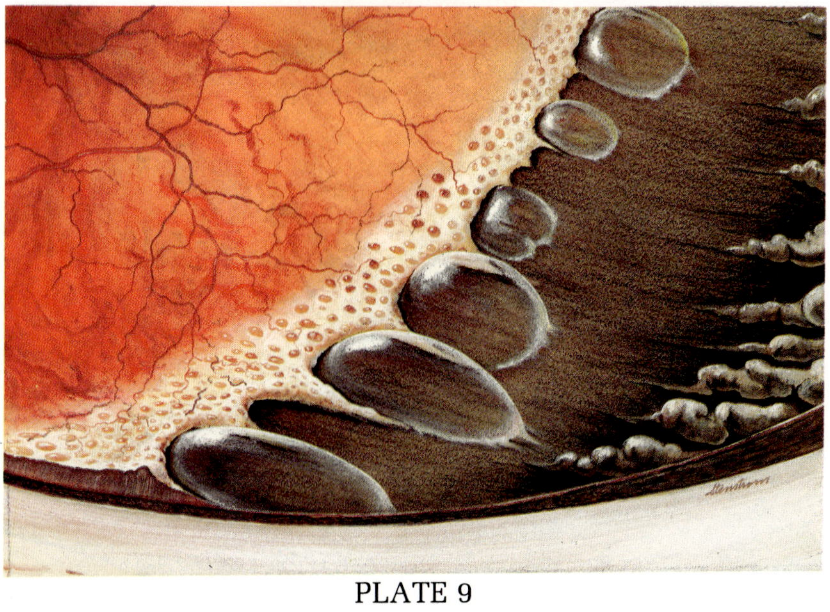

PLATE 9

LATTICE DEGENERATION WITHOUT BREAKS

Lattice degeneration is a distinctive and important retinal degeneration that appears as oval or elliptical areas of retinal thinning near the equator. These areas are oriented circumferentially parallel to the ora serrata. Lattice lesions occur in all meridians, but are slightly more frequent on either side of the 12 and 6 o'clock meridians, and are more common above than below.

The term lattice refers to the arborizing white lines seen in some lesions that represent attenuated and sheathed retinal vessels. However, only about 12 percent of lattice lesions have these visible white lines; more commonly retinal thinning and black clumps of pigment in the retina define areas of lattice degeneration. Fine white-to-yellow flecks can be seen within the margins of affected areas; these flecks are fragmented pieces of the inner retinal layers, which have undergone dissolution. The vitreous is liquefied directly over the lattice lesion, and there is a strong vitreoretinal adhesion surrounding the margins of lattice lesions that appears as a white halo on the retinal surface. Vitreous pull, or traction on these areas of firm adhesion may lead to retinal breaks and detachment.

Lattice degeneration is common, being present in about 8 percent of the general population. It becomes visible by the second decade of life and persists into the advanced years. It is equally common in males and females, and is bilateral in 50 percent of cases, usually with mirror symmetry. Although lattice degeneration may be common in certain families, no defined pattern of inheritance has been identified. It is more common in eyes with high myopia, and certain syndromes, such as Turner's, have a higher than expected incidence of lattice degeneration.

Beyer NE: Lattice degeneration of the retina. Surv Ophthalmol *23*:213–248, 1979

Boniuk M, Butler FC: An autopsy study of lattice degeneration, retinal breaks, and retinal pits. *In* McPherson A (ed): New and Controversial Aspects of Retinal Detachment. New York, Harper & Row, 1968, pp 59–75

Rutnin U, Schepens CL: Fundus appearance of normal eyes: III. Peripheral degenerations. Am J Ophthalmol *64*:1040–1062, 1967

Straatsma BR, Zeegen PD, Foos RY, et al: Lattice degeneration of the retina. Am J Ophthalmol *77*:619–649, 1974

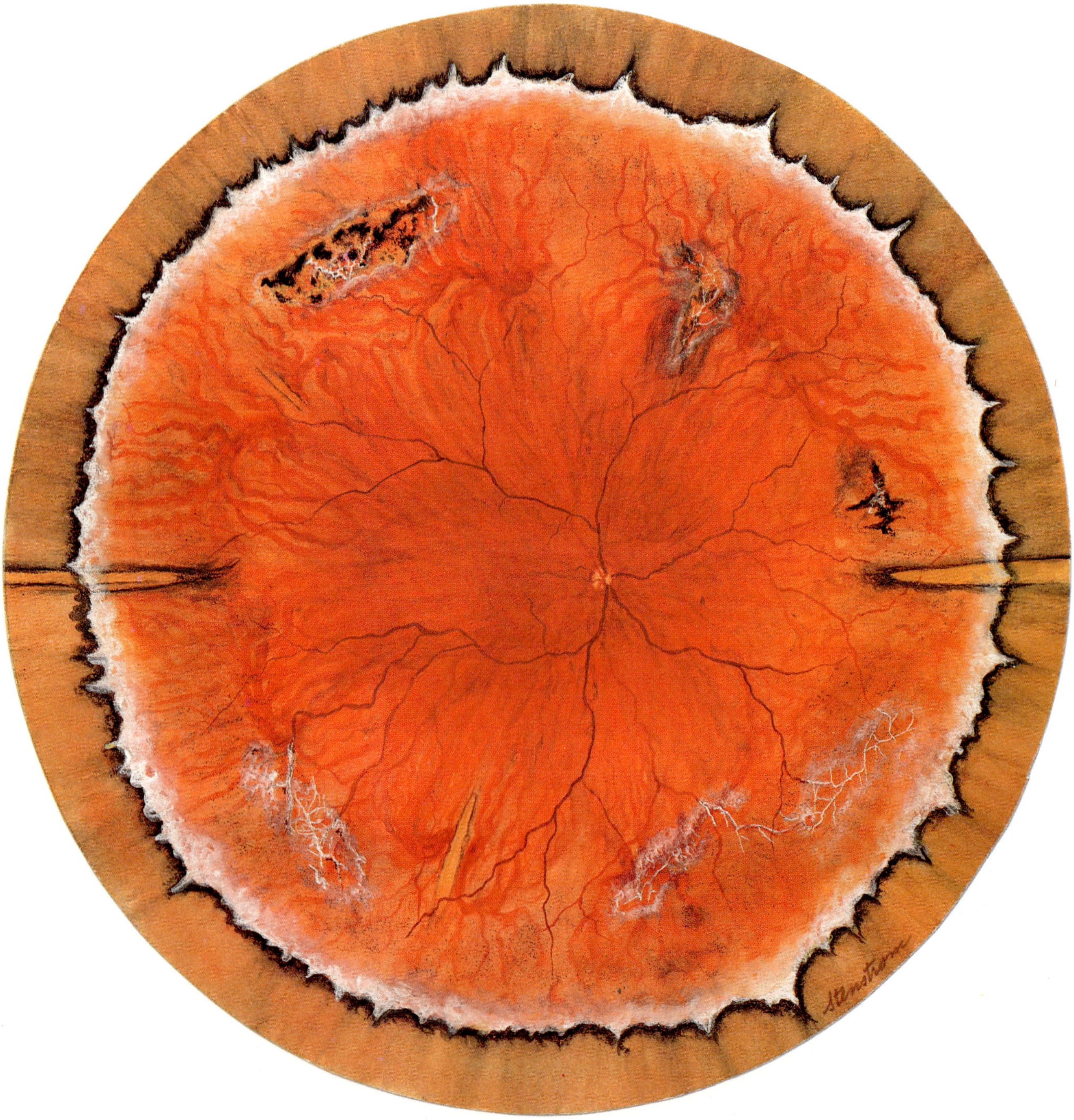

PLATE 10

LATTICE DEGENERATION WITH BREAKS

Lattice degeneration is also called palisade degeneration, equatorial degeneration, and snail track degeneration. Regardless of its name, one of the most characteristic features is the presence of small round holes within the lattice lesion itself. Such holes are shown in the 10:30, 11, and 1 o'clock lattice lesions in this illustration. The holes are typically small and round, and are easily visible by observation of the pigment epithelium, which is in bold contrast to the white appearance of the surrounding lattice. These breaks in lattice are atrophic, and may be either partial or full thickness. The vitreous overlying these lattice lesions is quite clear but is liquefied directly over each lattice lesion. These small round holes in lattice are generally quiescent and may be observed to be stationary for years without progressing to a retinal detachment. However, if the vitreous is disturbed, as in a spontaneous posterior vitreous detachment or during cataract removal, these holes in lattice may lead to a retinal detachment.

Another type of round retinal hole is portrayed in the 2 and 6 o'clock meridians. At 2 o'clock, the vitreous has detached and avulsed a small round piece of retina, leaving a round retinal hole. This avulsed piece of retina appears to float freely in the vitreous cavity, casting a shadow on the underlying retina. Such a free-floating piece of retina is called an operculum and is in reality attached to the detached posterior vitreous. The retinal hole is easily seen surrounded by a small area of detached retina. In the 6 o'clock meridian, no operculum is visible and it is believed that it has fragmented into particles too small to be visible. Although the round retinal holes in the 2 and 6 o'clock meridians are surrounded by small areas of detachment, these lesions are at low risk of progressing to a clinical retinal detachment.

Byer NE: Prognosis of asymptomatic retinal breaks. Arch Ophthalmol *92*:208–210, 1974

Byer NE: Changes in and prognosis of lattice degeneration of the retina. Trans Am Acad Ophthalmol Otolaryngol *78*:114–125, 1974

Davis MD: Natural history of retinal breaks without detachment. Arch Ophthalmol *92*:183–194, 1974

Dumas J, Schepens CL: Chorioretinal lesions predisposing to retinal breaks. Am J Ophthalmol *61*:620–630, 1966

Streeten BW, Bert M: Retinal surface in lattice degeneration of the retina. Am J Ophthalmol *74*:1201–1209, 1972

Tillery WV, Lucier AC: Round atrophic holes in lattice degeneration—an important cause of phakic retinal detachment. Trans Am Acad Ophthalmol Otolaryngol *81*:509–518, 1976

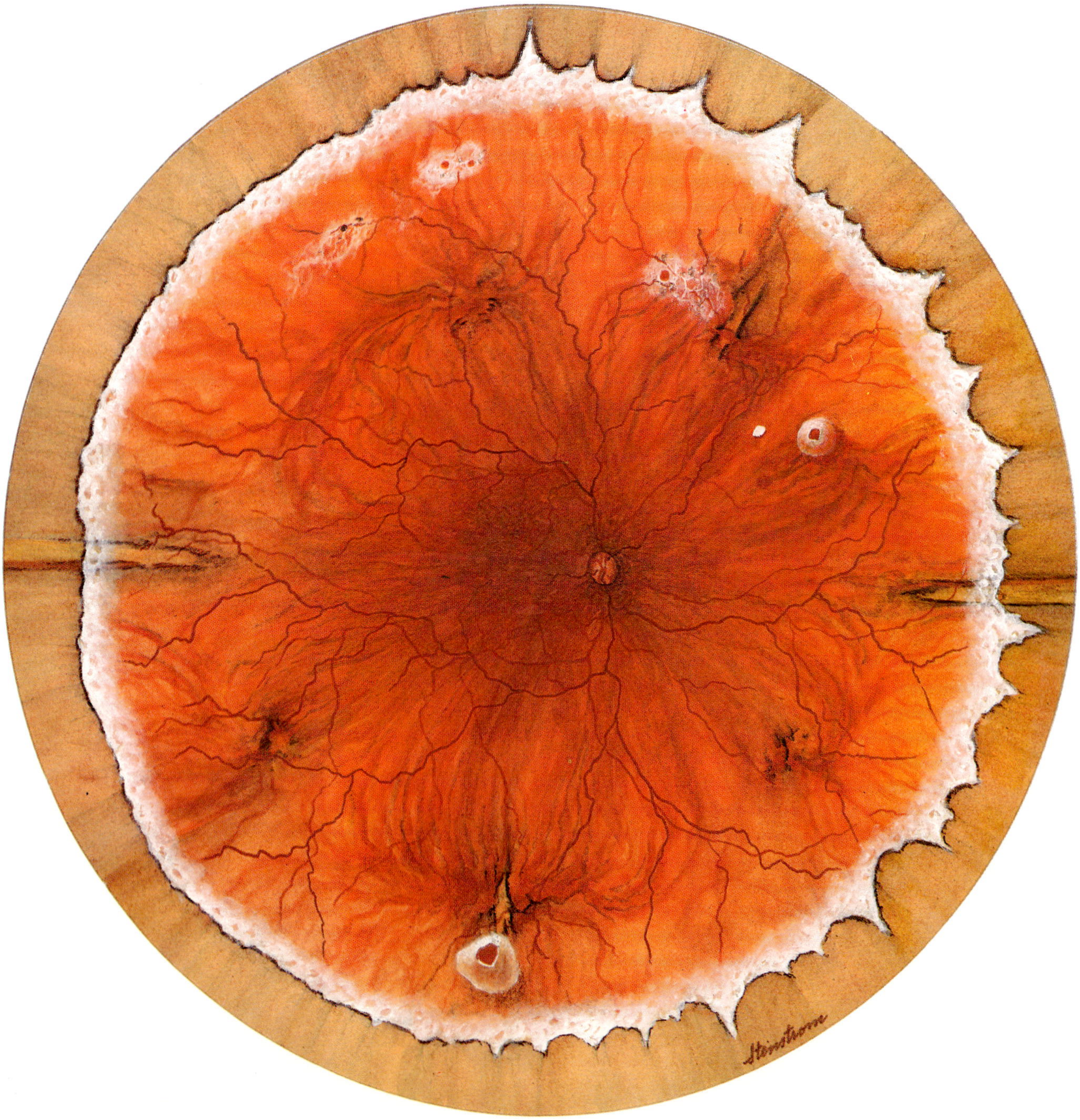

PLATE 11

VARIETIES OF LATTICE DEGENERATION

The broad spectrum of appearance of lattice degeneration is shown in these illustrations. At the upper left, typical lattice degeneration is shown; in the inset, scleral depression demonstrates retinal thinning and the small fragments of internal limiting membrane over the lattice lesion. At the upper right, pigmented spots are circumferentially arranged on either side of a short ciliary nerve. These pigmented spots are believed to be true lattice lesions but so much pigment is present that the typical lattice appearance is obscured. These pigmented spots usually adhere to the vitreous, so that if a vitreous detachment occurs, a retinal hole may be torn in the retina. For comparison, a typical lattice lesion is shown in the 2 o'clock meridian. In the lower left illustration, a typical lattice lesion with numerous round holes is shown. In the 11 o'clock meridian, the vitreous pull or traction on the lattice lesion has resulted in a horseshoe, or flap, tear. Note that the typical appearance of lattice degeneration is present on the elevated flap of the tear. At the anterior margin of the flap, the posterior margin of the vitreous base becomes visible as white lines parallel to the ora serrata. In the lower right illustration, a distinctive type of lattice degeneration is shown. The 1:00 o'clock lattice lesion is oriented radially perpendicular to the ora serrata rather than parallel to it. Many small round holes and pigmented spots are visible. The 2 o'clock lattice lesion is gently curved, with one end appearing to point posteriorly toward the optic nerve. Lattice lesions of this radial or curved configuration are found in Wagner's vitreoretinal syndrome, now considered part of the Stickler syndrome, which contains numerous systemic abnormalities. This distinctive radial type of lattice degeneration is inherited as an autosomal dominant and is notorious for leading to retinal detachments that may be difficult to repair.

Dumas J, Schepens CL: Chorioretinal lesions predisposing to retinal breaks. Am J Ophthalmol *61*:620–630, 1966

Hirose T, Lee KY, Schepens CL: Wagner's hereditary vitreo-retinal degeneration and retinal detachment. Arch Ophthalmol *89*:176–185, 1973

Jansen L: Degeneratio hyaloideo-retinalis hereditaria. Ophthalmologica *144*:458–464, 1962

Spencer LM, Foos RY: Paravascular vitreo-retinal attachments. Arch Ophthalmol *84*:557–564, 1970

Stickler GB, Belau PG, Farrell FJ, et al: Hereditary progressive arthro-ophthalmopathy. Mayo Clin Proc *40*:433–455, 1965

Wagner H: Ein bisher unbekanntes Erbleiden des Auges (Degeneratio hyaloideo-retinalis hereditaria) beobachtet im Kanton Zurich. Klin Monatsbl Augenheilkd *100*:840–856, 1938

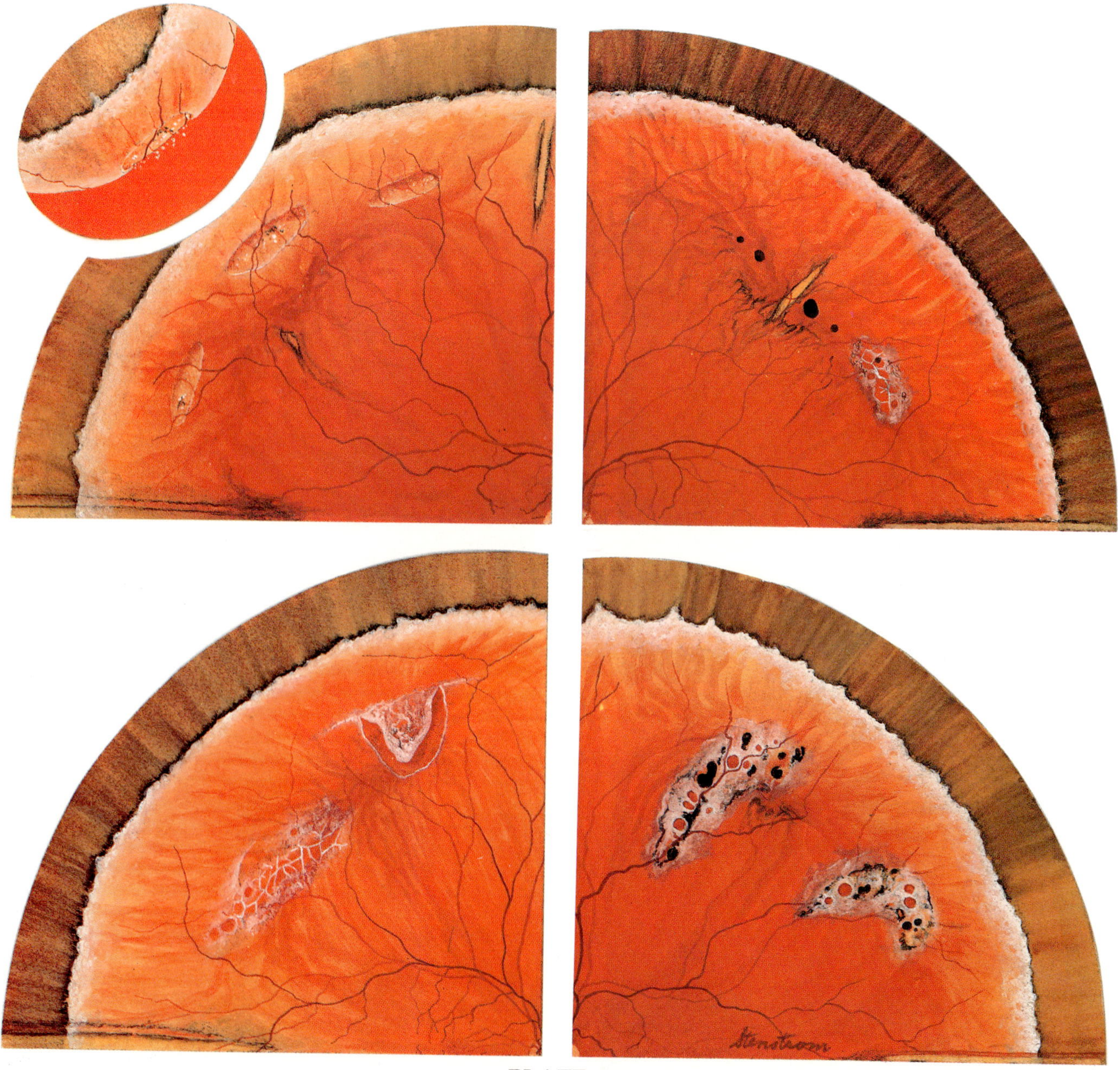

PLATE 12

Chapter 3

RETINAL DETACHMENTS

SHAFER'S SIGN

The presence of cells containing gold brown pigment granules in the anterior vitreous of a phakic eye suggests that a retinal break is present. This was pointed out by Shafer, who noted that in the absence of previous surgery or inflammation such pigment is almost pathognomonic of a retinal break.

These intracellular pigment granules, sometimes called "tobacco dust," are thought to represent displaced pigment epithelial cells. These cells have passed through a retinal break and migrated to the anterior vitreous, where they may be seen with the slit lamp. There is usually a posterior vitreous detachment present, and the retinal break may or may not have produced a retinal detachment.

Hamilton AM, Taylor W: Significance of pigment granules in the vitreous. Br J Ophthalmol 56:700–702, 1972

Shafer DM: *In* Schepens CL, Regan CDJ (eds): Controversial Aspects of the Management of Retinal Detachment. Boston, Little Brown, 1965, p 51

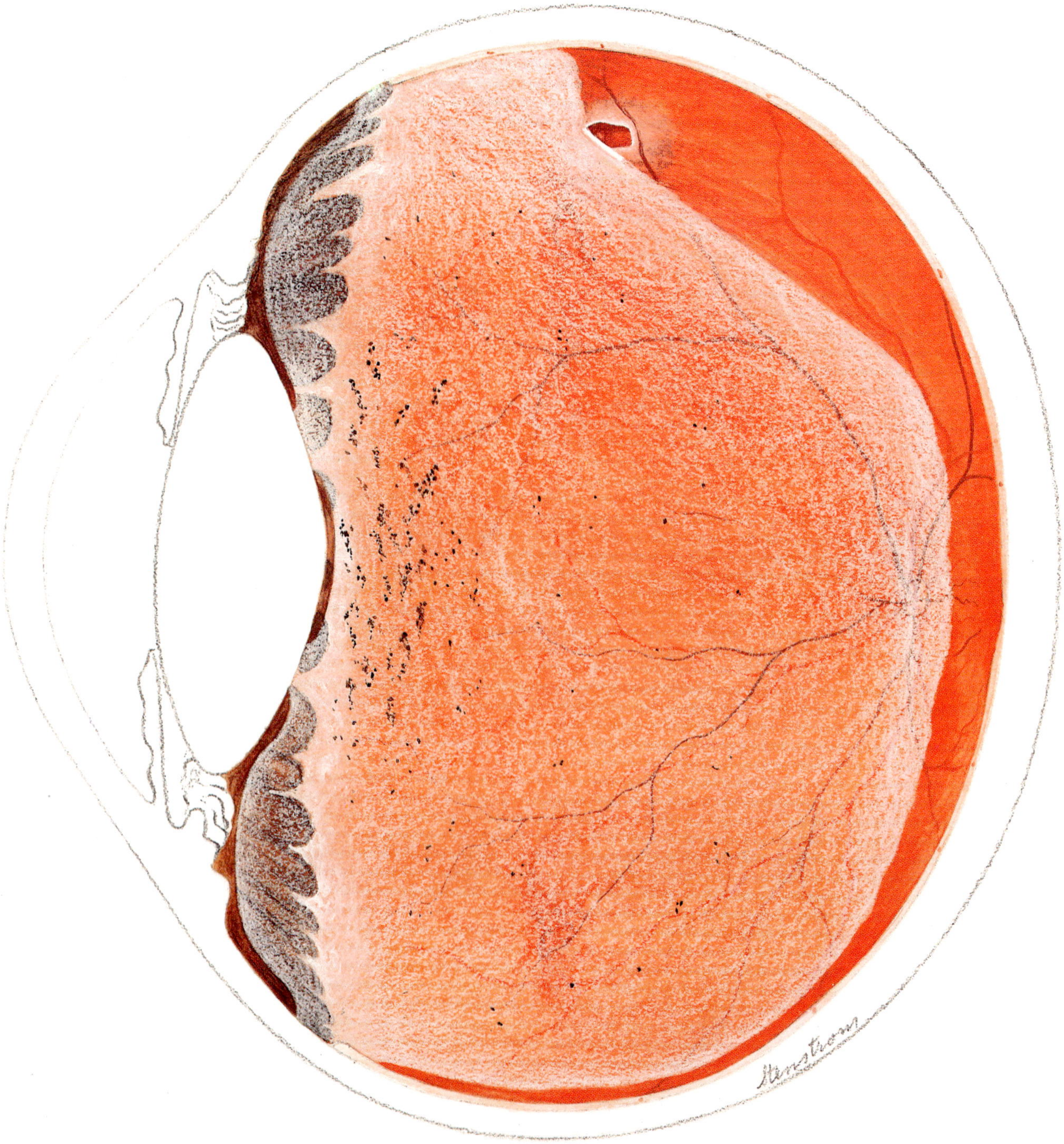

PLATE 13

MULTIPLE HORSESHOE TEARS WITHOUT DETACHMENT

The horseshoe tear, also called a flap tear, is a common and important type of full thickness retinal break. These tears are considered more likely to lead to retinal detachment than are round retinal holes because they have vitreous traction, or pull, on the flap of the tear. This traction makes it more likely that fluid passing through the tear will undermine the potential space between the retina and pigment epithelium, causing a retinal detachment. In this illustration, five horseshoe tears are present, all in the superior half of the retina. Horseshoe tears may also occur in the inferior quadrants. The elevated flap of the tear is always attached to the retina nearest the ora serrata, and the free end is attached to the vitreous. By indirect ophthalmoscopy it appears that the flap is projecting into the vitreous like a thumb sticking up, and careful observation with the fundus contact lens will reveal firm vitreous adhesion to the flap. Further evidence of vitreous pull or traction is seen as a white appearance of the peripheral retina. This is called "white without pressure" and should not be interpreted as a shallow retinal detachment.

Horseshoe tears occur when there is a posterior vitreous detachment in combination with a vitreoretinal adhesion. A posterior vitreous detachment is a common spontaneous occurrence in the older age groups. The initial symptoms are usually flashes of light and vitreous floaters. If there is a vitreoretinal adhesion, then a horseshoe tear is produced as the vitreous separates. Frequently, areas of lattice or other causes of vitreoretinal adhesion can be visualized on the flap of the tear. The vitreous is firmly attached to the globe at the vitreous base, which straddles the ora serrata. The hinge of the elevated flap is limited by the posterior margin of the vitreous base.

Foos RY: Posterior vitreous detachment. Trans Am Acad Ophthalmol Otolaryngol *76*:480–497, 1972

Foos RY: Vitreous base, retinal tufts, and retinal tears: Pathogenic relationships. *In* Pruett RC, Regan CDJ (eds): Retina Congress. New York, Appleton-Century-Crofts, 1972, pp 259–280

Jaffe NS: Complications of acute posterior vitreous detachment. Arch Ophthalmol *79*:568–571, 1968

Linder B: Acute posterior vitreous detachment and its retinal complications: A clinical biomicroscopic study. Acta Ophthalmol (Suppl) *87*:1–108, 1966

Spencer LM, Foos RY, Straatsma BR: Meridional folds, meridional complexes and associated abnormalities of the peripheral retina. Am J Ophthalmol *70*:697–714, 1970

Spencer LM, Foos RY: Paravascular vitreo-retinal attachments. Arch Ophthalmol *84*:557–564, 1970

Tasman W: Posterior vitreous detachment and peripheral retinal breaks. Trans Am Acad Ophthalmol Otolaryngol. *72*:217–224, 1968

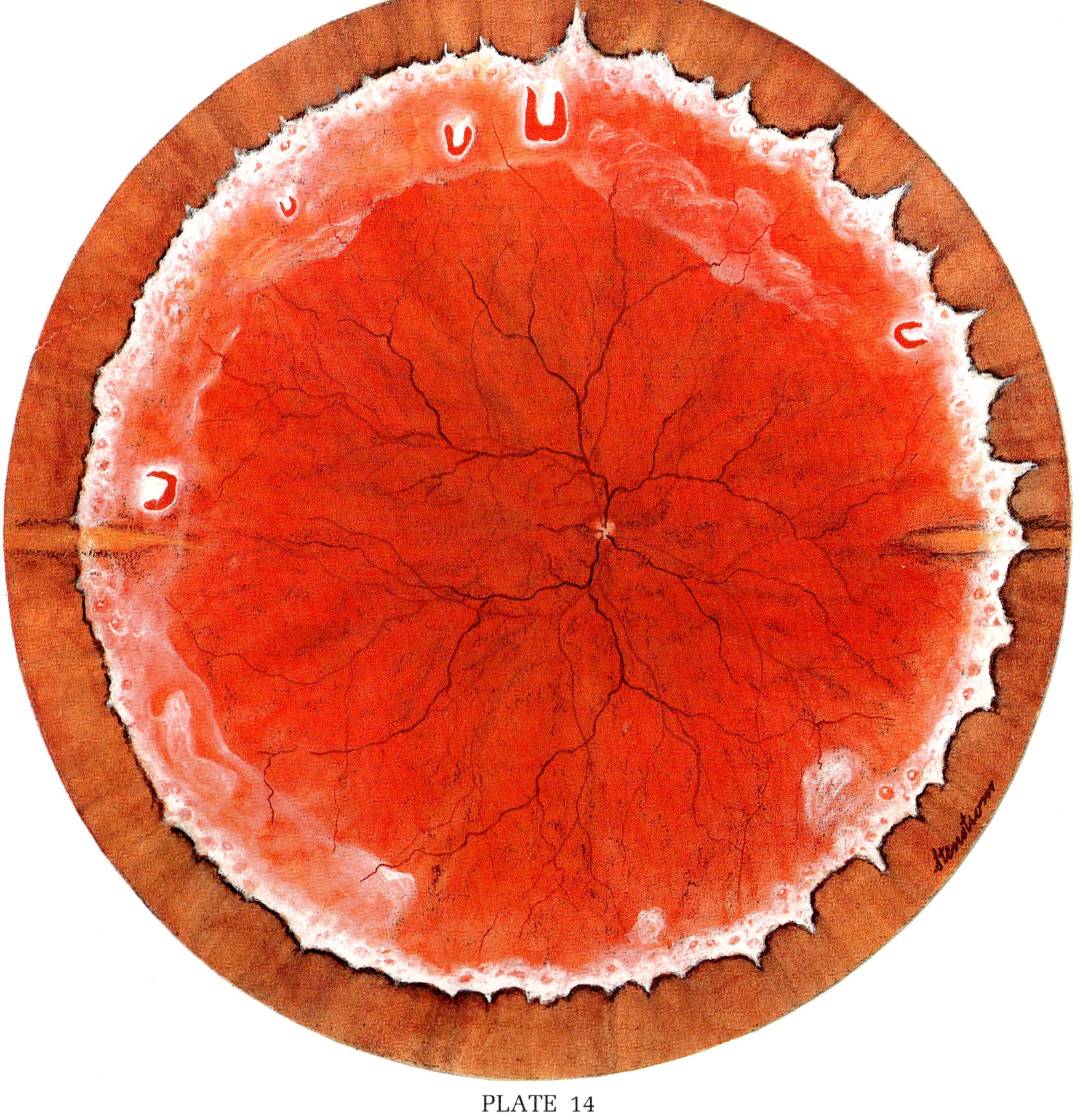

PLATE 14

HORSESHOE TEAR WITH HEMORRHAGE

Vitreous hemorrhage commonly occurs as a horseshoe tear is produced. The hemorrhage may obscure much of the retina and may obscure the retinal tear as well. Hemorrhage occurs as retinal vessels are torn during development of the tear. A bridging vessel traveling from the posterior lip of the retinal break to the flap can many times be visualized.

If the retinal tear can be visualized through the vitreous hemorrhage, treatment is recommended, as retinal tears in the presence of vitreous hemorrhage are particularly prone to progress to retinal detachment. When no retinal tear can be visualized, immobilization of the patient with the head elevated using bilateral patches is recommended, as many times the hemorrhage will settle sufficiently to allow visualization of the retinal tear. If the hemorrhage is so severe that no retinal details can be visualized, ultrasound studies may be of value. Small tears cannot be detected, but large tears with elevated margins can be revealed by ultrasound.

With the passage of several weeks the red blood is absorbed by the eye and the remaining hemorrhage slowly turns from red to white. Better visualization of retinal tears can be obtained but there is a tendency for fluid to collect beneath the retina, forming a retinal detachment.

Coleman DJ, Jack RL: B-Scan ultrasonography in diagnosis and management of retinal detachment. Arch Ophthalmol *90*:29–34, 1973

Colyear BH, Pischel DK: Clinical tears in the retina without detachment. Am J Ophthalmol *41*:773–793, 1956

Davis MD: The natural history of retinal breaks. Arch Ophthalmol *92*:183–194, 1974

Hyams SW, Meir E, Ivory M, et al: Chorioretinal lesions predisposing to retinal detachment. Am J Ophthalmol *78*:429–437, 1974

Jaffe NA: Complications of acute posterior vitreous detachment. Arch Ophthalmol *79*:568–571, 1968

Lincoff H: Guilty until proven innocent. Arch Ophthalmol *78*:271, 1967

Morse PH, Aminlari A, Scheie HG: Spontaneous vitreous hemorrhage. Arch Ophthalmol *92*:297–298, 1974

Robertson DM, Curtin VT, Norton EWD: Avulsed retinal vessels with retinal breaks. Arch Ophthalmol *85*:669–672, 1971

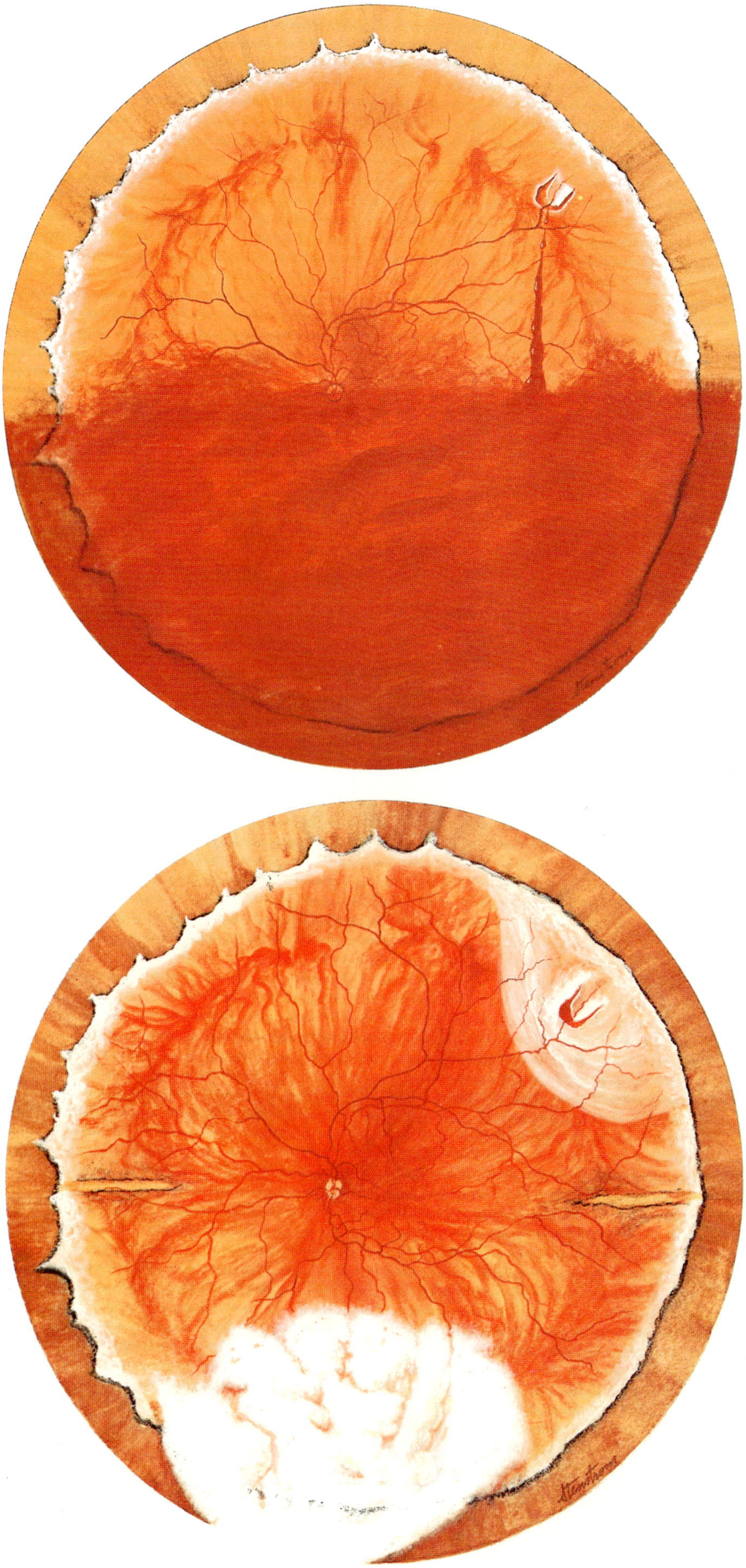

PLATE 15

LARGE HORSESHOE TEARS WITHOUT DETACHMENT

Two large horseshoe tears are present in the periphery of this eye at 1 o'clock and 5 o'clock. Typical symptoms of these tears would include flashes of light and vitreous floaters, but the central vision would remain excellent. The flap of the 1 o'clock tear is bifid, implying two closely spaced vitreoretinal adhesions. A thin rim of subretinal fluid is beginning to accumulate underneath the posterior margin of this tear, indicating that it will likely progress to a symptomatic retinal detachment.

Most authorities, but not all, would recommend prophylactic therapy for these two horseshoe tears, especially if they produce symptoms. If transconjunctival cryotherapy is performed, the treatment must be placed in fully attached retina surrounding the shallowly detached retina. If cryotherapy treatment is placed only underneath the shallowly elevated retina, no chorioretinal adhesion will be produced and extension of the detached area is likely to occur.

Benson WE: Prophylactic therapy of retinal breaks. Surv Ophthalmol *22*:41–47, 1977

Davis MD: Natural history of retinal breaks. Arch Ophthalmol *92*:183–194, 1974

Hosni FA: Management of peripheral retinal breaks. Ophthalmologica *166*:265–288, 1973

Morse PH, Scheie HG: Prophylactic cryotherapy of retinal breaks. Arch Ophthalmol *92*:204–207, 1974

Neumann E, Hyams BS, Feiler V, et al: The natural history of retinal holes with special reference to the development of retinal detachment and the time factor involved. Isr J Med Sci *8*:1424–1428, 1972

Robertson DM, Norton EWD: Long term follow-up of treated retinal breaks. Am J Ophthalmol *75*:395–404, 1973

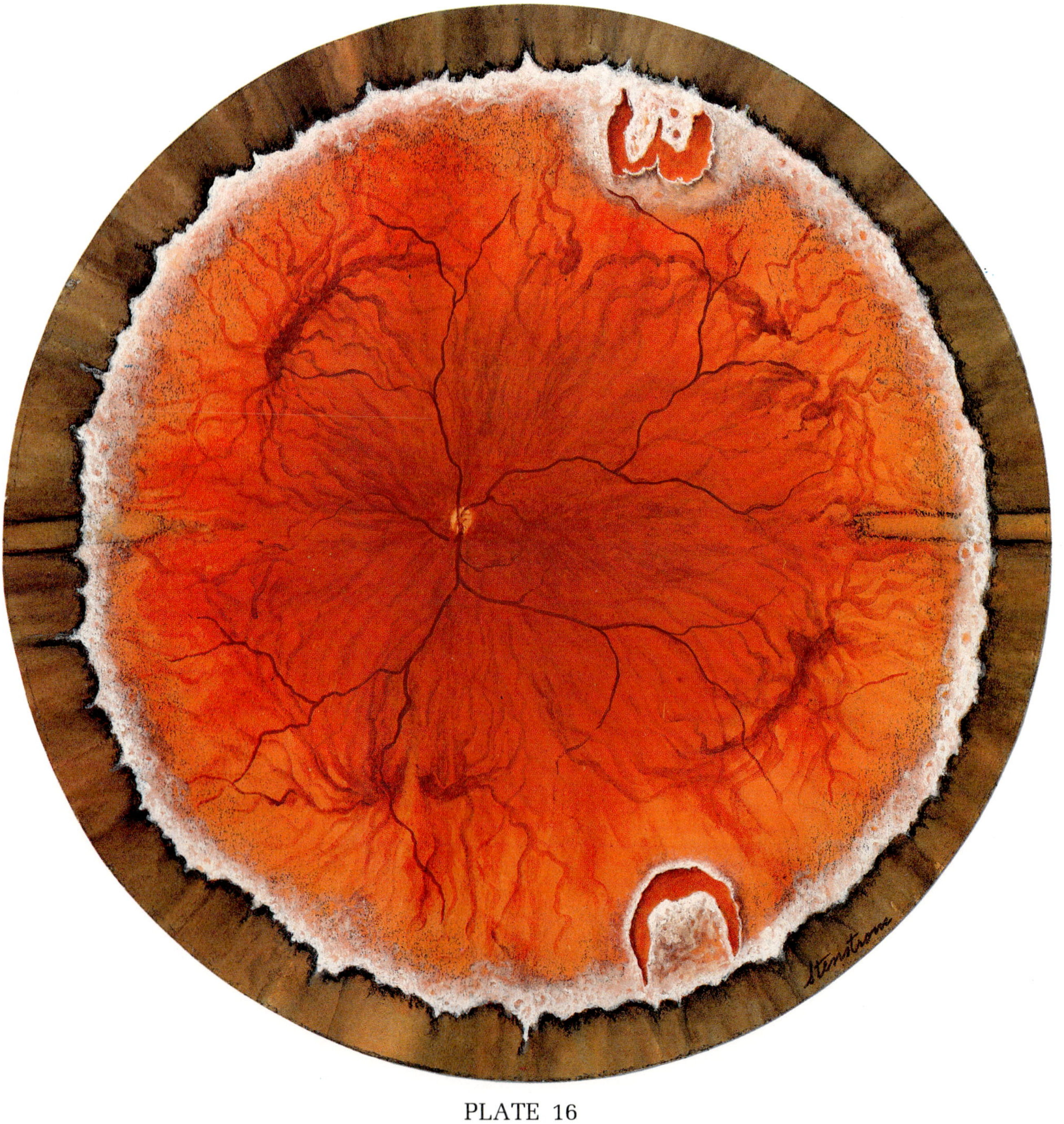

PLATE 16

HORSESHOE TEARS WITH DETACHMENT

This partial retinal detachment is typical of spontaneously occurring retinal detachments in either phakic or aphakic eyes. Horseshoe tears are noted in the 8 o'clock and 10:30 o'clock meridians, and a round hole is present at 11 o'clock with an operculum casting a shadow onto the underlying retina. The ora serrata is detached between 9 and 12 o'clock and there is a meridional fold in the 3 o'clock meridian. The detached retina shows multiple billowing elevations into the vitreous cavity that can be seen to undulate gently as the eye is moved slightly. The detachment has reached the optic nerve, detaching the macula, causing a profound visual loss. The border between detached and attached retina is well defined and visible as a slightly curved line between the disc and ora serrata.

This retinal detachment would be expected to respond well to any of the varieties of standard buckling techniques. With reattachment of the retina, marked improvement in central visual acuity and peripheral visual field can be expected to occur.

Aaberg TM, Wiznia RA: The use of solid soft silicone rubber exoplants in retinal detachment surgery. Ophthalmic Surg 7:98–105, 1976

Chignell AH: Retinal detachment surgery without drainage of subretinal fluid. Am J Ophthalmol 77:1–5, 1974

Lincoff H, Kreissig I: The treatment of retinal detachment without drainage of subretinal fluid. Trans Am Acad Ophthalmol Otolaryngol 76:1221–1233, 1972

Schepens CL: Diagnostic and prognostic factors as found in preoperative examination. Trans Am Acad Ophthalmol Otolaryngol 56:398–412, 1952

Schepens CL, Okamura ID, Brockhurst RJ: The scleral buckling procedures. I. Surgical technique and management. Arch Ophthalmol 58:797–811, 1957

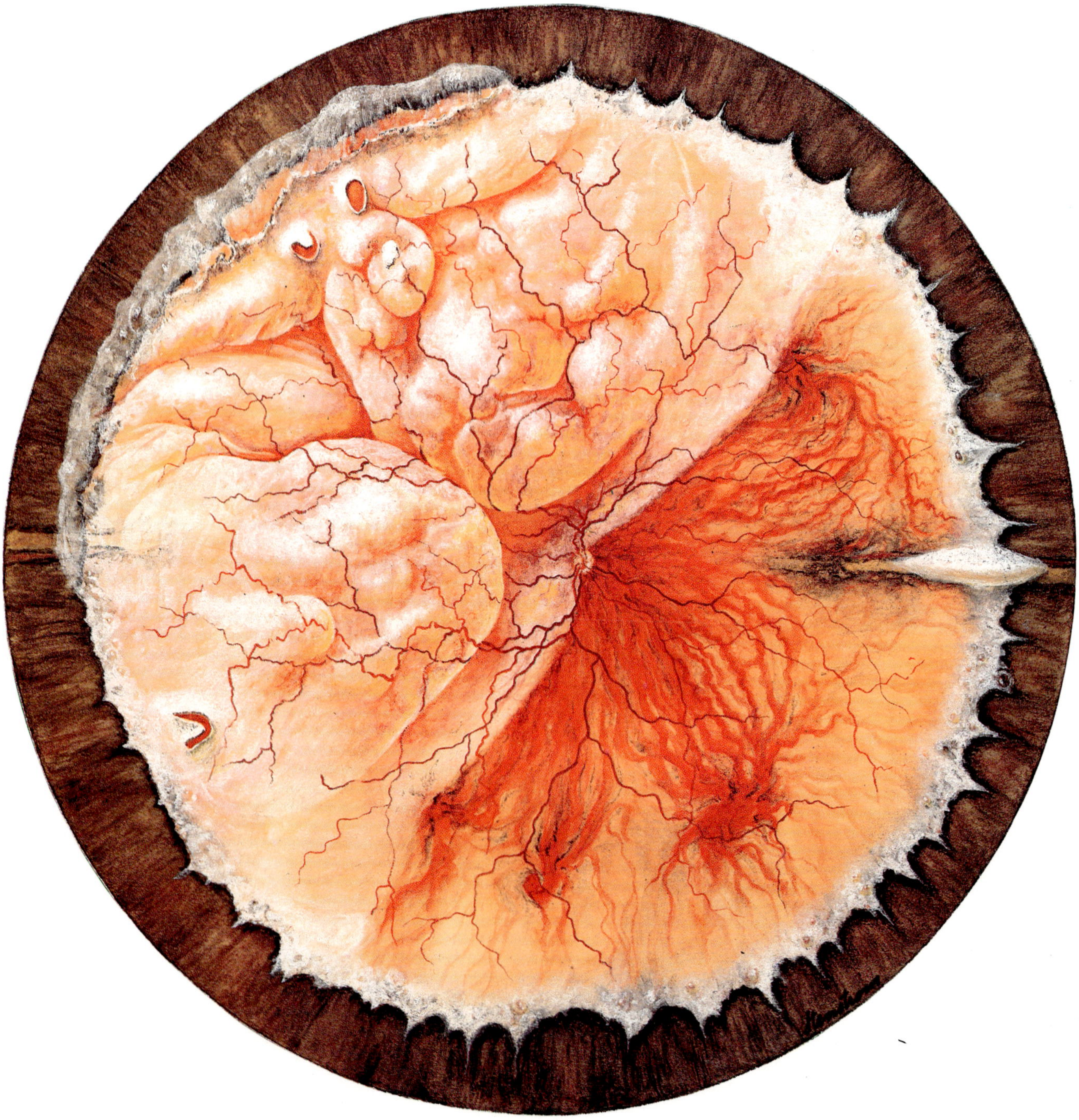

PLATE 17

TEARS IN POSTERIOR VITREOUS BASE WITH DETACHMENT

Three small retinal tears are present in the posterior vitreous base. Normally the vitreous base is not ophthalmoscopically visible, but in the presence of severe vitreous traction the posterior border of the vitreous base becomes visible as a slightly elevated thin ridge. The posterior vitreous base continues to be visible on either side of the detached area as a thin white line just posterior to the ora serrata. Another evidence of strong vitreous traction in the superior nasal quadrant is the detachment of the ora serrata between 9 and 12 o'clock. The detached retina involves only the superior nasal quadrant but has reached the optic nerve. The macula, however, is not detached and central visual acuity remains good.

The presenting symptom of this retinal detachment likely would be a curtain appearing in the inferior nasal visual field that progresses toward central vision. This retinal detachment is typical of those that occur after cataract extraction, particularly when vitreous is lost. Aphakic retinal detachments typically have obscure holes at the posterior vitreous base. Meticulous examination with scleral depression is required in order to discover all retinal holes present. It should always be assumed that more than one hole is present, as closure of all holes is required to achieve a cure of the retinal detachment.

Ashrafzadeh MT, Schepens CL, Elzeneiny IT: Aphakic and phakic retinal detachment. Arch Ophthalmol *89*:476–483, 1973

Benson WE, Grand MG, Okun E: Aphakic retinal detachment. Arch Ophthalmol *93*:245–249, 1975

Everett WG, Katzin D: Meridional distribution of retinal breaks in aphakic retinal detachment. Am J Ophthalmol *66*:928–932, 1968

Hauer Y, Barkay S: Vitreous detachment in aphakic eyes. Br J Ophthalmol *48*:341–343, 1964

Heller MD, Straatsma BR, Foos RY: Detachment of the posterior vitreous in phakic and aphakic eyes. Secondary detachment of the retina. Mod Prob Ophthalmol *10*:23–36, 1972

Norton EWD: Retinal detachment in aphakia. Trans Am Ophthalmol Soc *61*:770–789, 1963

Scheie HG, Morse PH, Aminlari A: Incidence of retinal detachment following cataract extraction. Arch Ophthalmol *89*:293–295, 1973

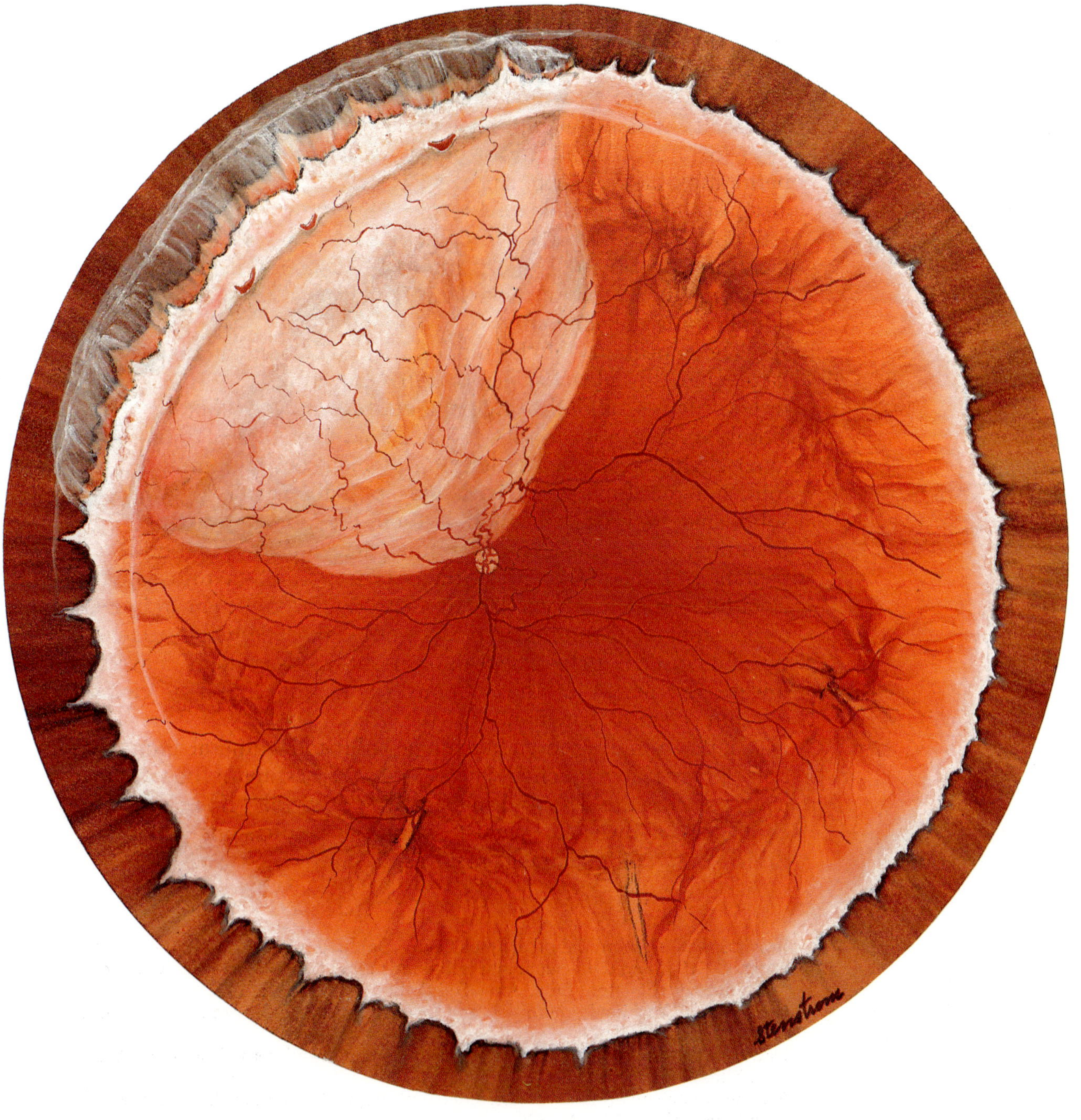

PLATE 18

KISSING CHOROIDAL DETACHMENTS

A choroidal detachment is a collection of clear fluid or blood between the choroid and sclera, producing a smooth, dome-shaped elevation of choroid and retina inside the eye. Choroidal detachments are found to a minimal extent after almost all intraocular surgery in which the intraocular pressure is drastically lowered even for a short time. Prolonged hypotony from a wound leak, perforation of the globe, or severe intraocular inflammation may also result in choroidal detachments. Sometimes a rhegmatogenous retinal detachment occurs in combination with choroidal detachment and hypotony. These combined detachments have a much worse prognosis than a rhegmatogenous retinal detachment without choroidal detachment.

The appearance of choroidal detachments is distinctive, with large, smoothly elevated, balloon-like elevations of retina visible in the fundus, and the pigment epithelium and choroid lying closely underneath the retina. The retina may appear to be separated slightly from the underlying pigment epithelium and choroid, but the appearance with the ophthalmoscope is that of a solid, smooth, broad elevation, without the large undulating folds present in a rhegmatogenous retinal detachment. The solid appearance of the intraocular bulges is important to differentiate from tumors such as a malignant melanoma, metastatic carcinoma or hemangioma. Another important ophthalmoscopic characteristic of choroidal detachment is that the ora serrata is elevated toward the center of the vitreous cavity and is easily visible without scleral depression.

In the example shown here, large nasal and temporal choroidal detachments have touched or "kissed" in the center of the vitreous cavity so that the disc and macula are not visible. If such retinal contact is allowed to persist, permanent adhesions and very difficult retinal detachment may result.

Brav SS: Serous choroidal detachment. Surv Ophthalmol *6*:395–415, 1961

Chignell AH: Choroidal detachment following retinal detachment surgery without drainage of subretinal fluid. Am J Ophthalmol *73*:860–862, 1972

Gottlieb F: Combined choroidal and retinal detachment. Arch Ophthalmol *88*:481–486, 1972

Hawkins WR, Schepens CL: Choroidal detachment and retinal surgery. Am J Ophthalmol *62*:813–819, 1966

Schepens CL: Importance of choroidal detachment in fundus diagnosis. Am J Ophthalmol *51*:333–334, 1961

Seelenfreund MH, Kraushar MF, Schepens CL, et al: Choroidal detachment associated with primary retinal detachment. Arch Ophthalmol *91*:254–258, 1974

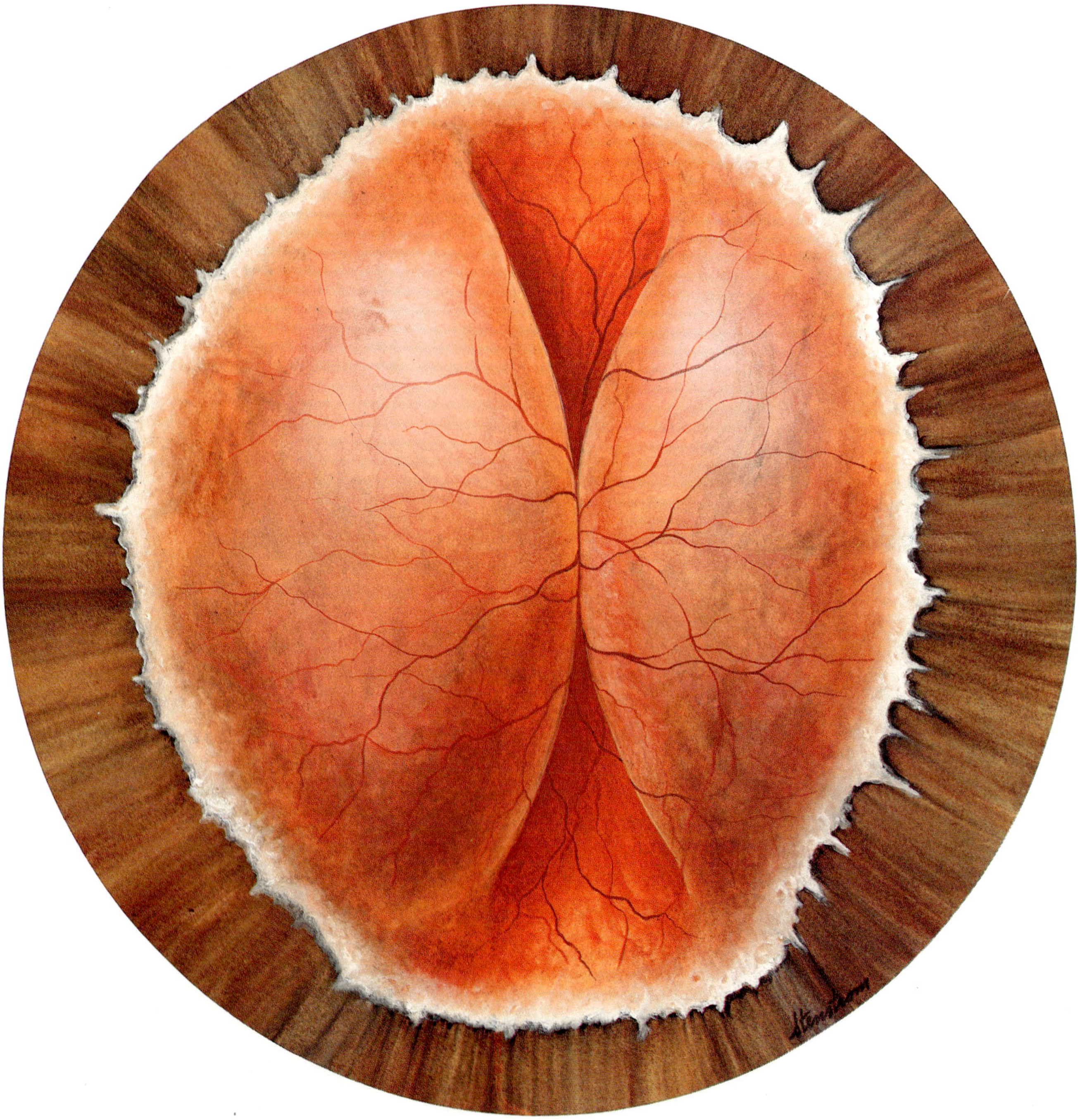

PLATE 19

HEMORRHAGIC CHOROIDAL DETACHMENT

A hemorrhagic choroidal detachment is the occurrence of hemorrhage between the scleral and choroidal layers of the eye. It may occur spontaneously during any intraocular operation in which the intraocular pressure is reduced. A large balloon-like bulge in the retinal periphery may be noted during the course of surgery, or the appearance of an elevated peripheral mass lesion may first be noted postoperatively. In the latter case, the smoothly elevated subretinal mass may be confused with a malignant melanoma or other tumor, but the urge to do immediate enucleation should be avoided until an adequate evaluation can be obtained.

Choroidal hemorrhage is more likely to occur in the elderly and in highly myopic eyes. In retinal detachment operations, choroidal hemorrhages are most likely produced at the time subretinal fluid is drained.

Several characteristic features differentiate a hemorrhagic choroidal detachment from simulating lesions. The most helpful sign is the presence of a rim of bright red blood along the margin of the dome-shaped elevation, shown here in the 6 o'clock meridian with a few drops of red blood on the retinal surface. This margin of red blood takes a few days to appear, but when present is suggestive of a hemorrhagic choroidal detachment. Another sign of choroidal hemorrhage is scleral icterus, which is localized to the affected area overlying the hemorrhage. Initially the vitreous is usually quite clear, but later blood may slowly diffuse into the vitreous, producing a slight haze.

Usually the hemorrhagic choroidal detachment will resolve over several weeks. If the hemorrhage extends far posteriorly into the macular area, a permanent decrease in visual acuity usually results. If several quadrants are involved with the hemorrhagic choroidal detachment, closure of the angle and secondary glaucoma may be produced, requiring surgical drainage.

Bietti GB: Hemorrhagic choroidal detachments. *In* McPherson A (ed): New and Controversial Aspects of Retinal Detachment, New York, Harper & Row, 1968, pp 471–472

Hawkins WR, Schepens CL: Choroidal detachment and retinal surgery: A clinical and experimental study. Am J Ophthalmol *62*:821–819, 1966

Tolentino FI, Brockhurst RJ: Unilateral scleral icterus due to choroidal hemorrhage. Arch Ophthalmol *70*:358–360, 1963

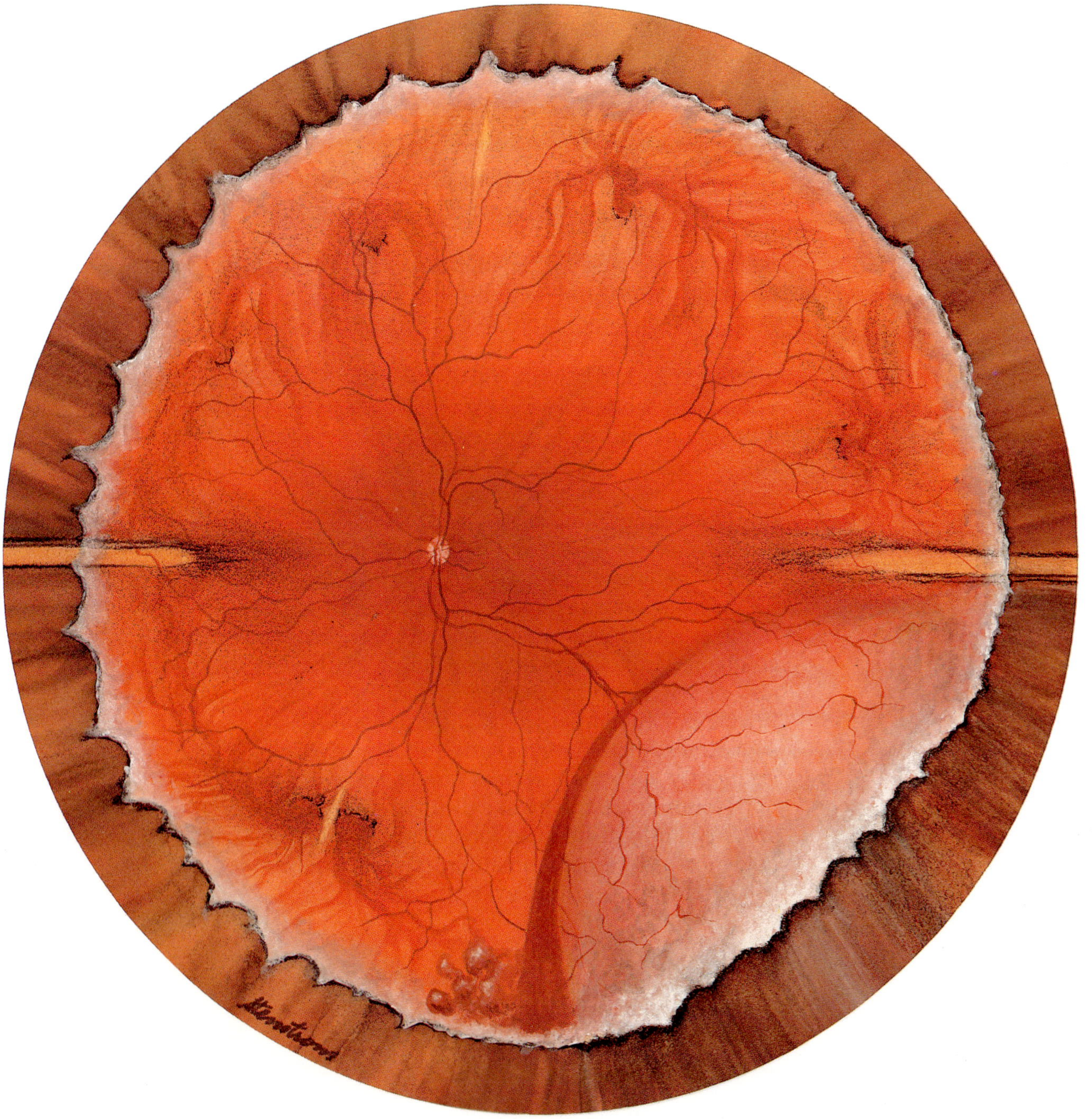

PLATE 20

COLOBOMA OF THE CHOROID WITH RETINAL DETACHMENT

Colobomas are congenital defects in the ocular structures due to imperfect closure of the optic cup during fetal development. Defects may occur in the sclera, choroid, retina, lens, zonule, and iris, and may be minimal or quite large in extent. Usually colobomatous defects occur inferonasally. Frequently, the eyes are microphthalmic and have limited vision.

Rhegmatogenous retinal detachments occur frequently in colobomatous eyes. The retinal breaks may occur in a number of locations and are frequently difficult to visualize because the underlying white sclera causes a lack of contrast with the overlying diaphanous and rudimentary retina. The sclera in the area of the coloboma may contain a staphyloma, while the rudimentary retina contains poorly formed retinal vessels. A retinal break within the staphylomatous area may be discovered more easily by using a fundus contact lens than by indirect ophthalmoscopy. The site of a break may be indicated by a small retinal hemorrhage. Retinal breaks also may occur at the margin of the staphyloma, where there is usually a pigmented margin sharply demarcating the coloboma from normal surrounding retina. Retinal breaks may also occur in the far periphery where the ora serrata would be if it were not encompassed by the coloboma. Giant retinal breaks are sometimes found in eyes with colobomas of the lens and zonule; frequently such giant retinal breaks are bilateral.

Not only are the breaks difficult to find but these detachments are frequently difficult to repair. The surgical prognosis for retinal detachment in a colobomatous eye is therefore much poorer than in anatomically normal eyes.

Hovland KR, Schepens CL, Freeman HM: Developmental giant retinal tears associated with lens coloboma. Arch Ophthalmol 80:325–331, 1968

Jesberg DO, Schepens CL: Retinal detachment associated with coloboma of the choroid. Arch Ophthalmol 65:1613–173, 1961

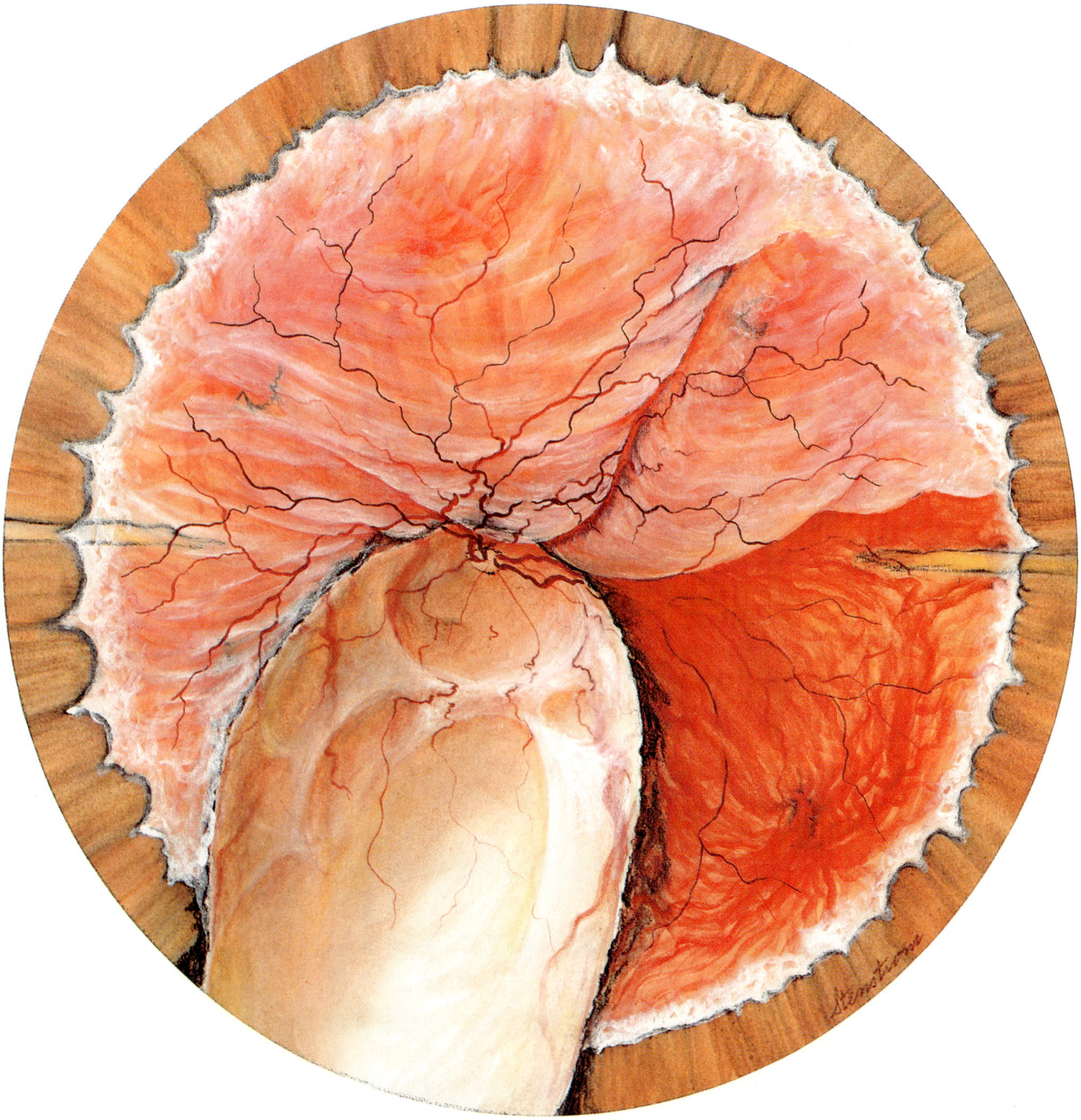

PLATE 21

RETINOSCHISIS WITH RETINAL DETACHMENT

Retinoschisis, a splitting of the retina into two layers, may be responsible in some instances for producing a retinal detachment. The retinoschisis is usually of the reticular degenerative type produced by the coalescence of cystic spaces in typical and reticular cystoid degeneration. The retinoschisis cavity appears as a smooth, rounded, bullous elevation usually in the inferior temporal quadrant between the equator and the ora serrata. The innermost of the two layers contains the retinal vessels, which frequently are sheathed, and may contain multiple small round holes. The outermost layer of the retinoschisis is closely applied to the pigment epithelium and frequently contains large round holes with rolled edges. These holes are usually found toward the posterior margin of the retinoschisis cavity.

Sometimes, as shown here, a true retinal detachment forms, with fluid flowing through the large outer layer holes to collect between the outer retinal layer and the pigment epithelium. These retinal detachments are very slowly progressive and may become symptomatic only when the detachment reaches the macula and central vision is lost. A retinal detachment occurring in combination with retinoschisis may show demarcation lines, a feature absent in retinoschisis alone. In surgical repair of a retinal detachment associated with retinoschisis, it is the outer layer holes that must be closed. The inner layer holes may be ignored, but, of course, the schisis cavity may persist.

Byer NE: Clinical study of senile retinoschisis. Arch Ophthalmol 79:36–44, 1968

Hagler WS, Woldoff HS: Retinal detachment in relation to senile retinoschisis. Trans Am Acad Ophthalmol Otolaryngol 77:99–113, 1973

Kurz OO, Reif J: Retinoschisis as prehole stage in the retinopathy of retinal detachment. Isr J Med Sci 8:1431–1433, 1972

Straatsma BR, Foos RY: Typical and reticular degenerative retinoschisis. Am J Ophthalmol 75:551–560, 1973

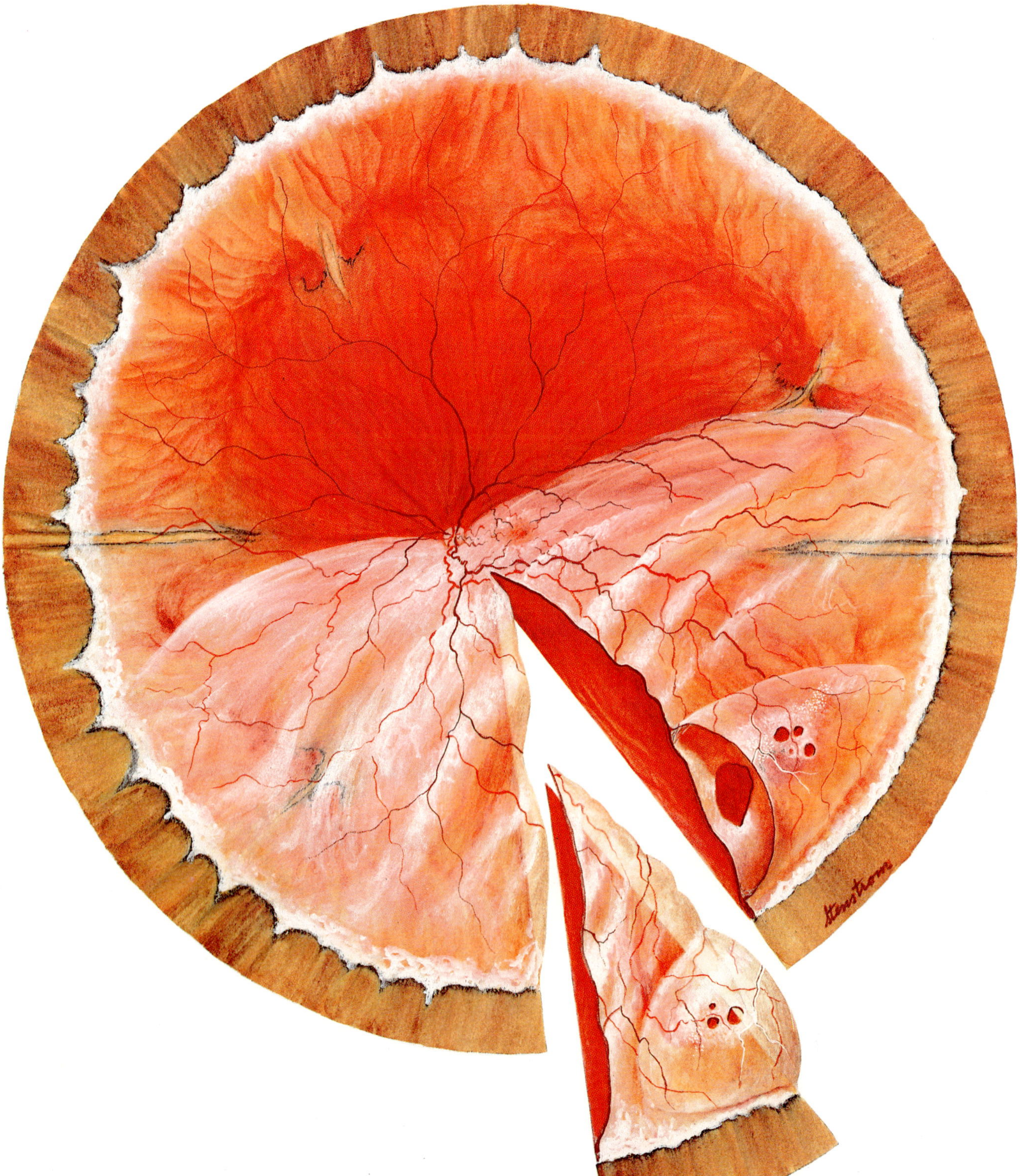

PLATE 22

DIALYSIS WITH DEMARCATION LINES

A retinal dialysis is a specific type of retinal break in which the retina tears neatly away at the posterior edge of the ora serrata. The size of the break in a retinal dialysis is frequently large but a dialysis should not be confused with a giant retinal tear. In a dialysis, there is no tendency for the retina to form a posteriorly rolled edge, and the prognosis is more favorable than in a giant tear.

Some retinal dialyses are spontaneous, as represented here, and some are produced by trauma (see Plate 24). Spontaneous retinal dialyses are thought to be a genetically determined condition. Most patients are young adults with no past history of eye trauma. There is an equal incidence in both sexes. Frequently, spontaneous dialyses are bilateral, and a careful study of the opposite eye must be made to search for an asymptomatic, occult dialysis. The inferior temporal quadrant is most commonly affected. The resulting retinal detachment progresses slowly, and many patients do not complain until the detachment reaches the macula and central vision is lost.

One characteristic finding in retinal dialysis is the presence of demarcation lines. A demarcation line is a white, brown, or black line that is gently concentric with the retinal break. These lines are subretinal and can be seen to pass underneath the retinal vessels. They represent a form of subretinal proliferation and may limit the mobility and unfolding of the detached retina.

The presence of a demarcation line indicates that the edge of the retinal detachment was stable at that point for at least six weeks. Multiple demarcation lines roughly parallel to each other indicate continuing progression of the detachment even though there have been periods of stability. It is obvious that a demarcation line gives no protection against the extension of a retinal detachment.

Benson WE, Nantawan P, Morse PH: Characteristics and prognosis of retinal detachments with demarcation lines. Am J Ophthalmol *84*:641–644, 1977

Hagler WS, North AW: Retinal dialyses and retinal detachment. Arch Ophthalmol *79*:376–388, 1968

Hilton GF, Norton EWD: Juvenile retinal detachment. Mod Prob Ophthalmol *8*:325–341, 1969

Hudson JR: Retinal detachment in children. Trans Ophthalmol Soc UK *85*:79–91, 1965

Tasman W: Peripheral retinal changes following blunt trauma. Trans Am Ophthalmol Soc *70*:190–198, 1972

Verdaguer TJ, Rojas B, Lechuga M: Genetical studies in nontraumatic retinal dialyses. Mod Probl Ophthalmol *15*:34–39, 1975

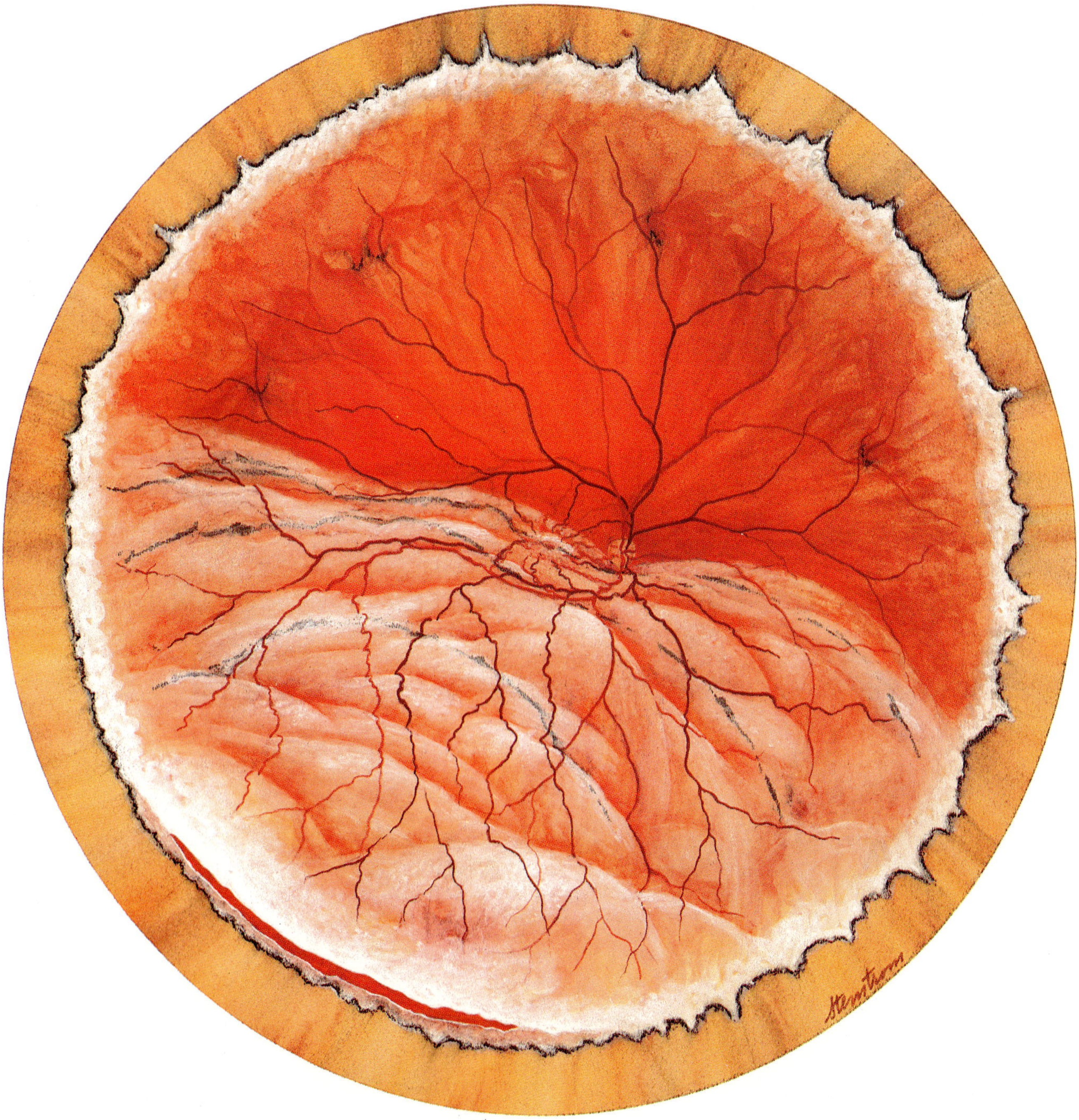

PLATE 23

DIALYSIS WITH RETINAL DETACHMENT

A retinal dialysis may be caused by trauma or it may occur spontaneously (see Plate 23). Traumatic dialyses occur most commonly in young males. Frequently, a missile such as a ball, rock, or fist is responsible for the injury.

A retinal dialysis is the most common type of retinal break caused by blunt trauma. Tasman believes that traumatic dialyses are produced at the time of injury, but clinical dialyses with detachment commonly present months or years after the trauma has occurred. The dialysis may not be visible immediately after the injury because of hemorrhage or edema.

If trauma to the eye occurs from straight ahead, a superior nasal dialysis is most commonly produced. If the traumatic insult is from an angle, the inferior temporal quadrant is most commonly affected, as this is the least protected quadrant of the eye.

The clinical appearance of a traumatic dialysis reveals the free edge of the torn retina bowing forward into the vitreous, revealing a large expanse of pigment epithelium and choroidal pattern. Despite the dramatic appearance of a retinal dialysis, there is little traction on the retina and the retinal break, although large, can usually be successfully closed. The large size of many dialyses should not cause them to be confused with giant retinal tears, which have a much worse prognosis.

Black RK, Davies EWG: The management of retinal dialysis. Trans Ophthalmol Soc UK *87*:317–333, 1967

Chignell AH: Retinal dialysis. Br J Ophthalmol *57*:572–577, 1972

Cox MS: Retinal breaks caused by nonperforation trauma at the point of impact. Tr Am Ophthalmol Soc *78*:413–466, 1980

Cox, MS, Schepens CL, Freeman HM: Retinal detachment due to ocular contusion. Arch Ophthalmol *76*:678–685, 1966

Tasman W: Retinal dialysis following blunt trauma. In Freeman, HM (ed.): Ocular Trauma. New York, Appleton-Century-Crofts, 1979, pp. 295–299

Weidenthal DT, Schepens CL: Peripheral fundus changes associated with ocular contusion. Am J Ophthalmol *62*:465–477, 1966

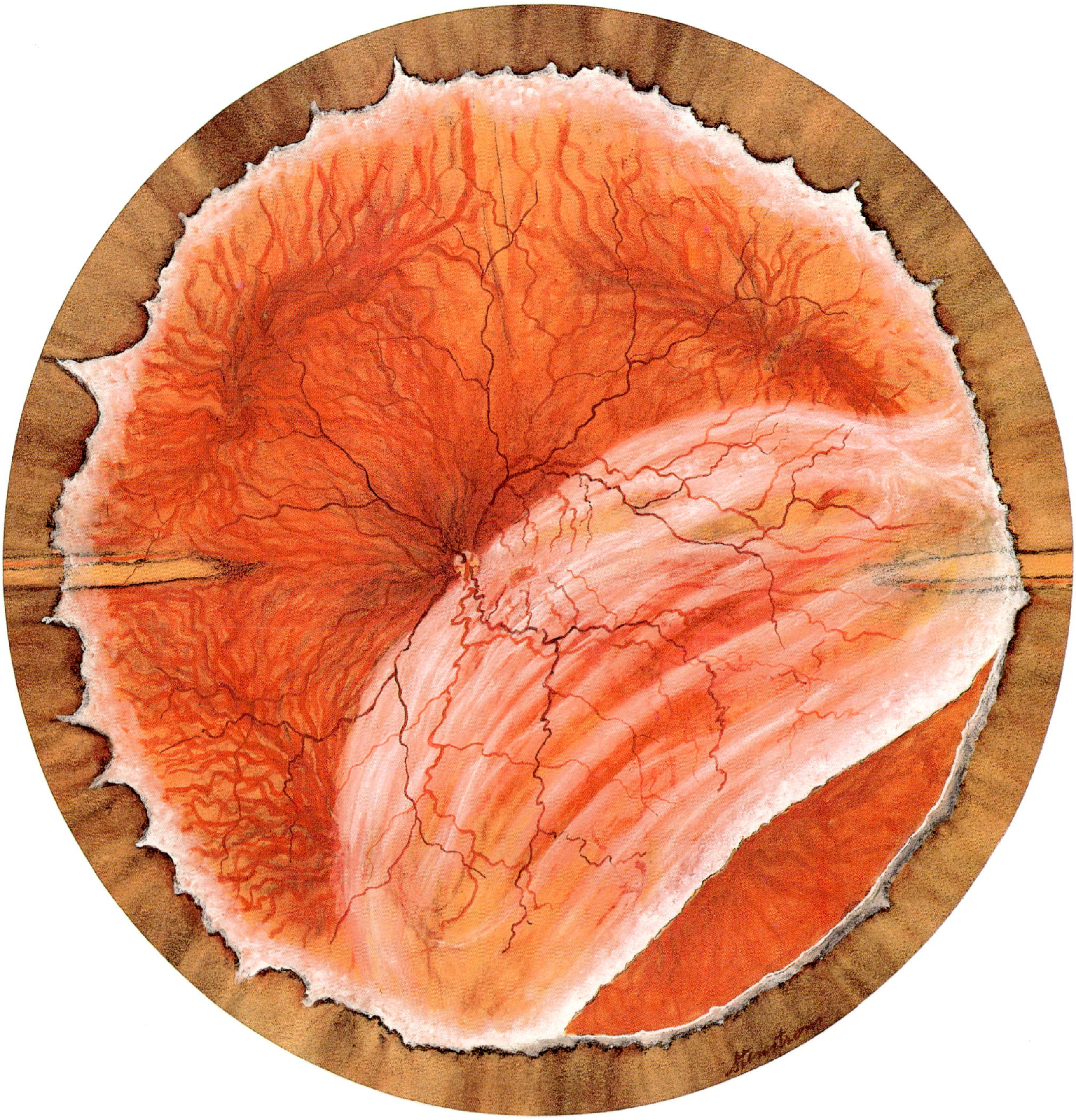

PLATE 24

BERLIN'S EDEMA

Berlin's edema, also called commotio retinae, is a milky white edema of the retina caused by blunt injury to the globe. It becomes visible within 24 hours of the injury and subsides over several days. The border between the white edematous retina and adjacent normal retina is quite sharp, producing a dramatic effect. The retinal vessels stand out in bold relief against the white background. If the macula is involved, a cherry-red spot is visible in the fovea. The pattern of involvement is quite variable, and either the posterior pole or the periphery may be involved. Sometimes there are islands of normal retina completely surrounded by Berlin's edema. The white areas give the subjective illusion of retinal elevation, and this must not be confused with a retinal detachment.

The concussion injury that leads to Berlin's edema may also produce other ocular injuries as well. Histologically, there is edema of all retinal layers, and there may be associated retinal, subretinal, choroidal, or vitreous hemorrhage. Over several days, the dramatic white retinal edema gradually fades and the retina may either resume its normal function or undergo atrophy and necrosis. The visual prognosis is therefore dependent upon the area of retina involved and the severity of the injury.

Blight R, Hart JCP: Structural changes in the outer retinal layers following blunt mechanical non-perforating trauma to the globe. An experimental study. Br J Ophthalmol *61*:573–587, 1977

Delori F, Pomerantzeff O, Cox MS: Deformation of the globe under high-speed impact: Its relation to contusion injuries. Invest Ophthalmol *8*:290–301, 1969

Sipperley JO, Quigley HA, Gass JDM: Traumatic retinopathy in primates: The explanation of commotio retinae. Arch Ophthalmol *96*:2267–2273, 1978

Tasman W: Peripheral retinal changes following blunt trauma. Trans Am Ophthalmol Soc *70*:190–198, 1972

Weidenthal DT, Schepens CL: Peripheral fundus changes associated with ocular contusion. Am J Ophthalmol *62*:465–477, 1966

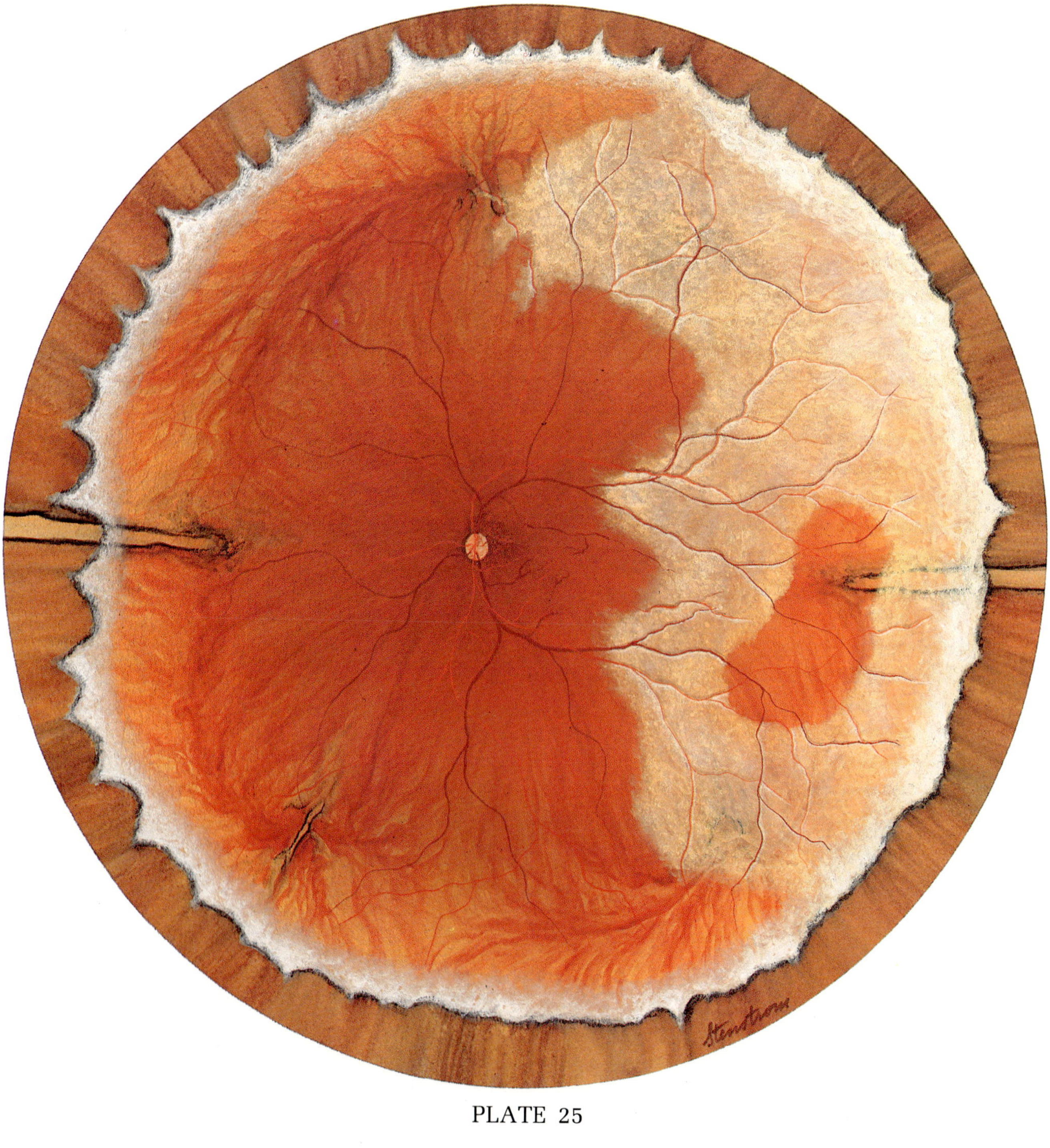

PLATE 25

CHOROIDAL RUPTURE

Choroidal rupture occurs as a result of severe blunt trauma to the anterior eye. A shock wave is transmitted to the posterior pole, producing crescent-shaped ruptures in the choroidal layers. The choroid breaks much as a hard-boiled egg shell does. The ruptures typically occur in the posterior pole and curve around the optic nerve. The ruptures are long and thin, with the white sclera appearing in the base of the rupture. The retinal vessels can be seen passing over the choroidal rupture. Curiously, the retina appears to be able to stretch so that a retinal break is infrequently produced and retinal detachments rarely occur. Generally there is no rupture of the globe, but a combination of other traumatic injuries to the globe may be present.

Immediately after the injury, the intraocular pressure may be low or entirely normal. As the retinal and vitreous hemorrhages absorb, repair occurs by extensive glial proliferation, with pigmentation occurring at the margins of the rupture. The visual prognosis depends on whether or not the macular area is involved. Even if the choroidal rupture does not pass directly through the macula, there may be late development of subretinal neovascularization growing in from the scar, leading to late hemorrhagic detachment of the macula and loss of central vision.

Eagling EM: Ocular damage after blunt trauma. Br J Ophthalmol 58:126–140, 1974

Fuller B, Gitter KA: Traumatic rupture with late serous detachment of the macula: Report of successful argon laser treatment. Arch Ophthalmol 89:354–355, 1973

Gitter KA, Slusher M, Justice J: Traumatic hemorrhagic detachment of the pigment epithelium. Arch Ophthalmol 79:729–732, 1968

Ingram DV, Lewkonia I: Ocular hazards of playing squash rackets. Br J Ophthalmol 57:434–438, 1973

Richards RD, West CE, Neisels AA: Chorioretinitis sclopetaria. Am J Ophthalmol 66:852–860, 1968

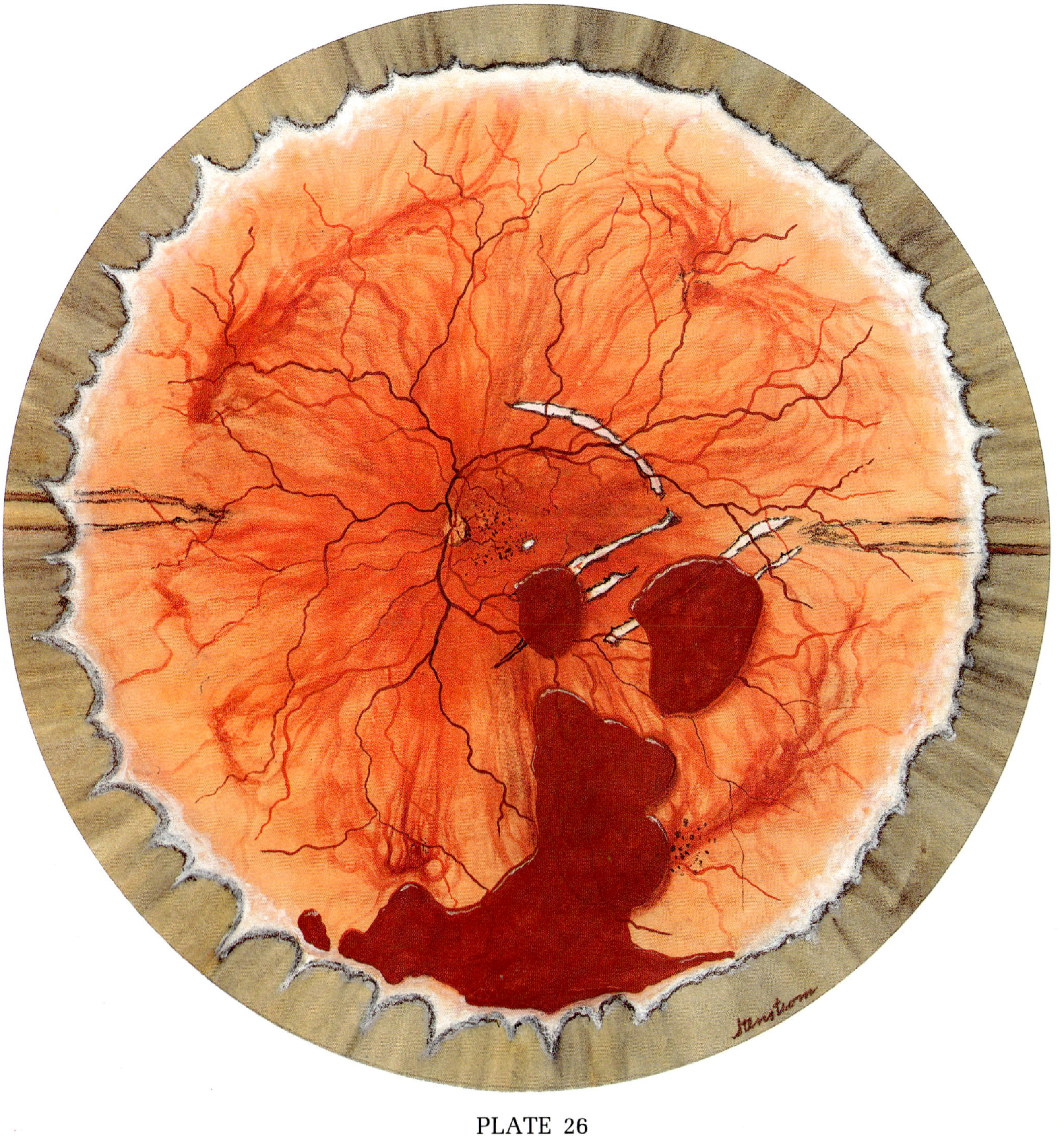

PLATE 26

AVULSION OF THE VITREOUS BASE

Avulsion of the vitreous base occurs after severe blunt trauma to the eye. The vitreous base is firmly attached to the nonpigmented ciliary epithelium overlying the pigmented pars plana epithelium. A severe blow can tear loose the vitreous base, and with it a strip of non-pigmented epithelium that may dangle as a festoon in the vitreous cavity. This occurs most commonly in the superior nasal quadrant. When present, this finding is considered definitive evidence of prior ocular trauma. The retina is almost always torn at the time of avulsion, producing retinal breaks at the site of the former attachment of the anterior or posterior vitreous base.

Here, the festoon is more visible to the patient and observer than is the retinal detachment, which is relatively flat. Frequently, the retinal break is obscured by retinal or vitreous hemorrhage. When a festoon such as this is visualized, careful scleral depression of the far periphery must be done in order to find retinal breaks before they progress to complete retinal detachment. Other late effects include peripheral chorioretinal atrophy at the site of the avulsion and also a later traumatic macular hole.

Delori F, Pomerantzeff O, Cox MS: Deformation of the globe under high-speed impact: Its relation to contusion injuries. Invest Ophthalmol *8*:290–301, 1969

Schepens CL: Pathogenesis of traumatic rhegmatogenous retinal detachment. *In* Freeman HM (ed): Ocular Trauma. New York, Appleton-Century-Crofts, 1979, pp 273–284

Tasman W: Peripheral retinal changes following blunt trauma. Trans Am Ophthalmol Soc *70*:190–198, 1972

Weidenthal DT, Schepens CL: Peripheral fundus changes associated with ocular contusion. Am J Ophthalmol *62*:465–477, 1966

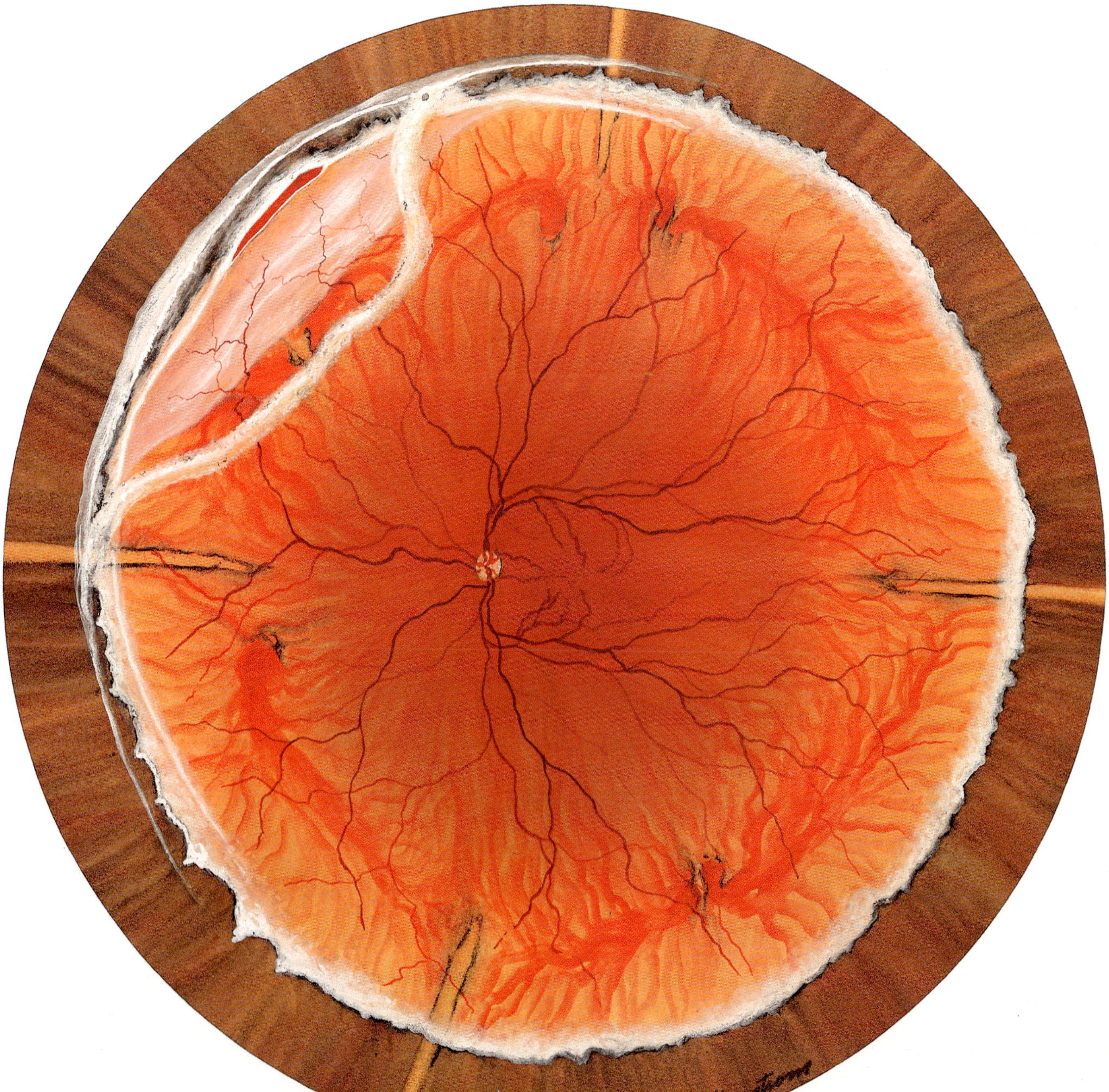

PLATE 27

TRAUMATIC RETINAL TEAR IN THE ANTERIOR VITREOUS BASE

Severe blunt ocular trauma frequently produces a tear or dialysis of the retina at either the anterior or posterior vitreous base. Typically, the trauma occurs to a young male engaged in athletic pursuits, or in an industrial setting. There may be a latent interval between the trauma and the symptomatic detachment, but there is a definite history of trauma. This long, thin linear dialysis of the retina is quite typical of traumatic retinal breaks. In this particular instance the dialysis is at the anterior vitreous base, but dialyses occur more frequently at the posterior vitreous base. It is believed that the dialysis may be produced immediately at the time of trauma but frequently is obscured by vitreous hemorrhage and the difficulty of examining the far periphery in a painful and swollen eye. It is also possible that such a dialysis may occur as a late effect of contusion injury, produced by progressive vitreous contraction and traction on the retina. Other late findings may include peripheral chorioretinal atrophy and pigmentation.

This total retinal detachment could have been produced by a break anywhere in the retina. Frequently much time is expended searching in vain for a break at the equator or posterior pole. An ophthalmoscopic clue to the location of the dialysis is the detachment extending to the pars plana. When the pars plana is detached, a careful study with scleral depression must be made to rule out retinal breaks of this type.

Cox MS: Retinal breaks caused by blunt nonperforating trauma at the point of impact. Tr Amer Ophthamol Soc *78*:413–466, 1980

Cox MS, Schepens CL, Freeman HM: Retinal detachment due to ocular contusion. Arch Ophthalmol *76*:678–685, 1966

Freeman HM, Cox MS, Schepens CL: Traumatic retinal detachments. Int Ophthalmol Clin *14*(4):151–170, 1974

Schepens CL: Pathogenesis of traumatic rhegmatogenous retinal detachment. *In* Freeman HM (ed): Ocular Trauma. New York, Appleton-Century-Crofts, 1979, pp 273–284

Tasman W: Peripheral retinal changes following blunt trauma. Trans Am Ophthalmol Soc. *70*:190–198, 1972

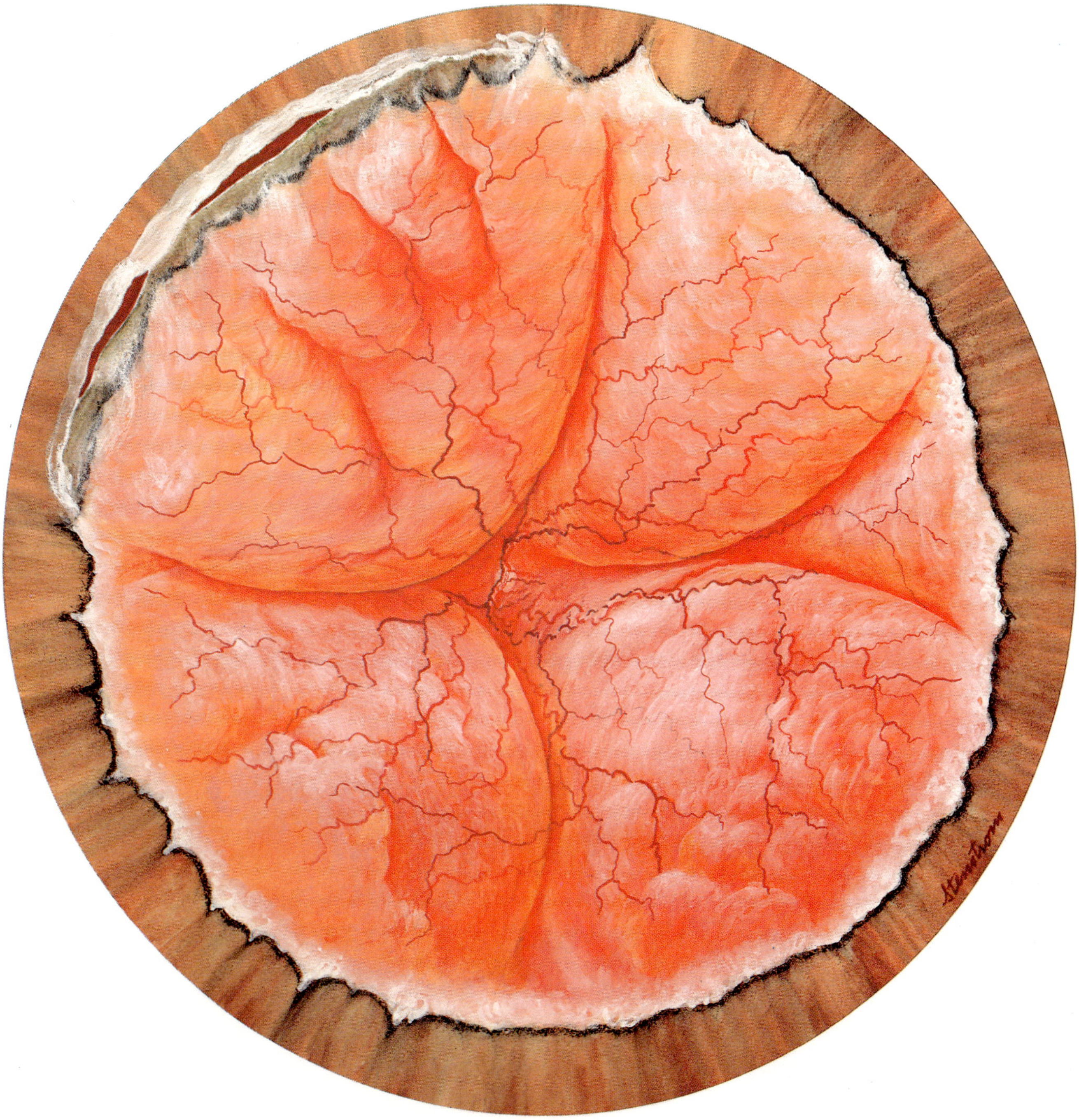

PLATE 28

TOTAL RETINAL DETACHMENT, HORSESHOE TEARS, STAR FOLD

This total retinal detachment is of some duration, as shown by the white, thinned appearance of the retina. Two typical horseshoe tears are present in the 10 o'clock and 4 o'clock meridians. The posterior margin of the vitreous base is visible on either side of both tears as a white line that is dragged somewhat posteriorly by the contracting vitreous. A star fold is present in the 5:30 o'clock meridian. This star fold contains several smaller radiating folds, as though the retina were grabbed on the underside with a slight twisting motion. In reality, there are usually both preretinal and subretinal proliferations of glial and pigment epithelial cells that proliferate on the retinal surfaces. With time, these cellular proliferations contract to produce star folds and other fixed retinal folds. The vitreous is usually strongly adherent to the retina in the area of star folds and may be incarcerated in the depths of the fold. Abundant pigment is usually present at the base of the fold along with the membranes, which may attach to one another.

Star folds are most common in the inferior half of a retinal detachment of some duration. The star fold represents an early stage of the development of massive periretinal proliferation.

Clarkson JG, Green WR, Massof D: A histopathological review of 168 cases of preretinal membrane. Am J Ophthalmol *84*:1–17, 1977

Constable IJ, Tolentino FI, Donovan RH, et al: Clinico-pathologic correlation of vitreous membranes. *In* Pruett RC, Regan CDJ (eds.): Retina Congress. New York, Appleton-Century-Crofts, 1974, pp 245–257

Machemer R: Removal of pre-retinal membranes. Trans Am Acad Ophthalmol Otolaryngol *81*:420–425, 1976

Machemer R: Pathogenesis and classification of massive periretinal proliferation. Br J Ophthalmol *62*:737–747, 1978

Machemer R, Laqua H: Pigment epithelial proliferation in retinal detachment (Massive periretinal proliferation). Am J Ophthalmol *80*:1–23, 1975

Morse PH: Fixed retinal star folds in retinal detachment. Am J Ophthalmol *77*:760–761, 1974

Van Horn DL, Aaberg TM, Machemer R, et al: Glial cell proliferation in human retinal detachment with massive periretinal proliferation. Am J Ophthalmol *84*:383–393, 1977

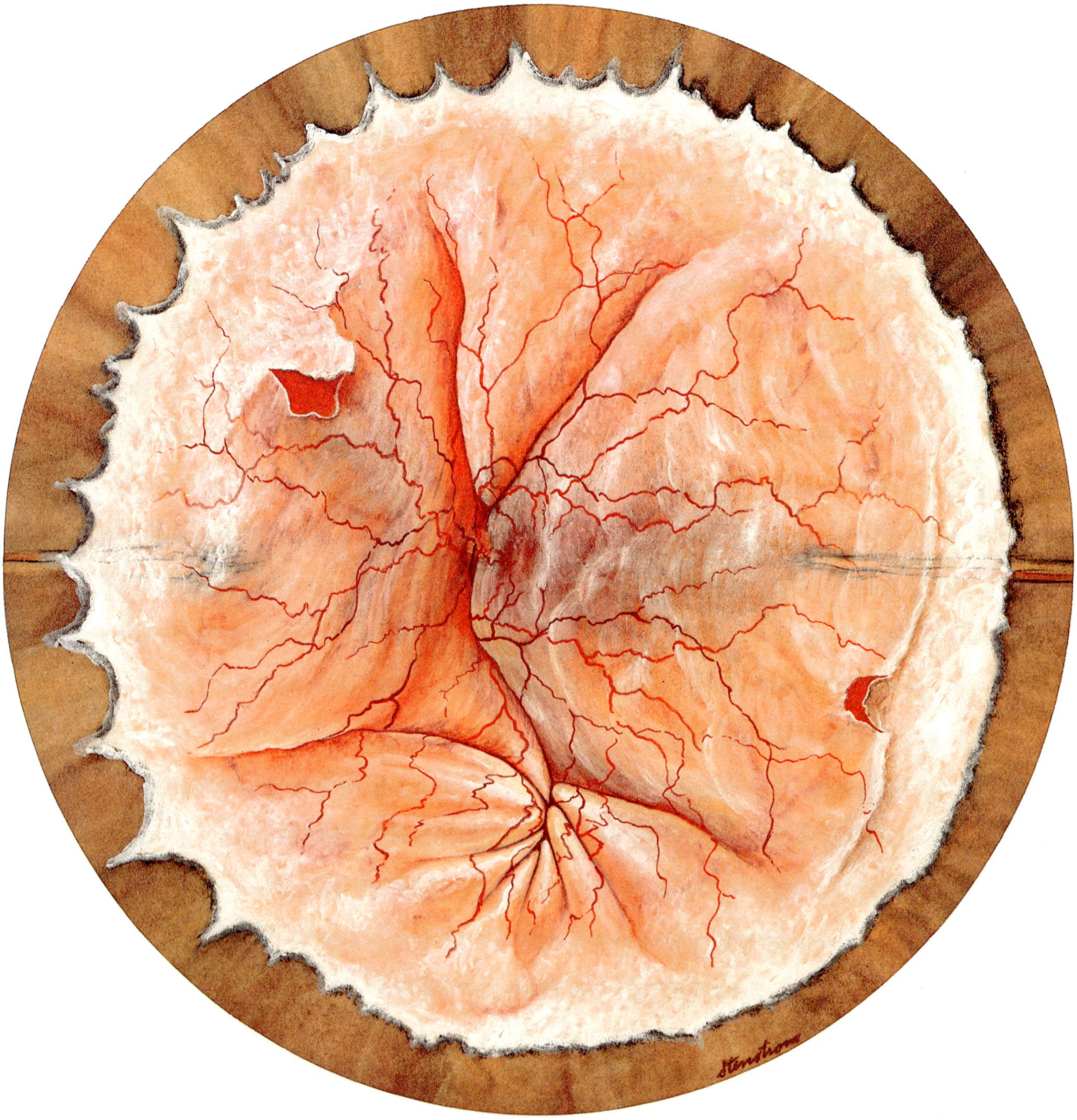

PLATE 29

LONG-STANDING TOTAL RETINAL DETACHMENT WITH TRAUMATIC LARGE HOLE AND INTRARETINAL MACROCYSTS

This total retinal detachment, which occurred after blunt trauma, illustrates several important features. The large, irregular retinal break is typically produced directly at the impact site of severe trauma. The retina and choroid may undergo immediate fragmentation and dissolution, but the later atrophy of large retinal areas is also documented to produce large retinal holes. Retinal and vitreous hemorrhages are prominent at the time of injury, but in this example the hemorrhage has long since been absorbed. The presence of extensive vitreous hemorrhage may obscure even large retinal breaks for considerable time, and clinically, many detachments are not diagnosed until weeks or months after the injury.

Note that the optic nerve is not visible; the retina has gathered into a funnel shape posteriorly as a result of massive preretinal membranes growing on the anterior retinal surfaces, binding the detached retina to itself in fixed folds.

Several macrocysts of the retina have formed near the retinal break. These macrocysts are actually a splitting of the retina in the outer plexiform layer and are found in retinas that have been chronically detached. In rare instances, hemorrhage may occur into macrocysts. Retinal macrocysts do not require drainage or puncture, as they will resolve spontaneously with closure of all retinal breaks and reattachment of the retina.

Cox MS: Retinal breaks caused by nonperforating trauma at the point of impact. Trans Am Ophthalmol Soc *78*:413–466, 1980

Cox MS, Freeman HM: Traumatic retinal detachment. *In* Freeman HM (ed): Ocular Trauma. New York, Appleton-Century-Crofts, 1979, pp 285–293

Cox MS, Schepens CL, Freeman HM: Retinal detachment due to ocular contusion. Arch Ophthalmol *76*:678–685, 1966

Hagler WS, North AW: Intraretinal macrocysts and retinal detachment. Trans Am Acad Ophthalmol Otolaryngol *71*:442–454, 1967

Ruiz RS: Hemorrhagic macrocyst of the retina. Arch Ophthalmol *83*:588–590, 1970

Schepens CL: Pathogenesis of traumatic rhegmatogenous retinal detachment. *In* Freeman HM (ed): Ocular Trauma. New York, Appleton-Century-Crofts, 1979, pp 273–284

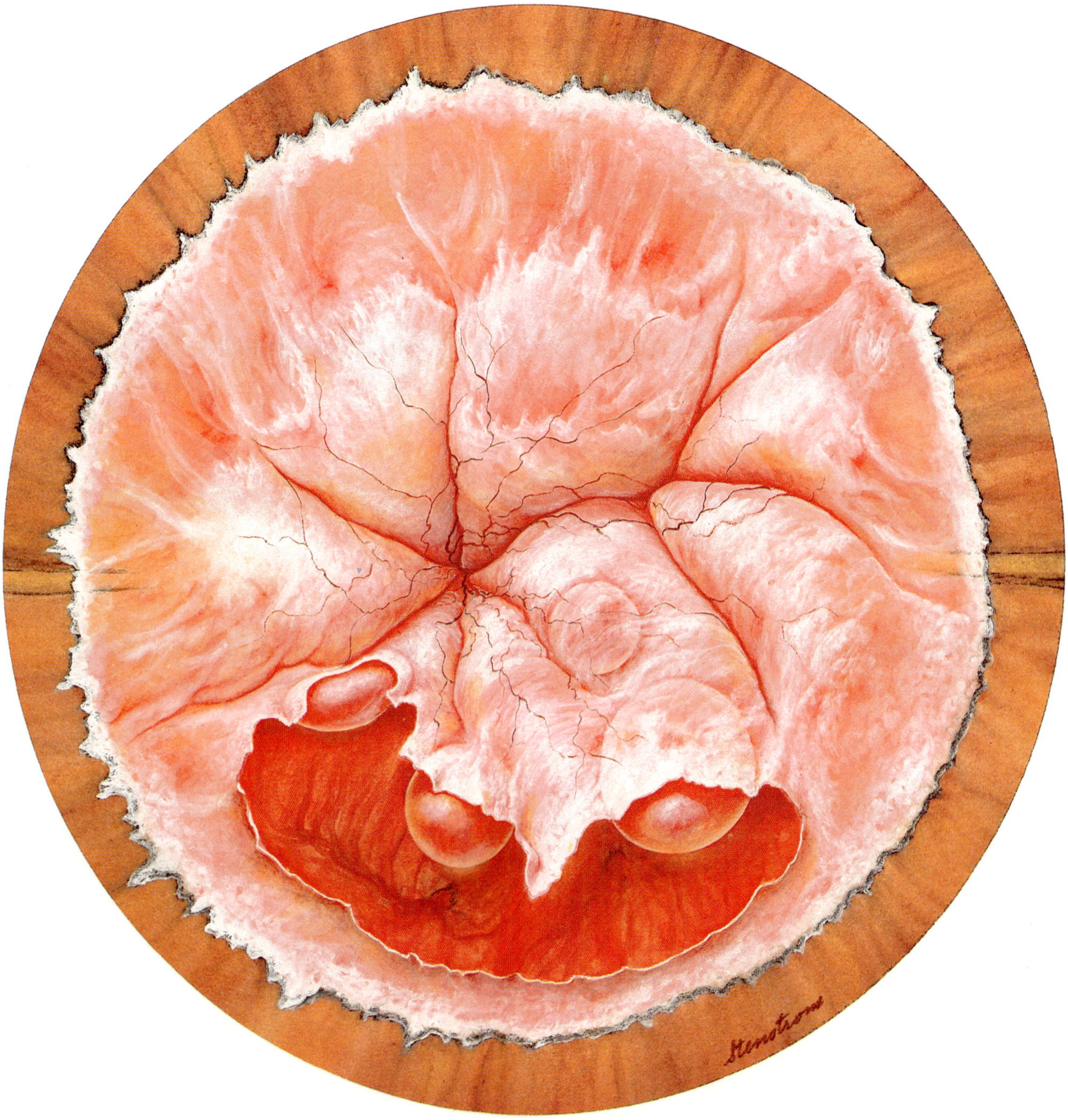

PLATE 30

TOTAL RETINAL DETACHMENT BREAKS WITH POSTERIOR ROLLED EDGES

This total retinal detachment contains several breaks, any one of which could have produced the total detachment. The breaks are large, and all must be closed completely in order to achieve successful reattachment. The posterior margin of each retinal break shows a tendency to curve posteriorly, a sign of severe retinal traction. When posteriorly rolled edges of the retinal break are noted in the preoperative examination, difficulty in achieving complete closure of the break at operation may be anticipated. Frequently such breaks exhibit the fish-mouth phenomenon, in which the retina does not lie flat on the elevation produced by the buckle, but rather, a tented-up portion of the retina allows communication between the vitreous cavity and the subretinal space.

Surgical techniques that aid in avoiding the fish-mouth phenomenon include high, localized buckling of the sclera, radial buckling, and the avoidance of excessive circumferential constriction. The injection of intravitreal air or gas may also be of assistance.

Lincoff HA, Kreissig I: Advantages of radial buckling. Am J Ophthalmol 79:955–957, 1975

Lincoff HA, Baras I, McLean JM: Modifications to the Custodis procedure for retinal detachment. Arch Ophthalmol 73:160–163, 1965

Lincoff H, McLean JM: Modifications to the Custodis procedure II. A new silicone implant for large tears. Am J Ophthalmol 64:877–879, 1967

Norton EWD: Intraocular gas in the management of selected retinal detachments. Trans Am Acad Ophthalmol Otolaryngol 77:85–98, 1973

Pruett RC: The fishmouthing phenomenon. Arch Ophthalmol 95:1777–1787, 1977

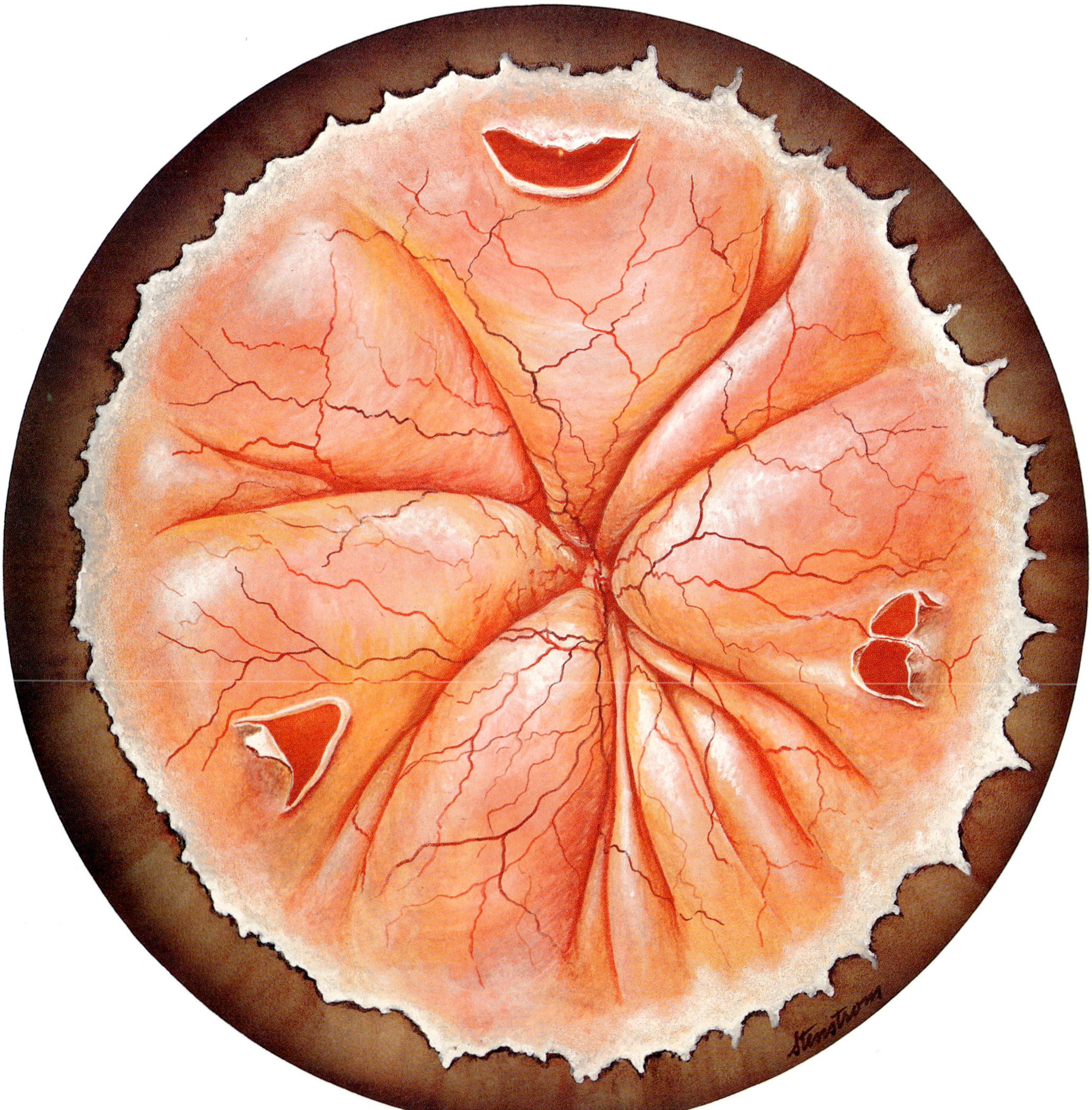

PLATE 31

MASSIVE PERIRETINAL PROLIFERATION

A small but definite percentage of all retinal detachments progress to massive intraocular scarring with the retina pulled into a funnel configuration. The view with the indirect ophthalmoscope reveals taut, rigid folds radiating from the periphery into a central, white, fibrotic sheet of tissue that completely overlies the mouth of the funnel. In far advanced cases vascularization may be noted in this fibrotic tissue. It is believed that this tissue is derived from glial and pigment epithelial cells that proliferate on both sides of the retina and along vitreous strands. These membranes then contract, dragging the retina into the funnel-shaped configuration shown here.

Operative approaches to this difficult problem include conventional scleral buckling, vitrectomy and membranectomy procedures, and the injection of intraocular gases and silicone oil. Although some eyes may be salvaged by these procedures, the overall prognosis remains rather poor.

Charles S: Vitrectomy for retinal detachment. Trans Ophthamol Soc UK *100*:542–549, 1980

Grizzard WS, Hilton GF: Scleral buckling for retinal detachments complicated by periretinal proliferation. Arch Ophthalmol *100*:419–422, 1982

Machemer R: Massive periretinal proliferation: A logical approach to therapy. Trans Am Ophthalmol Soc *75*:556–585, 1977

Machemer R, Laqua H: A logical approach to the treatment of massive periretinal proliferation. Ophthalmol *85*:584–593, 1978

Norton EWD: Intraocular gas in the management of selected retinal detachments. Trans Am Acad Ophthalmol Otolaryngol *77*:85–98, 1973

Okun E, Arribas NP: Therapy of retinal detachment complicated by massive preretinal fibroplasia. *In* Symposium on Retina and Retinal Surgery. Transactions of the New Orleans Academy of Ophthalmology. St. Louis, C V Mosby, 1969, pp 278–293

Scott JD: The treatment of massive vitreous retraction. Trans Ophthalmol Soc UK *93*:417–423, 1973

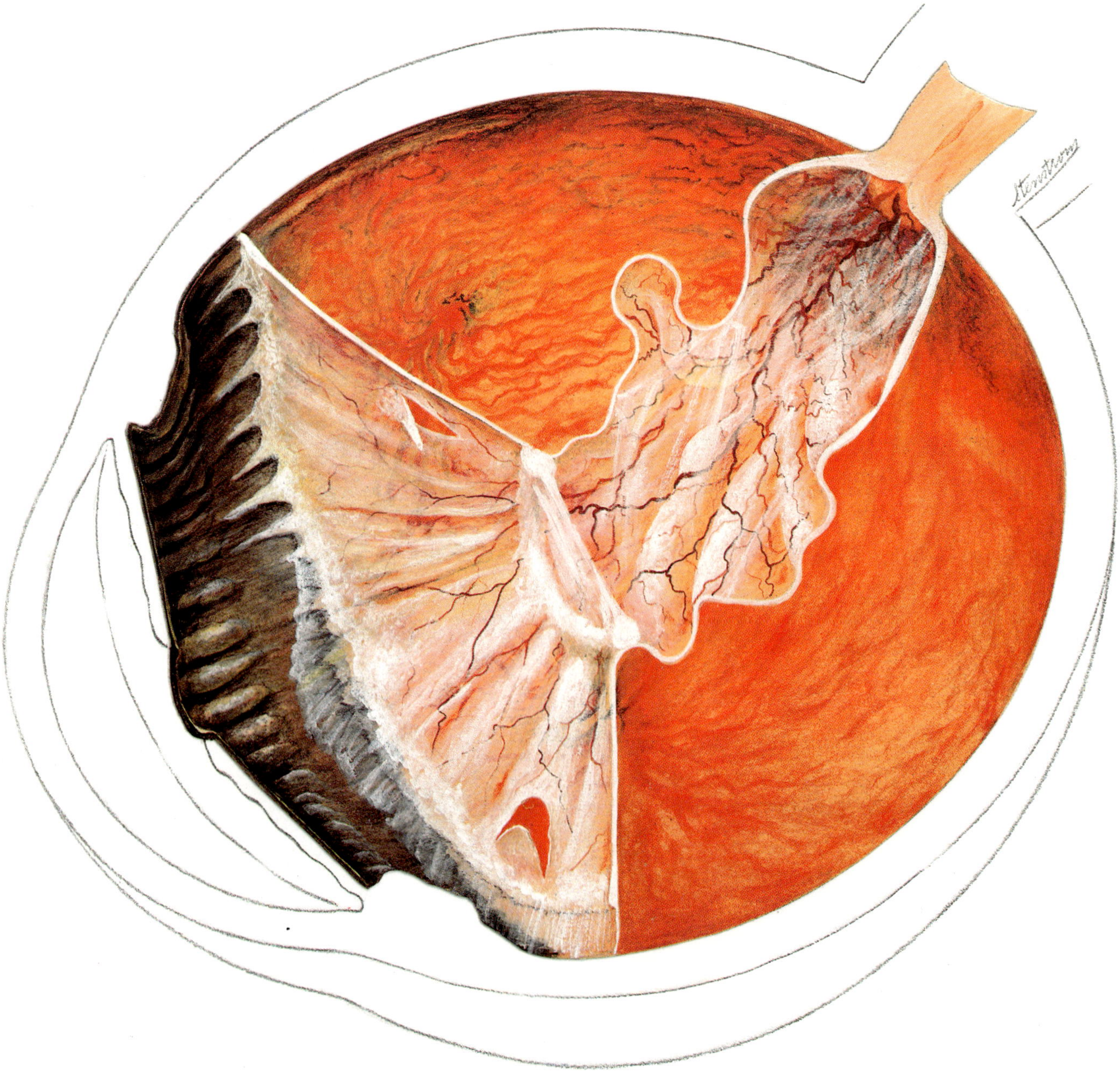

PLATE 32

GIANT RETINAL TEAR

A giant retinal tear is defined as a tear that extends through 90 degrees or greater of the retinal circumference. Many cases are spontaneous, occurring without warning, typically in young males. Post-traumatic giant tears also occur, as do giant tears associated with congenital colobomas of the lens and zonule.

The retina tears just posterior to the ora serrata, and there is typically a skirt of retina remaining at the ora that is tented upward due to vitreous traction. There is a tendency for the free edge of the retinal tear to roll up like a scroll, producing a detachment that is very difficult to repair. Giant retinal tears have a poor surgical and visual prognosis, and a number of special operative techniques frequently are necessary to achieve successful reattachment.

The giant retinal tear is a specific type of retinal tear that should not be confused with a retinal dialysis, in which the peripheral break may also be quite large. In a retinal dialysis, there is no tendency for the free edge of the torn retina to roll posteriorly, and the surgical prognosis is quite good.

There may be no recognizable pre-existing retinal degeneration at the site of a giant tear. Since it is quite common for a spontaneous giant tear to develop in the second eye, prophylactic treatment of the opposite eye is considered indicated even if the retina appears ophthalmoscopically normal.

Freeman HM: Current management of giant retinal breaks. *In* Symposium on Retina and Retinal Surgery. Transactions of the New Orleans Academy of Ophthalmology. St. Louis, C V Mosby, 1969, pp 171–183

Glasspool MG, Kanski JJ: Prophylaxis in giant tears. Trans Ophthalmol Soc UK *93*:363–371, 1973

Hovland KR, Schepens CL, Freeman HM: Developmental giant tears associated with lens coloboma. Arch Ophthalmol *80*:325–331, 1968

Norton EWD, Aaberg TM, Fung W, et al: Giant retinal tears. Am J Ophthalmol *68*:1011–1021, 1969

Schepens CL, Freeman HM: Current management of giant retinal breaks. Trans Am Acad Ophthalmol Otolaryngol *71*:474–487, 1967

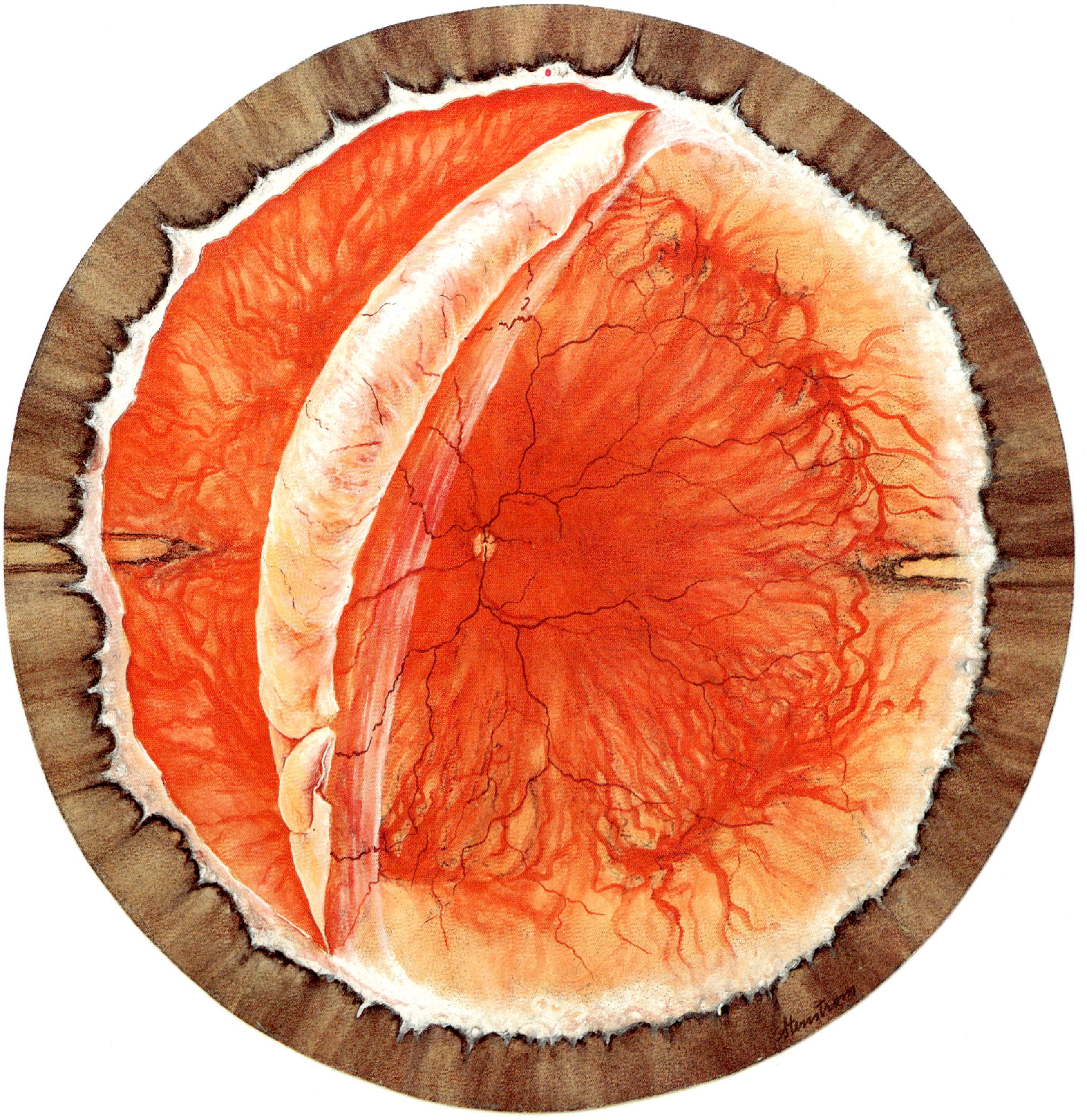

PLATE 33

GIANT RETINAL TEAR

This giant retinal tear has produced a detachment extending into the macular area. The free edge of the tear curves posteriorly toward the disc so that the posterior retinal surface is easily seen. The tented up peripheral skirt of retina has extended over the ora serrata so that there is a pars plana detachment as well. A large area of bare choroid and pigment epithelium is visible through the break, allowing excellent visualization of the temporal long posterior ciliary nerve and artery, and also the vortex vein collection systems.

Giant retinal breaks frequently extend circumferentially from both ends rather rapidly, so immediate operation is advised to limit progression. The vitreous is quite clear, allowing excellent visualization of the retina, but the vitreous body may become trapped posterior to the rolled edge of detachment, making unrolling of the detachment at operation difficult. Operative injection of air or gas is frequently of benefit in aiding the unrolling of the free edge of the retina. It is generally advisable to use a low rather than a high scleral buckle in large tears to avoid radial folds and leakage over the buckle. Despite the fact that initial operative success may be achieved, there is a great tendency for giant tears to redetach in the postoperative period, and the difficulty of these detachments should never be underestimated.

Kanski J: Giant retinal tears. Am J Ophthalmol *79*:846–852, 1975

Lincoff HA, Kreissig I, LaFranco F: Large retinal tears. Am J Ophthalmol *84*:501–508, 1977

Norton EWD: Intra-ocular gas in the management of selected retinal detachments. Trans Am Acad Ophthalmol Otolaryngol *77*:85–98, 1973

Schepens CL, Freeman HM: Current management of giant retinal breaks. Trans Am Acad Ophthalmol Otolaryngol *71*:474–487, 1967

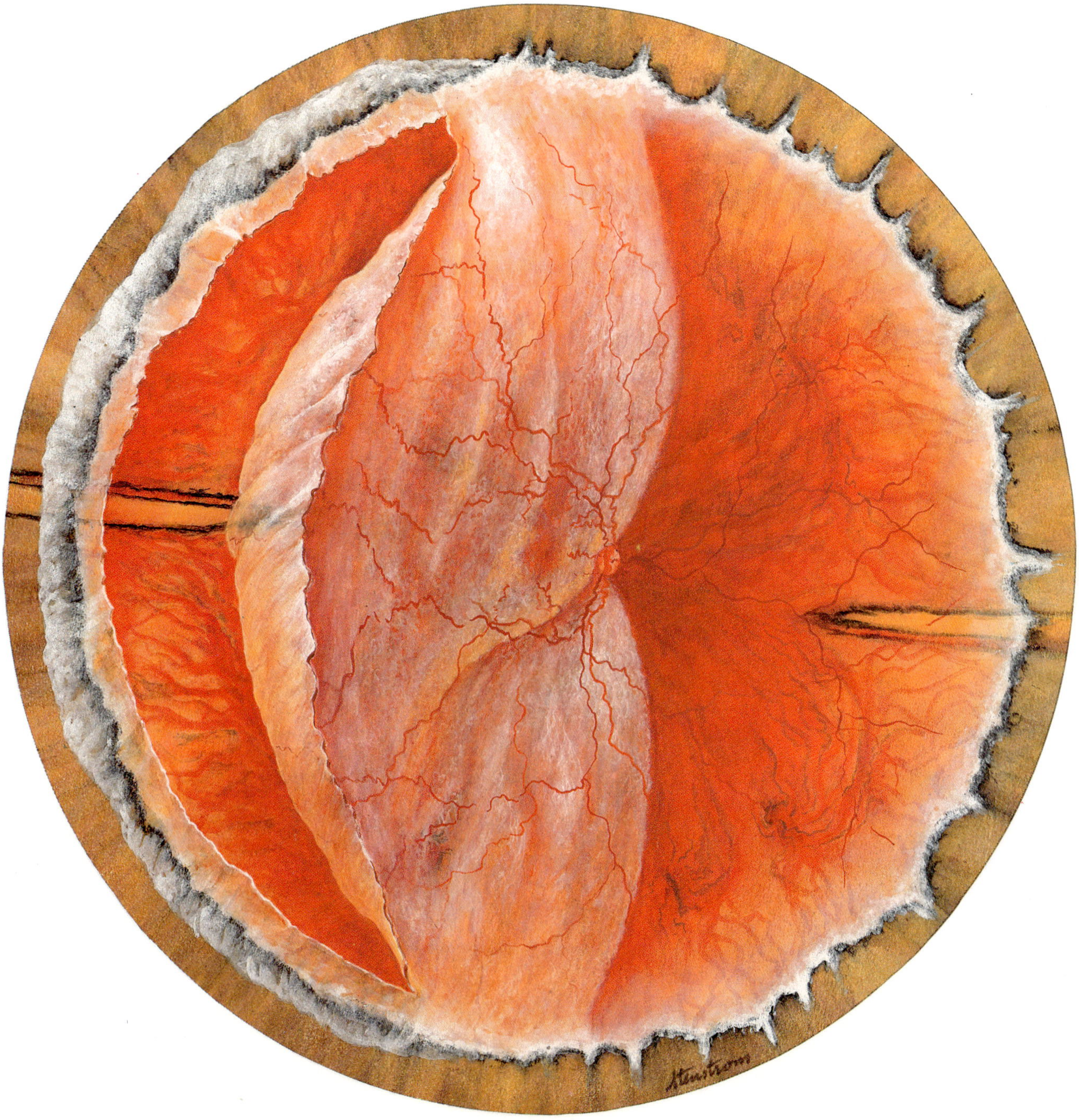

PLATE 34

GIANT RETINAL TEAR

This giant retinal tear has extended almost 300 degrees around the circumference, and the retina is rolled tightly upon itself so as to obscure the optic nerve and macula. In giant tears, there is a rapid formation and contraction of surface preretinal membranes. These preretinal membranes are almost invisible ophthalmoscopically, but they produce firm adhesions to one another, causing the retina to be difficult, if not impossible, to unroll. Special operative techniques, including vitrectomy procedures, the cutting of vitreous membranes, injection of intraocular air or gas, and in extreme cases, the injection of silicone oil are sometimes necessary. Special positioning during surgery using inverted operating room tables assists in unrolling the retina. Even with these extraordinary techniques, the surgical prognosis remains very poor.

Freeman HM: Current management of giant retinal breaks, *In* Symposium on Retina and Retinal Surgery. Transactions of the New Orleans Academy of Ophthalmology. St. Louis, CV Mosby, 1969, pp 171–183

Freeman HM: Vitreous surgery. X. Current status of vitreous surgery in cases of rhegmatogenous retinal detachment. Trans Am Acad Ophthalmol Otolaryngol *77*:202–215, 1973

Machemer R, Allen AW: Retinal tears 180 degrees and greater. Management with vitrectomy and intravitreal gas. Arch Ophthalmol *94*:1340–1346, 1976

Scott JD: Equatorial giant tears affected by massive vitreous retraction. Trans Ophthalmol Soc UK *96*:309–312, 1976

Scott JD: A rationale for the use of liquid silicone. Trans Ophthalmol Soc UK *97*:235–237, 1977

Watzke R: Silicone retinopoiesis for retinal detachment. Arch Ophthalmol *77*:185–196, 1967

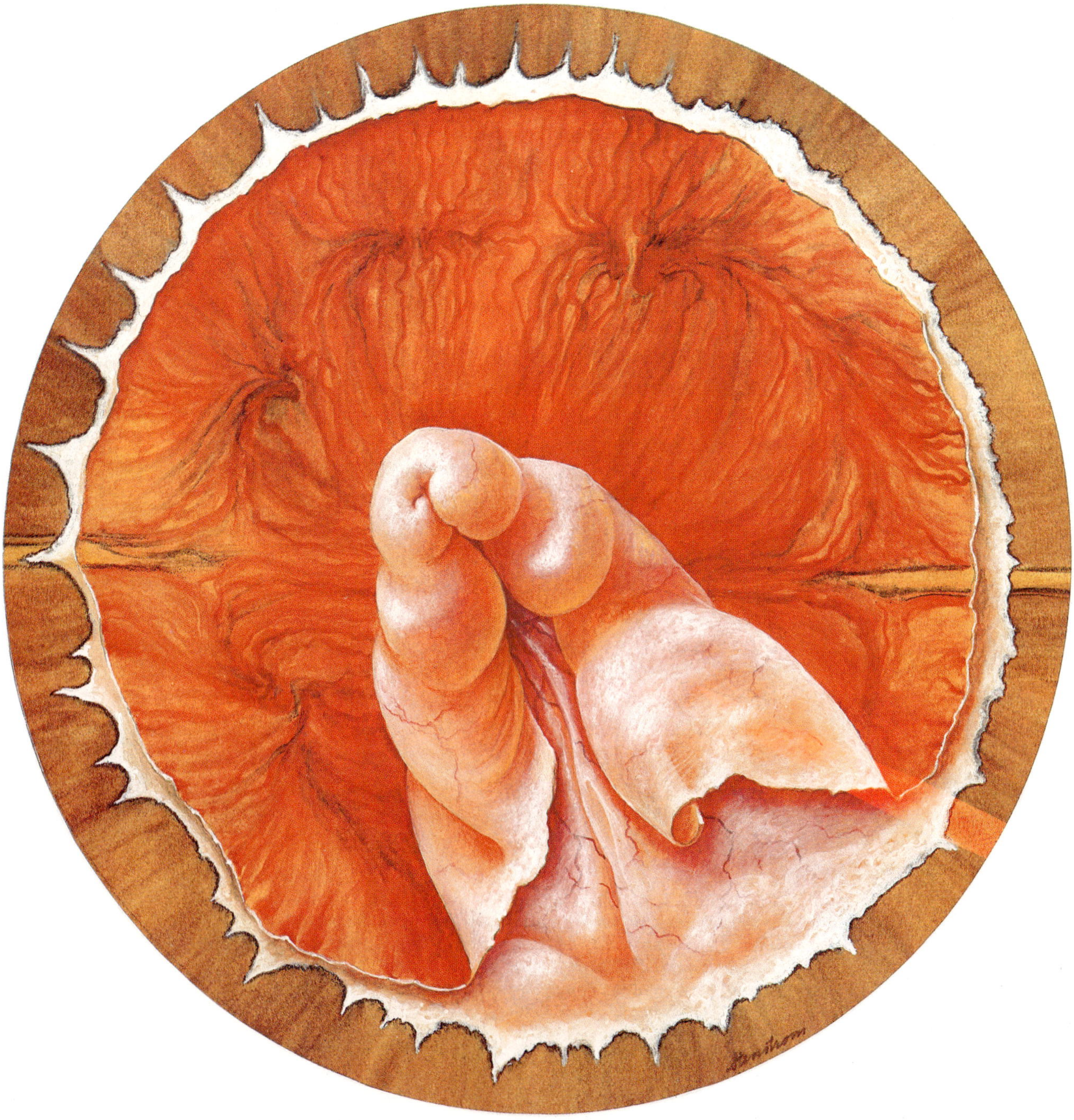

PLATE 35

REPAIRED RETINAL DETACHMENT

The clinical appearance of a successfully repaired retinal detachment should be recognized in order to avoid confusion with pathologic conditions. This retinal detachment has been successfully repaired, as shown by the fact that the pigment epithelium and choroid can be seen closely beneath all areas of the retina. In the superior temporal periphery, a horseshoe tear can be seen in the 10:30 o'clock meridian surrounded by a ring of cryotherapy. The ring of cryotherapy appears as a slightly pigmented circle around the horseshoe tear that contains pepper-like pigment clumping. In the ring of cyrotherapy treatment, the retina and underlying structures are fused into a single layer that heals into a watertight seal surrounding the tear. A segmental scleral buckle is visible running from 9 to 12 o'clock, indenting the outer layers of the globe inward toward the previously detached retina. This indentation into the vitreous cavity is permanent and should not be misinterpreted as a scleritis, choroidal hemorrhage, or tumor. An encircling element is seen gently indenting the equator around the remainder of the circumference of the eye.

The optic nerve, retinal vessels, and macula appear anatomically normal. If the macula is detached preoperatively, the postoperative visual acuity may never be as good as before the detachment occurred. There are a number of reasons for this, including the presence of cystoid macular edema, pigment fallout into the macular area from cryotherapy, and postoperative macular striae from preretinal membranes. It is axiomatic to prevent the macula from detaching if it has not already done so, and to reattach a recently detached macula as soon as practically possible. It is generally agreed that rapid operative reattachment gives the best visual prognosis.

Chisholm IA, McClure E, Foulds WS: Functional recovery of the retina after retinal detachment. Trans Ophthalmol Soc UK *95*:167–172, 1975

Cleary PE, Leaver PK: Macular morphology in the reattached retina. Mod Prob Ophthalmol *18*:400–407, 1977

Crews SJ: Macular changes following retinal detachment procedures. Mod Prob Ophthalmol *7*:337–347, 1968

Grupposo SS: Visual acuity following surgery for retinal detachments. Arch Ophthalmol *93*:327–330, 1975

Hilton GF: Subretinal pigment migration following cryosurgical retinal detachment. Mod Prob Ophthalmol *12*:64–70, 1964

Kreissig I: Prognosis of return of macular function after retinal detachment. Mod Prob Ophthalmol *18*:415–429, 1977

Meredith TA, Reeser FH, Topping TM, et al: Cystoid macular edema after retinal detachment surgery. Ophthalmol *87*:1090–1095, 1980

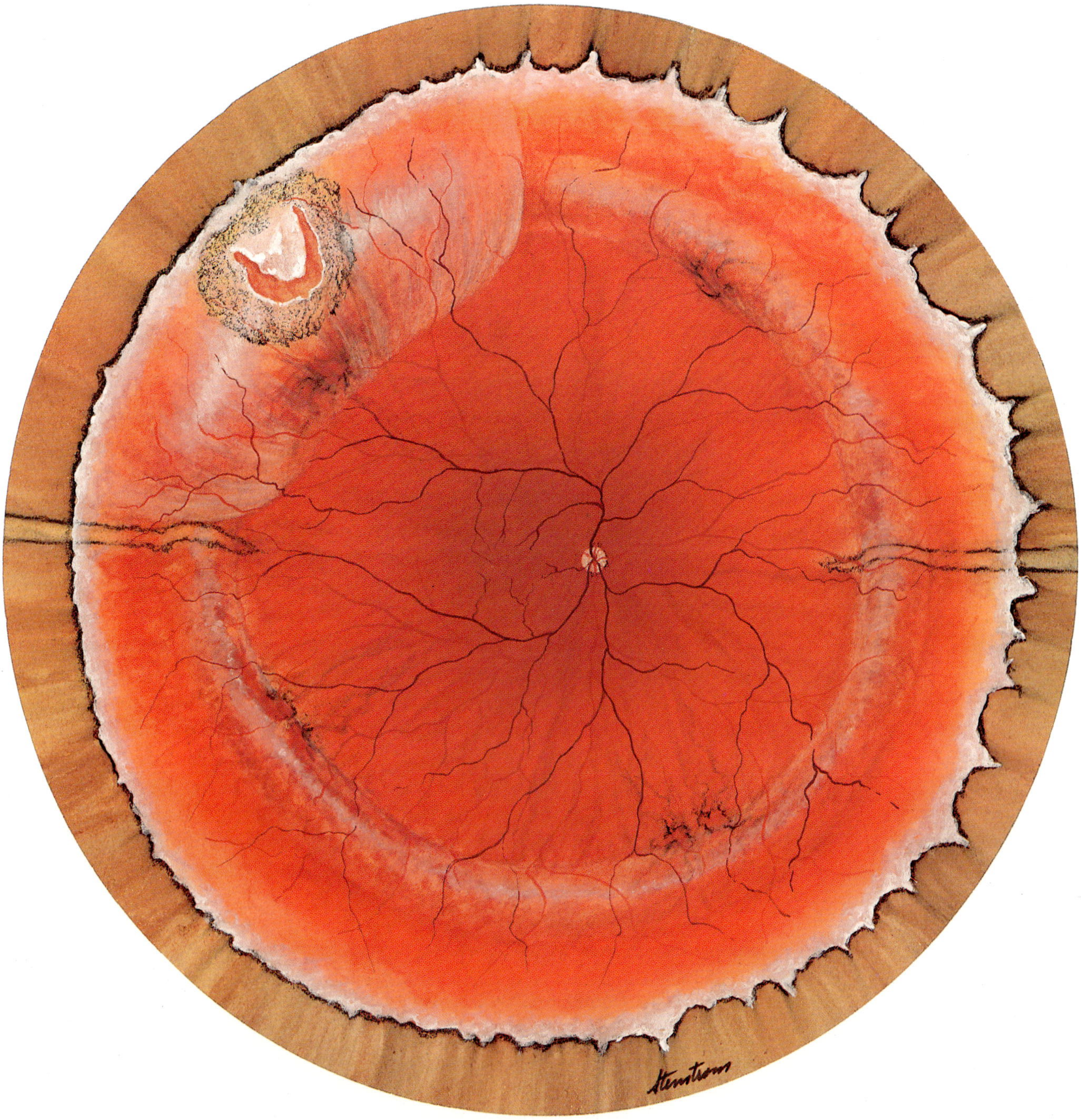

PLATE 36

SCLERAL BUCKLE WITH CHOROIDAL DETACHMENT

It is common to have choroidal detachments appear one to two days after a scleral buckle is performed. The choroidal detachments present as smooth, broadly elevated, solid-appearing elevations of retina with underlying pigment epithelium and choroid. They tend to occur in the fundus periphery, particularly to either side of a segmental buckle. The ora serrata is quite elevated and usually can be seen easily without scleral depression. Sometimes circumferential folds may be present.

Postoperative choroidal detachments are more common in elderly patients and in those with myopia and aphakia. Other factors are also thought to contribute to choroidal detachments, including the use of extensive diathermy or cryotherapy, prolonged hypotony, and the compression of vortex veins by tight encircling elements or broad posterior buckles. Postoperative positioning with the head dependent may also contribute to the development of choroidal detachments.

Usually the accumulation of suprachoroidal fluid causing the choroidal detachments is serous in nature, and it usually resolves without difficulty in one to two weeks. No great harm seems to be done by small choroidal detachments, although coarse granular pigmentation may result from longstanding choroidal detachments. There is no known way to completely prevent the development of choroidal detachments, and steroid therapy has no beneficial effect. A rare complication is for 360° choroidal detachments to produce angle closure glaucoma. Also, a hemorrhagic choroidal detachment occasionally occurs, producing a dark mass beneath the retina that slowly leaks blood at its margins into the vitreous cavity.

Burton BC, Stevens TS, Harrison TJ: The influence of subconjunctival depot corticosteroids on choroidal detachment following retinal detachment surgery. Trans Am Acad Ophthalmol Otolaryngol 79:845–849, 1975

Chignell AH: Choroidal detachment following retinal detachment surgery without drainage of subretinal fluid. Am J Ophthalmol 73:860–862, 1972

Hawkins WR, Schepens CL: Choroidal detachment and retinal surgery. Am J Ophthalmol 62:813–819, 1966

Hayreh SS, Baines JAB: Occlusion of the vortex veins—an experimental study. Br J Ophthalmol 57:217–238, 1973

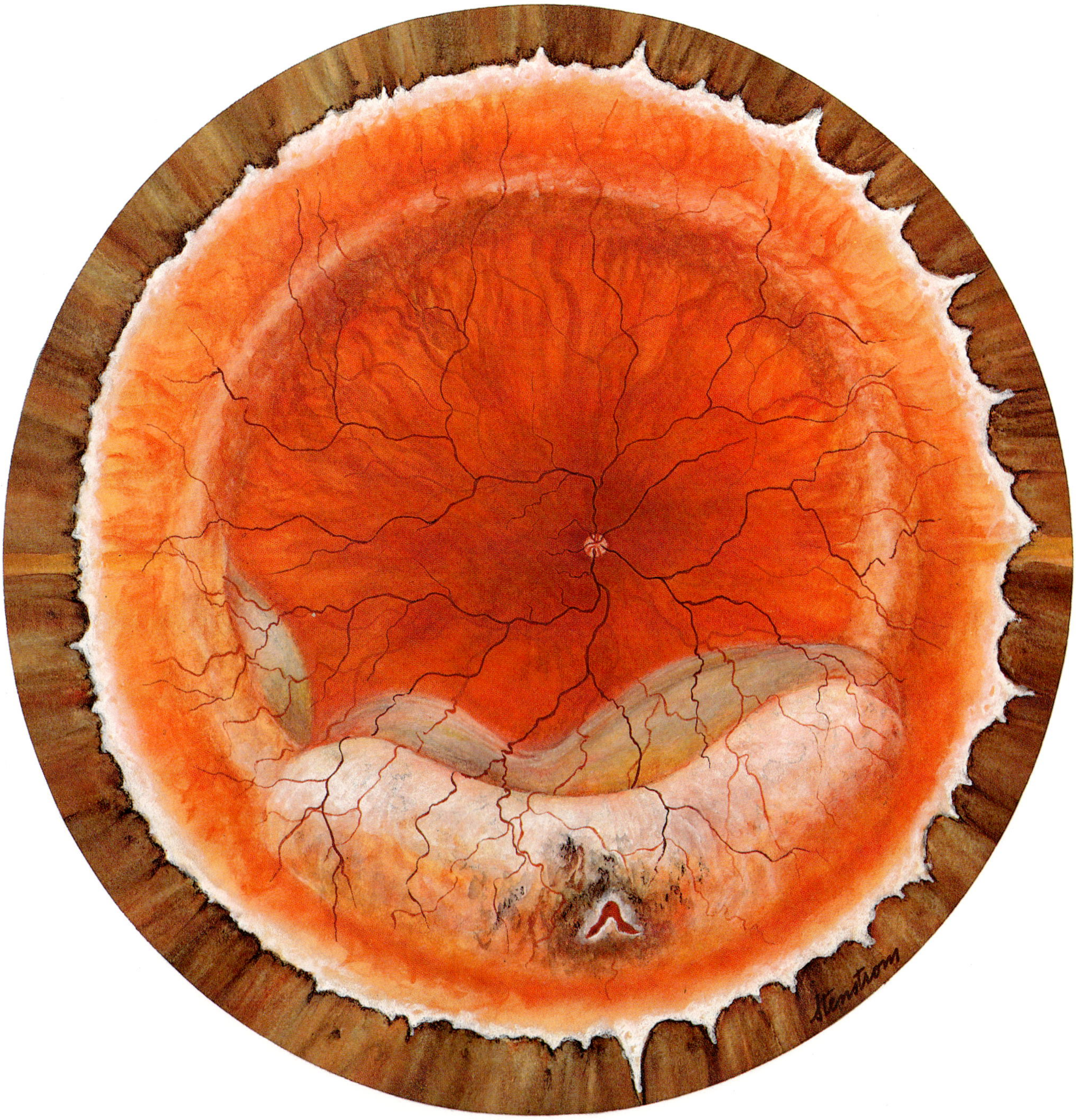

PLATE 37

XENON ARC

Xenon arc is sometimes used in place of laser treatment when particularly destructive photocoagulation is desired. In the plate on the left, three xenon arc photocoagulations have been applied to small vascular lesions. There is extensive destruction of the retina, pigment epithelium, and choroid, allowing the white sclera to be visible in the base of the lesion. A prominent rim of pigmentation appears at the margin of each application. Such lesions should not be confused with old chorioretinitis scars. Xenon arc photocoagulation is also used postoperatively as a noninvasive method of supplementing the chorioretinal reaction surrounding a retinal hole. Using additional xenon arc photocoagulation in this manner may prevent the necessity of performing a second operation.

Curtin VT, Norton EWD, Gass JDM: Photocoagulation: Its use in the prevention of reoperation after scleral buckling operations. Trans Am Acad Ophthalmol Otolaryngol 71:432–441, 1967

L'Esperance FA: Clinical comparison of xenon-arc and laser photocoagulation of retinal lesions. Arch Ophthalmol 75:61–67, 1966

Wallow IHL: Retinal repair after experimental xenon arc photocoagulation. Am J Ophthalmol 75:32–52, 1973; II. Am J Ophthalmol 75:610–626, 1973; III. Am J Ophthalmol 75:957–972, 1973

DIATHERMY

The characteristic appearance of diathermy treatment of retinal detachment is shown on the right. Multiple pigmented subretinal and intraretinal spots are seen spaced at regular intervals. Diathermy is best used only after scleral flaps have been dissected, as it is not advisable to treat through full thickness sclera. The retina between the diathermy applications appears entirely normal. Schepens has emphasized the advantages of using diathermy for retinal detachment operations, placing special emphasis on the correct instrumentation and technique of application.

Elzeneiny I, deGuillebon HF: Scleral damage in diathermy. Am J Ophthalmol 69:754–762, 1970

deGuillebon HF, Elzeneiny I: Electrical impedance of ocular coats during diathermy applications. Voltage and time of application. Arch Ophthalmol 83:489–503, 1970

Hilton GF, Norton EWD, Curtin VT, et al: Retinal detachment surgery: A comparison of diathermy and cryosurgery. Mod Prob Ophthalmol 8:440–448, 1969

Schepens CL: Methods of producing a chorioretinal scar: I. Diathermy. *In* Schepens CL: Retinal Detachment and Allied Diseases. Philadelphia, W B Saunders, 1983, pp 289–299

Swan KC, Christensen L: Scleral changes induced by diathermy in retinal detachment. Arch Ophthalmol 53:664–670, 1955

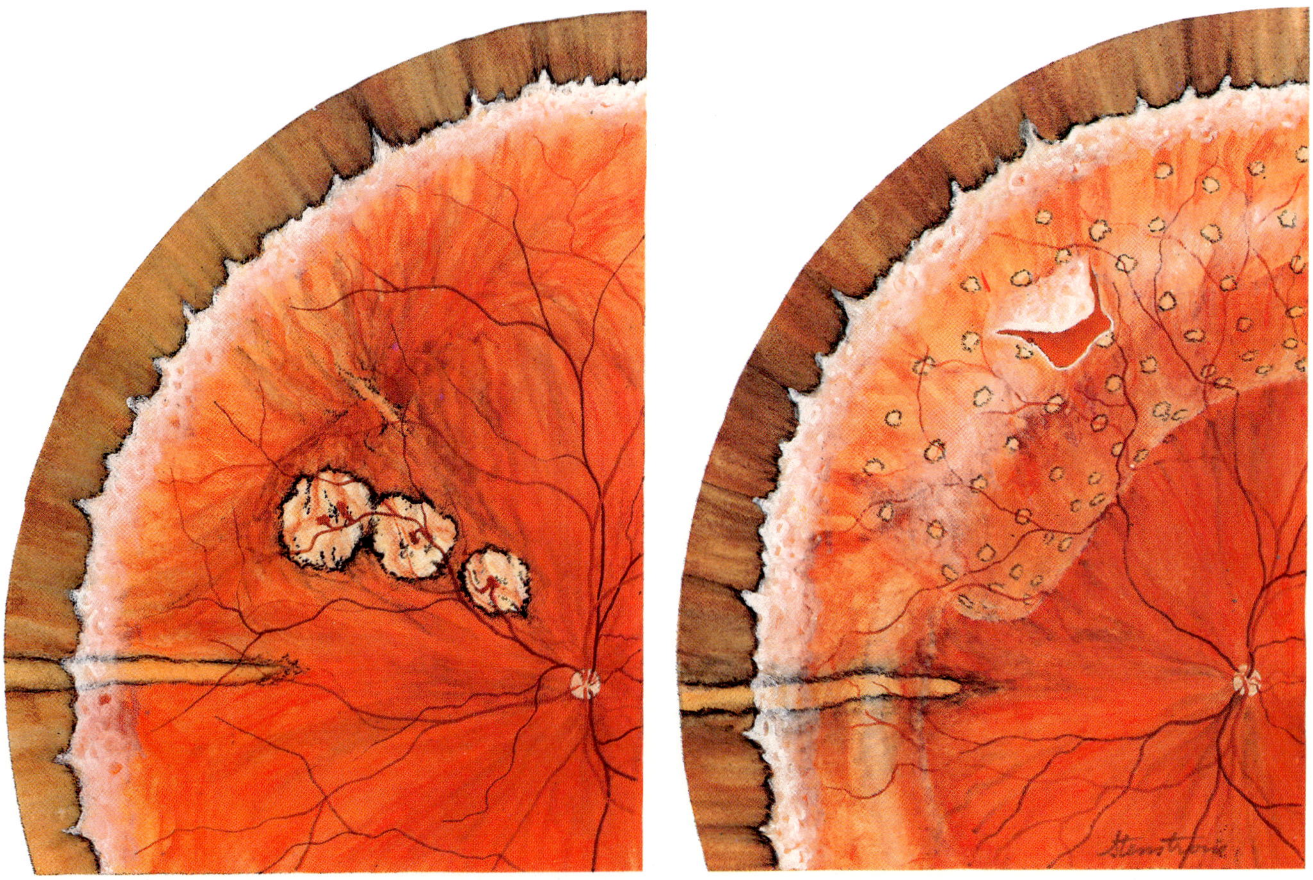

PLATE 38

CRYOTHERAPY OF LATTICE DEGENERATION

Transconjunctival cryotherapy has been applied to the numerous areas of lattice degeneration in the peripheral retina. Cryotherapy tends to produce depigmentation of heavily pigmented fundi, while lightly pigmented fundi may show an accumulation of dark pigment. In either case clumps of pepper-like granules may accumulate in the treated areas.

Note that all lattice lesions are completely surrounded with cryotherapy treatment. When there is a small ring of subretinal fluid surrounding a round retinal hole, care is taken to apply cryotherapy to the surrounding retina, which is in full apposition to the pigment epithelium and choroid. Only in this way is a watertight chorioretinal adhesion formed. It is not necessary to apply cryotherapy so strongly that extensive necrosis of the pigment epithelium and choroid is produced, creating an intensely white area. The proper intensity of cryotherapy leaves the pigment epithelium and choroid basically intact, while at the same time producing a watertight chorioretinal adhesion.

Abraham RK, Shea M: Avoidance of depigmentation and retinal atrophy following cryoretinopexy. J Cryosurg *1*:190–192, 1968

Chignell AH, Revie HS, Clemett RS: Complications of retinal cryotherapy. Trans Ophthalmol Soc UK *91*:635–651, 1971

Laqua H, Machemer R: Repair and adhesion mechanism of the cryotherapy lesion in experimental retinal detachment. Am J Ophthalmol *81*:833–846, 1976

Lincoff H, McLean JM: Mechanism of the cryosurgical adhesion. Am J Ophthalmol *67*:477–493, 1969

Lincoff H, Kreissig I: The mechanism of the cryosurgical adhesion. IV. Electron microscopy. Am J Ophthalmol *71*:674–689, 1971

Lincoff H, Kreissig I, Jakobiec F, et al: Remodeling of the cryosurgical adhesion. Arch Ophthalmol *99*:1845–1849, 1981

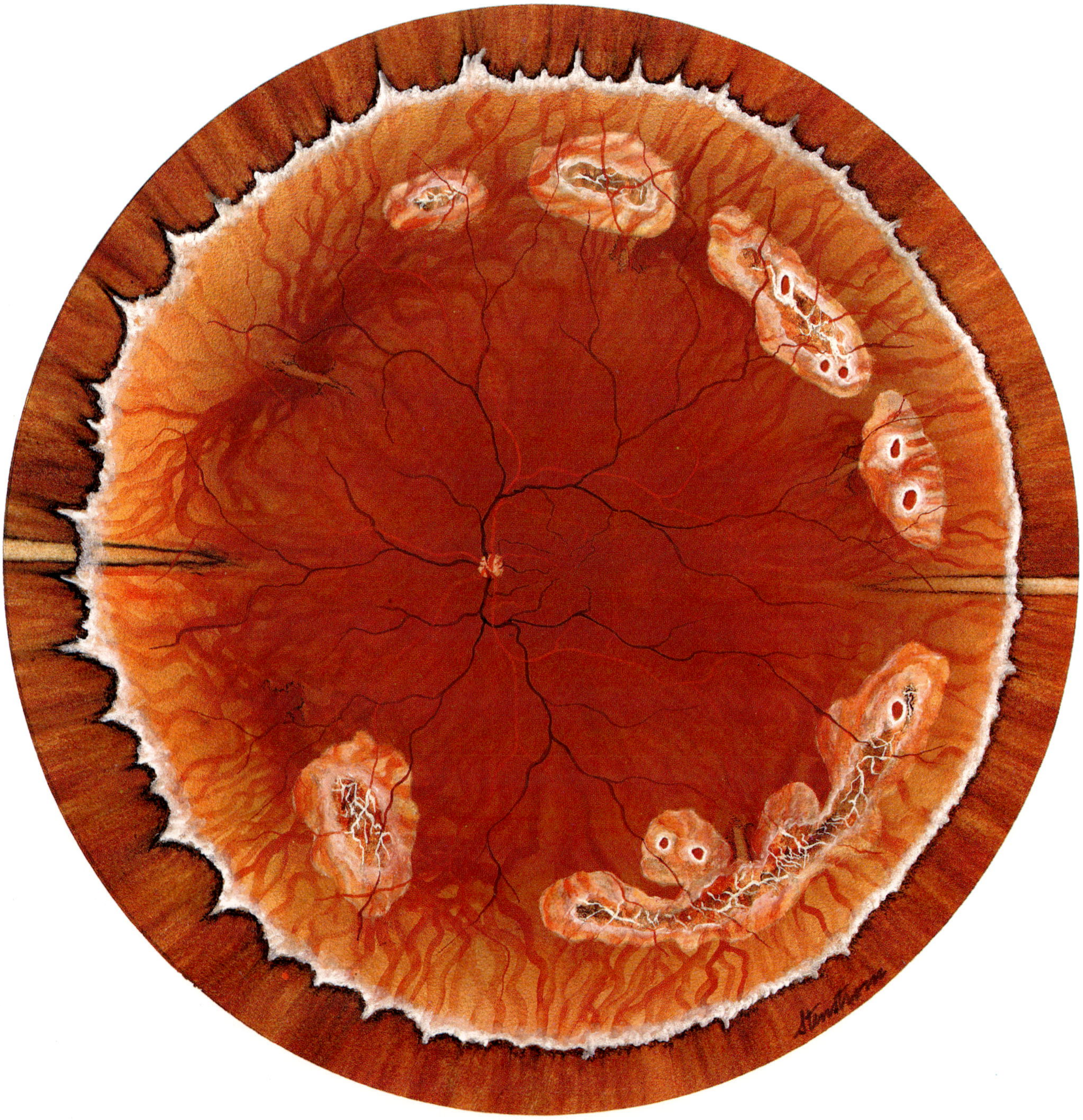

PLATE 39

CRYOPEXY: EXCESSIVE AND CORRECT

The appearance of the retina and pigment epithelium after cryotherapy treatment depends on the intensity of the treatment. Lincoff and others have described three intensities. Light cryotherapy is defined as cryotherapy treatment terminated just as the choroid blanches. Medium treatment is produced when the treatment is stopped just as the retina first turns white, and heavy treatment is defined as treatment stopped after the retina has turned white for three seconds. Although the heavier the treatment the stronger the chorioretinal adhesion, in most clinical instances only light or medium intensity cryotherapy should be applied. These treatments produce a well demarcated area of treated retina with a fine, stippled salt and pepper clumping. With medium intensity cryotherapy, shown in the inferior fundus, there is more depigmentation of the pigment epithelium and some larger clumps of dark pigment. Heavy cryotherapy, shown in the superior fundus, produces a totally white sclera in the treated area with preservation of only the largest choroidal vessels. The margins of the treated area are heavily pigmented and there are large clumps of pigment scattered over the treated area. With heavy cryotherapy in a detached retina, there is frequently pigment fallout that migrates to areas not treated. If this pigment fallout reaches the macula, diminished vision may result.

Bloch D, O'Conner P, Lincoff H: The mechanism of cryosurgical adhesion. III. Statistical analysis. Am J Ophthalmol *71*:666–673, 1971

Chignell AH, Revie HS, Clemett RS: Complications of retinal cryotherapy. Trans Ophthalmol Soc UK *91*:635–651, 1971

Hilton G: Subretinal pigment migration: Effects of cryosurgical retinal reattachment. Arch Ophthalmol *91*:445–450, 1974

Lincoff H, Long R, Marquardt J, et al: The cryosurgical adhesion. Trans Am Acad Ophthalmol Otolaryngol *72*:191–202, 1968

Lincoff H, O'Connor P, Bloch D, et al: Mechanism of the cryosurgical adhesion. II. Trans Am Acad Ophthalmol Otolaryngol *74*:98–107, 1970

Lincoff H, Kreissig I: The mechanism of the cryosurgical adhesion. IV. Electron microscopy. Am J Ophthalmol *71*:674–689, 1971

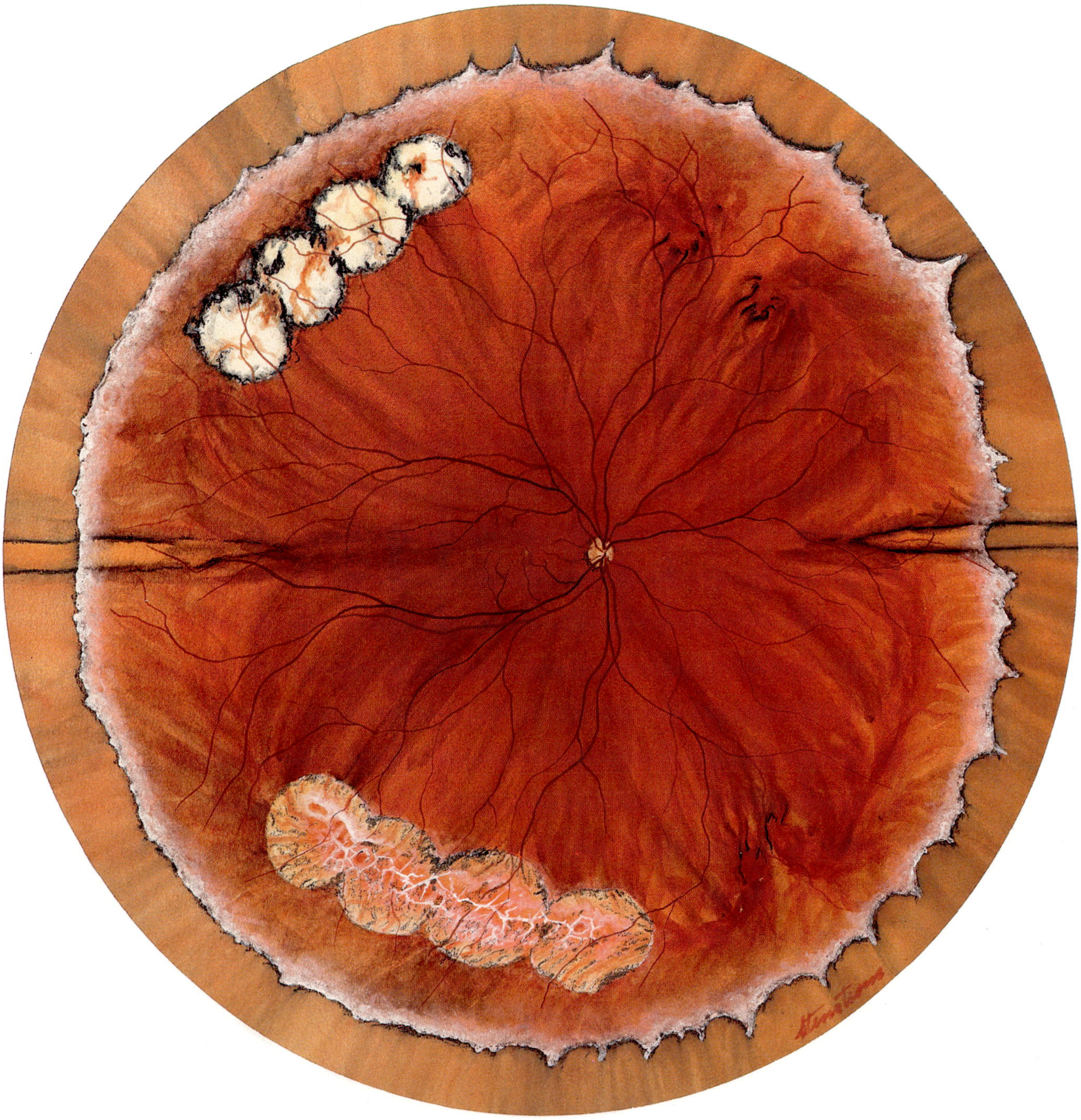

PLATE 40

Chapter Four

BENIGN AND MALIGNANT TUMORS

CHOROIDAL NEVI

Choroidal nevi are small round pigmented subretinal lesions. They range in size from less than one to four or more disc diameters; rarely, larger nevi occur. Nevi are flat or very slightly elevated, but if their thickness becomes more than two millimeters, the possibility of malignant melanoma must be considered. The most common color is slate gray, but variations from almost white to jet black are seen. The margins of a nevus are not as well defined as an area of hypertrophy of the retinal pigment epithelium; the nevus imperceptibly blends into the surrounding fundus pigmentation without a well defined boundary.

Gass has found nevi to be common lesions that can be identified in 30% of the population. Nevi tend to grow most rapidly during adolescence, but become more pigmented and visible during adulthood. They are much more common in caucasians than in the more heavily pigmented races. There is no sex predilection.

Some nevi produce changes in the overlying pigment epithelium such as pigment clumping or, rarely, the orange pigment frequently found over malignant melanomas. Drusen, visible as multiple white spots that may be either multiple and pinpoint or larger and coalescent, are frequently found in nevi. Drusen frequently enlarge very slowly and sometimes produce decompensation of the overlying pigment epithelium, so that a serous detachment of the retina develops. If there is further degeneration under a nevus so that there is an actual break in Bruch's membrane, subretinal neovascularization may occur. Neovascular vessels leak large amounts of subretinal fluid and frequently produce a yellow carcinate ring of exudate. Bleeding may also occur, producing subretinal hemorrhage that may clinically suggest rapid enlargement of melanoma.

Nevi are benign lesions although great care must be taken to distinguish them from malignant melanomas. Sometimes nevi may show very slow growth. Ganley estimates that malignant transformation from nevus to malignant melanoma will occur in one of every five thousand nevi. Nevertheless, most nevi are benign lesions and will remain so.

Ganley LP, Comstock GW: Benign nevi and malignant melanomas of the choroid. Am J Ophthalmol *76*:19–25, 1973

Gass JDM: Problems in the differential diagnosis of choroidal nevi and malignant melanomas. The XXXIII Edward Jackson Memorial Lecture. Am J Ophthalmol *83*:299–323, 1977

Naumann G, Hellner K, Naumann LR: Pigmented nevi of the choroid. Clinical study of the secondary changes in the overlying tissues. Trans Am Acad Ophthalmol Otolaryngol *75*:110, 123, 1971

Tamler E, Maumanee AE: A clinical study of choroidal nevi. Arch Ophthalmol *62*:196–202, 1959

Tamler E: A clinical study of choroidal nevi. A follow up report. Arch Ophthalmol *84*:29–32, 1970

Waltman DD, Gitter KA, Yanuzzi L, et al: Choroidal neuovascularization associated with choroidal nevi. Am J Ophthalmol *85*:704, 1978

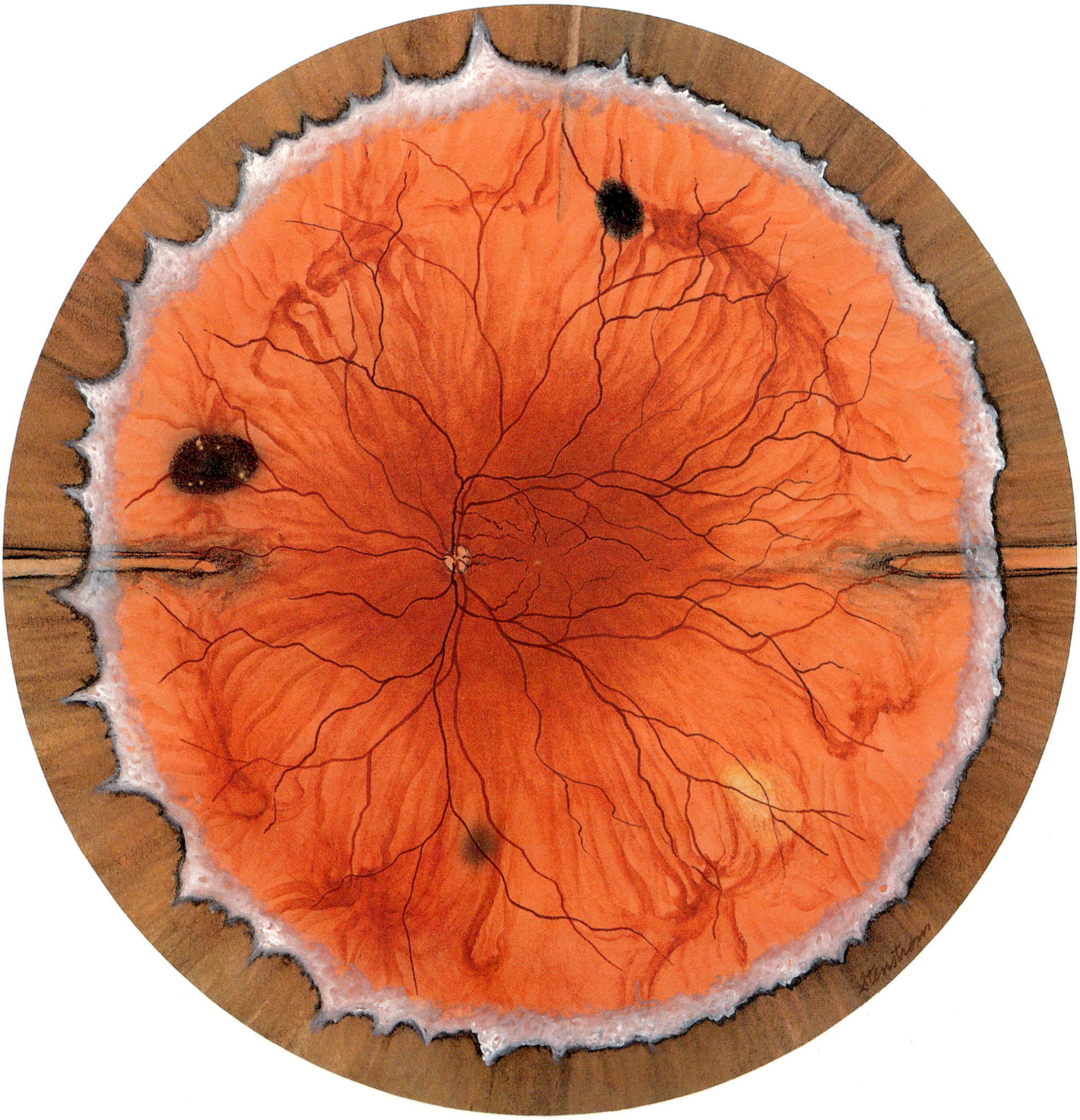

PLATE 41

HYPERTROPHY OF RETINAL PIGMENT EPITHELIUM

Hypertrophy of the retinal pigment epithelium appears as a round, dramatically dark pigmented lesion one to several disc diameters in size. The surface is flat, and the edges are distinctive, with very sharply defined margins surrounded by a depigmented halo. Small punched out holes, or lacunae, are frequently present, through which choroidal vessels may be seen. Drusen and orange pigment do not characteristically appear in these lesions. The retinal vessels are usually normal. Retinal function is normal and a visual field defect is not usually noted by the patient but may be detected by sensitive examining techniques.

These asymptomatic lesions are usually unilateral and solitary, and may occur in any position in the fundus. Their recognition is important, for they should not be confused with nevi or malignant melanomas, as they are not thought to have malignant potential. They have, however, been documented to enlarge very slowly.

Boldrey EE, Schwartz A: Enlargement of congenital hypertrophy of the pigment epithelium. Am J Ophthalmol *94*:64–66, 1982

Buettner H: Congenital hypertrophy of the retinal pigment epithelium. Am J Ophthalmol *79*:177–190, 1975

Cleary PE, Gregor Z, Bird AC: Retinal vascular changes in congenital hypertrophy of the retinal pigment epithelium. Br J Ophthalmol *60*:499–503, 1976

Kurz GH, Zimmerman LE: Vagaries of the retinal pigment epithelium. Int Ophthalmol Clin *2*:441–464, 1962

Purcell JJ, Shields JA: Hypertrophy with hyperpigmentation of the retinal pigment epithelium. Arch Ophthalmol *93*:1122–1126, 1975

Reese AB, Jones IS: Benign melanomas of the retinal pigment epithelium. Am J Ophthalmol *42*:207–212, 1956

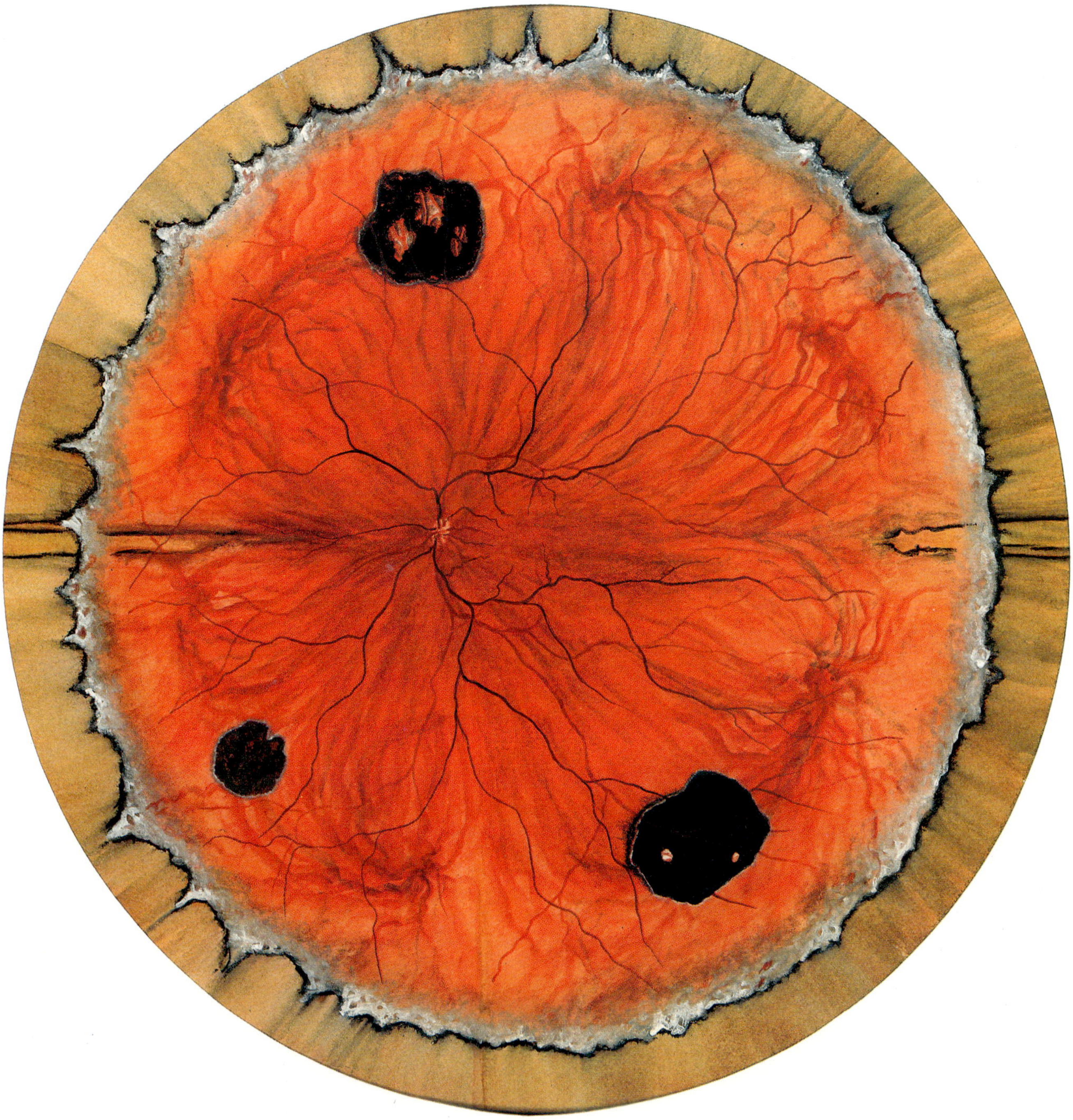

PLATE 42

SMALL MALIGNANT MELANOMA

There may be considerable difficulty in making the clinical distinction between a nevus and a small malignant melanoma. A nevus is defined as a histologically and biologically benign pigmented lesion, while a small malignant melanoma contains histologically and biologically malignant cells that can endanger life. Small malignant melanomas are defined as those melanomas that are 10 mm or less in diameter and 2 mm or less in elevation. The color of the lesion is typically slate gray, but may vary from white to black. The surface is smoothly and gently convex, but not highly elevated. The surface of the tumor beneath the retina may also show many white or yellow drusen, golden brown pigment, yellow exudates, or rarely subretinal hemorrhage. The tumor margins are not sharply demarcated but rather blend into the surrounding normal retina.

Small malignant melanomas frequently contain cells of low but definite malignant potential. Studies have shown that cell type is the most important determinant of whether a specific lesion will exhibit malignant potential, but size, mitotic activity, location of the tumor in the eye, and the presence or absence of transscleral extension and optic nerve invasion are also important factors. It is not always possible to clinically differentiate a benign nevus from a small malignant melanoma, and ancillary diagnostic tests may be useful. Future studies hopefully will reveal more accurate methods of clinically distinguishing these lesions.

Davidorf H, Lang JR: The natural history of malignant melanoma of the choroid: Small vs. large tumors. Trans Am Acad Ophthalmol Otolaryngol 79:310–320, 1975

McLean IW, Foster WD, Zimmerman LE: Prognostic factors in small malignant melanomas of choroid and ciliary body. Arch. Ophthalmol 95:48–58, 1977

Shields JA, Hagler WS, Federman JL, et al: The significance of the 32P uptake test in the diagnosis of posterior uveal melanoma. Trans Am Acad Ophthalmol Otolaryngol 79:297–306, 1975

Shields JA, Rodrigues MM, Sarin LK, et al: Lipofuscin pigment over benign and malignant choroidal tumors. Trans Am Acad Ophthalmol Otolaryngol 81:871–881, 1976

Zimmerman LE, McLean IW: Changing concepts in the prognosis and management of small malignant melanomas of the choroid. *In* Peyman GA, Apple DJ, Sanders DR: Intraocular Tumors. New York, Appleton-Century-Crofts, 1977, pp 63–74

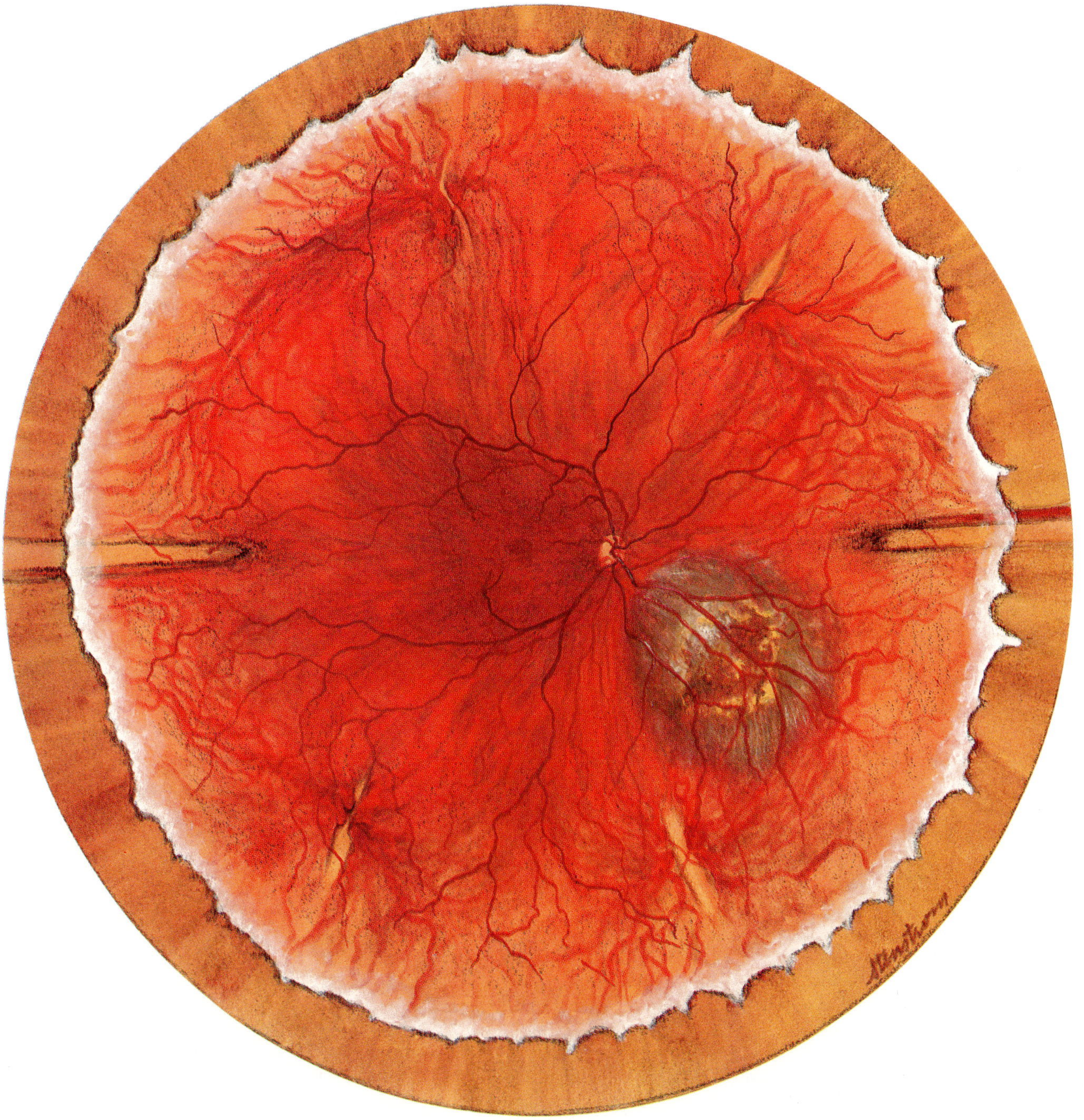

PLATE 43

MALIGNANT MELANOMA AND CHOROIDAL FOLDS

Choroidal folds, or striae, appear as alternating light and dark parallel lines in the retina. They are usually horizontal or obliquely oriented and typically occur temporal to the optic nerve, frequently passing through the macula. With foveal involvement, symptoms of blurred vision and distortion are noted by the patient.

There are many causes of choroidal folds. Most commonly orbital masses such as tumors or thyroid exophthalmos are associated with choroidal folds. Diseases of the sclera such as scleritis or conditions within the eye such as malignant melanoma, as shown here, prolonged hypotony, and papilledema are all possible causes. Abnormalities of the shape of the globe after scleral buckling and also marked hypermetropia are known to produce choroidal folds. Finally, choroidal folds may be of completely unknown etiology.

It is important to distinguish choroidal folds from folds of the retina alone produced by inflammatory scars or preretinal membranes. Retinal folds are thinner and less prominent and are more likely to show a radiating pattern. Retinal folds do not show the typical fluorescein angiographic pattern characteristic of choroidal folds. Fluorescein angiography of choroidal folds shows alternating light and dark lines in the early stages of the angiogram, with the lighter lines identified as the crests while the valleys are dark. This pattern apparently occurs because the pigment epithelium is stretched at the crests of the folds while it is compressed in the valleys, blocking more of the transmitted choroidal fluorescence. This corrugated appearance disappears in the late stages of the angiogram and there is no fluorescein leakage.

Bird AC, Sanders MD: Choroidal folds in association with papilledema. Br J Ophthalmol 57:89–97, 1973

Hedges TR, Leopold IH: Parallel retinal folds. Their significance in orbital space taking lesions. Arch Ophthalmol 62:353–355, 1959

Kroll AJ, Norton EWD: Regression of choroidal folds. Trans Am Acad Ophthalmol Otolaryngol 74:515–526, 1970

Newell FW: Choroidal folds. Am J Ophthalmol 75:930–942, 1973

Norton EWD: A characteristic fluorescein angiographic pattern in choroidal folds. Proc R Soc Med 62:119–128, 1969

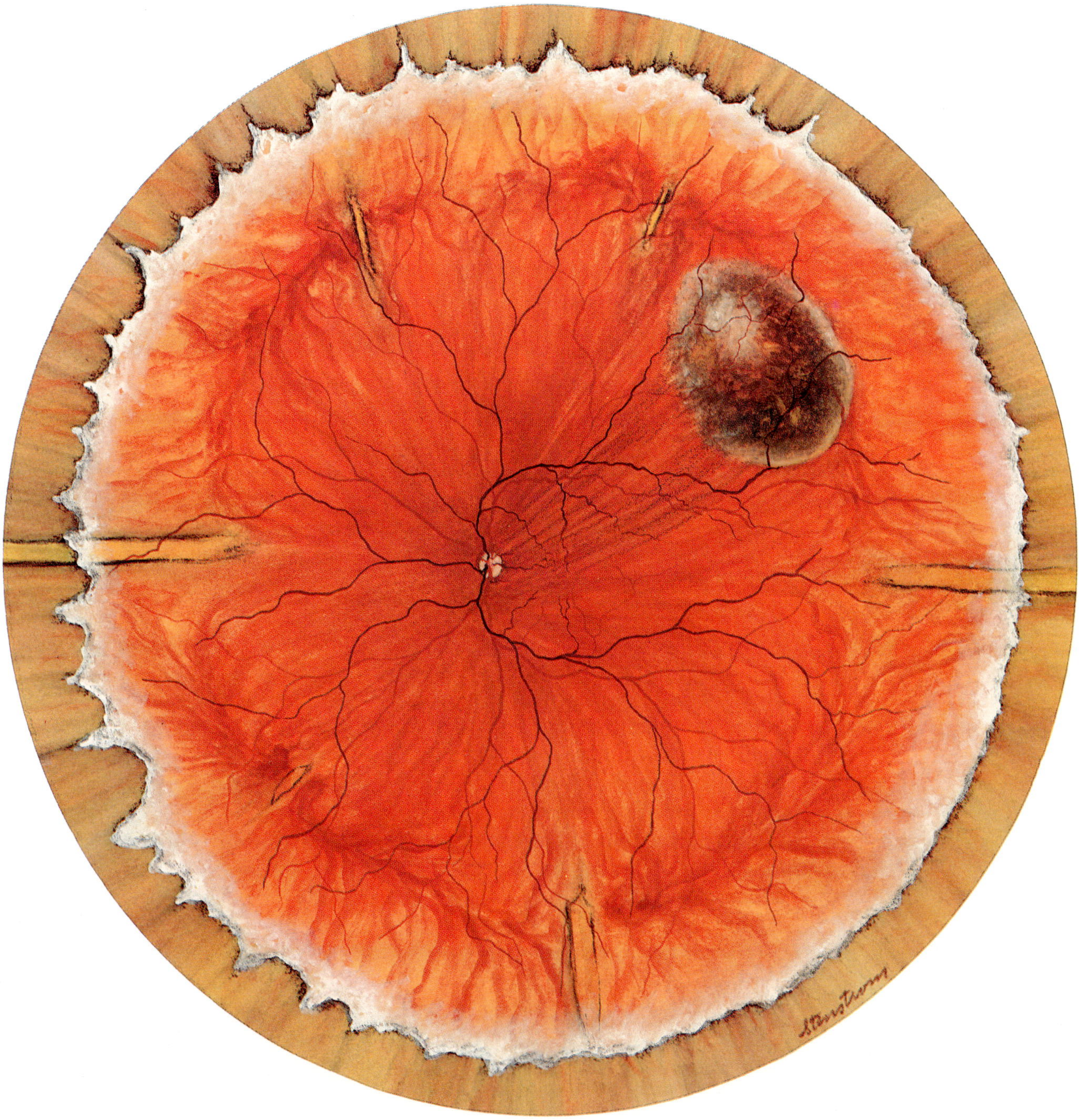

PLATE 44

MALIGNANT MELANOMA BREAKING THROUGH BRUCH'S MEMBRANE

Malignant melanomas of the choroid are typically round, convex, bulging subretinal mass lesions. They may be minimally to markedly pigmented, and range in size from several disc diameters to huge masses occupying much of the vitreous cavity. Malignant melanomas may occur in the posterior pole or in the periphery of the fundus. Although malignant melanomas have occurred in teen-age and younger people, they are most commonly found in individuals in the fifth to seventh decade. There is a marked racial preference for whites although melanomas are known to occur in blacks. There is no marked sex predilection.

Certain ophthalmoscopically visible features of these lesions may suggest malignant melanoma. It is important to remember, however, that there are no absolute clinical or ophthalmoscopic criteria for distinguishing a malignant melanoma from a simulating lesion.

With continuing growth of a malignant melanoma, the tumor may break through Bruch's membrane toward the center of the eye, and appear as a mushroom-like mass beneath the retina. In rare cases the melanoma may extend also through the retina, appearing as a dome-shaped mass in the vitreous cavity. Rapidly growing melanomas may also erode through the sclera, producing a pigmented mass that may be visible beneath the conjunctiva. Any of these appearances are strong evidence of malignancy. With growth of melanomas, pigment is usually released from the pigment epithelium and may clump in varying patterns between the retina and the surface of the tumor. The degree and pattern of the pigment is of no help in determining the nature and malignant potential of the lesion. Some pigment epithelial cells may undergo proliferation and appear as an irregular, cream-colored to dirty gray membrane between the retina and the surface of the subretinal mass lesion. Subretinal and vitreous hemorrhage is not typically produced by malignant melanomas, but the presence of hemorrhage should never be used to exclude the possibility of malignancy. Melanomas may sometimes produce intraocular inflammation as a result of ischemic necrosis. The clinical picture may vary from that of a mild uveitis to severe inflammation suggestive of infectious endophthalmitis.

Gass JDM: Differential Diagnosis of Intraocular Tumors. A stereoscopic presentation. St. Louis, CV Mosby, 1974

Gass JDM: Problems in the differential diagnosis of choroidal nevi and malignant melanomas. The XXXIII Jackson Memorial Lecture. Am J Ophthalmol *83*:299–323, 1977

Jacobiec FA: Ocular and Adnexal Tumors. Birmingham, Alabama, Aesculapius Publishing Company, 1978

Reese AB: Tumors of the Eye. 3rd ed. Hagerstown, Md, Harper & Row, 1976

Ressequie LJ, Marks SJ, Winkelmann RK, et al: Malignant melanoma in the resident population of Rochester, Minnesota. Mayo Clin Proc *2*:191–195, 1977

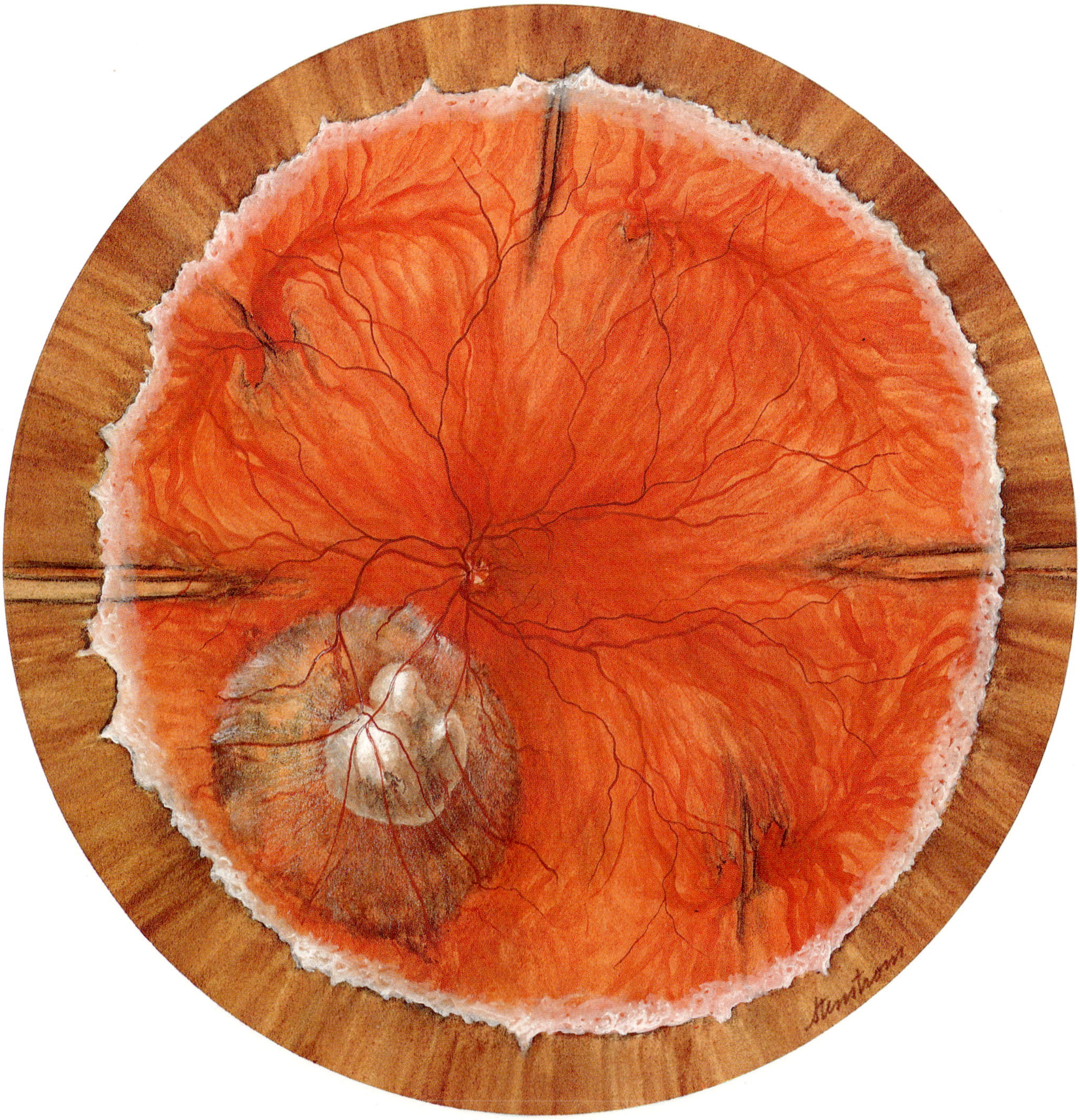

PLATE 45

LARGE MALIGNANT MELANOMA

Large choroidal melanomas usually present as pigmented or nonpigmented convex mass lesions beneath the retina. They may occur in any portion of the fundus, and be so large as to fill almost the entire vitreous cavity. The overlying retina typically shows cystoid degeneration, and sometimes the retina shows traction lines or striae. Clear serous fluid frequently is present surrounding the tumor elevation, and accumulates in a pattern defined by gravity. This patient is in the upright position and if the head position is changed, the serous fluid would shift to assume an inferior location. Note also that the fluid does not extend all the way to the ora serrata as it would in a rhegmatogenous retinal detachment. There may be a change in the pigment epithelium over the surface of the tumor, with drusen appearing, and also a lipofuscin pigment appearing in subretinal clumps. An abnormal vascular pattern of intrinsic vascularization of the tumor may be noted, and can sometimes be further delineated by fluorescein angiography.

Large malignant melanomas generally present fewer diagnostic dilemmas than small melanomas. But other, less common presentations of malignant melanomas may produce confusion. These include a flat diffuse tumor with little elevation but broad extent, and tumors that show spontaneous subretinal or vitreous hemorrhage or inflammatory signs in the eye due to tumor necrosis. Although clinical examination with the binocular indirect ophthalmoscope remains the most important diagnostic method, atypical presentations frequently require other diagnostic measures.

Coleman DJ: Reliability of ocular tumor diagnosis with ultrasound. Trans Am Acad Ophthalmol Otolaryngol *77*:677–686, 1973

Font RL, Zimmerman LE, Armaly MF: The nature of the orange pigment over a choroidal melanoma: Histochemical and electron microscopal observations. Arch Ophthalmol *91*:359–362, 1974

Reese AB: Tumors of the Eye. 3rd ed., Hagerstown, Maryland, Harper & Row, 1976, pp. 193–223

Shields JA, McDonald PR: Improvements in the diagnosis of posterior uveal melanomas. Arch Ophthalmol *91*:259–264, 1974

Shields JA, Zimmerman LE: Lesions simulating malignant melanoma of the posterior uvea. Arch Ophthalmol *89*:466–471, 1973

Shields JA, Hagler WS, Federman JL, et al: The significance of the P32 uptake test in the diagnosis of posterior uveal melanomas. Trans Am Acad Ophthalmol Otolaryngol *79*:297–306, 1975

Shields JA: Current approaches to the diagnosis and management of choroidal melanomas. Surv Ophthalmol *21*:443–463, 1977

Zimmerman LE: Problems in the diagnosis of malignant melanomas of the choroid and ciliary body. Am J Ophthalmol *75*:917–929, 1970

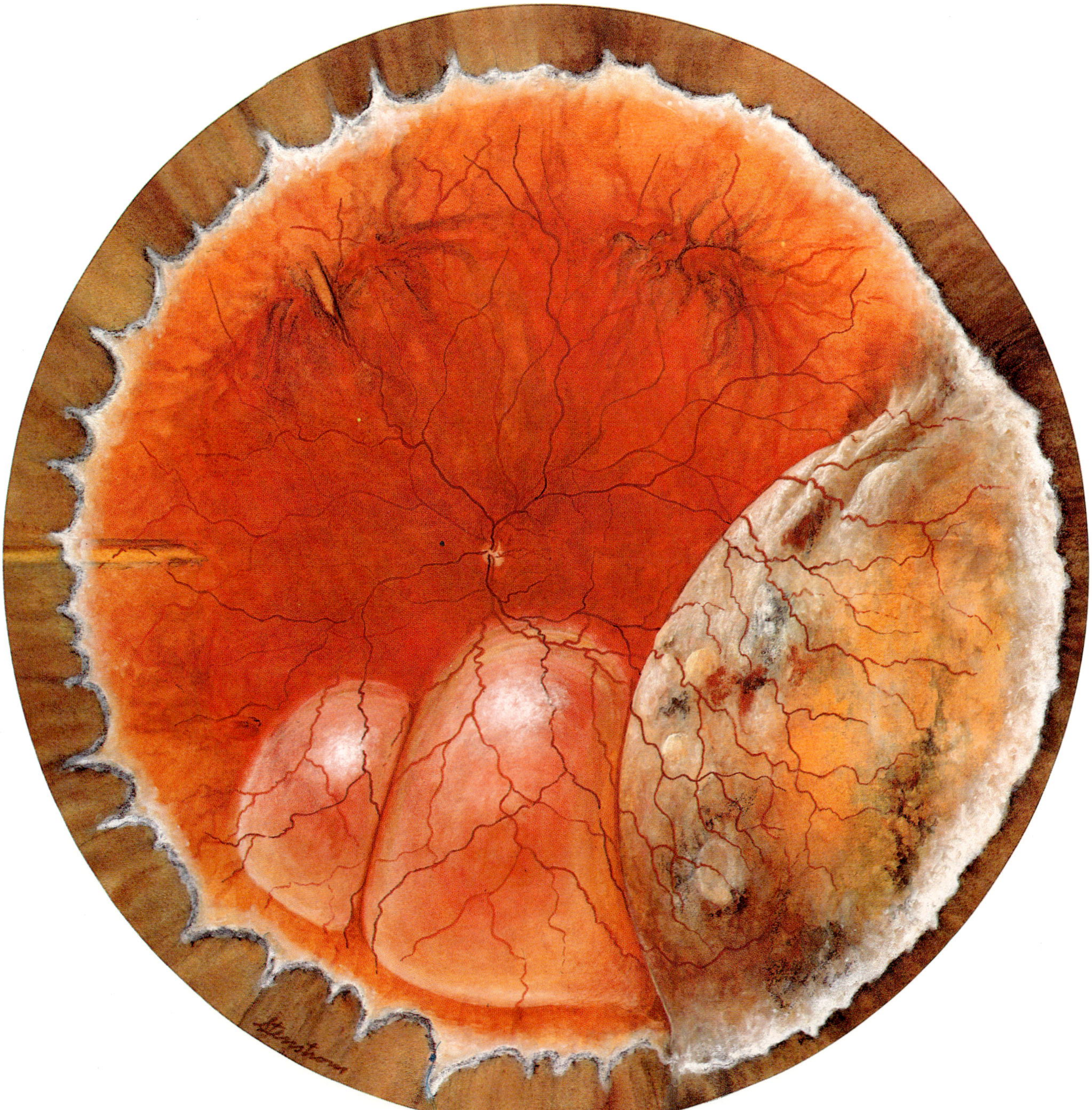

PLATE 46

METASTATIC CARCINOMA OF THE CHOROID

Metastatic carcinoma of the choroid, once thought to be a rare entity, is in fact a common intraocular tumor. A metastatic carcinoma of the choroid may be the presenting sign of malignancy or it may appear any time during the course of a documented tumor. Adults in the fifth decade or later are usually affected, and the incidence seems to be slightly higher in females than males. Approximately 25 per cent of the tumors are bilateral.

Metastatic tumors may occur anywhere in the fundus, but usually occur in the posterior portion of the eye. They occur most frequently just temporal to the macula, probably because of greater blood flow in this area. The most common primary tumor site in males is the lung and in females the breast. However, any malignant tumor that produces blood-borne metastases may metastasize to the choroid.

Initially, choroidal metastasis appears as a faint, white, ill defined subretinal patch, with no disturbance of the overlying pigment epithelium or retina. There is usually no visual disturbance until subretinal fluid is produced, creating a shallow blister-like retinal detachment. The metastasis grows rapidly to become visible beneath the retina as a flat, fluffy plaque with ill defined margins. Typically, metastases grow by lateral extension rather than in thickness. An occasional metastatic tumor will, however, develop as a convex mass and be very difficult to distinguish from an amelanotic melanoma. Larger tumors have a mottled appearance as the pigment epithelium degenerates and accumulates in clumps over the surface of the tumor. There is, however, no pigment in the substance of the tumor itself. Blood vessels may sometimes be seen within the substance of the tumor. The subretinal fluid may be clear or somewhat cloudy. Rarely hemorrhage may occur in the tumor and produce a hemorrhagic detachment of the pigment epithelium and retina. This may lead to the mistaken impression of a degenerative disciform lesion or to bleeding in a malignant melanoma. Although metastatic carcinoma of the choroid usually can be readily identified by its characteristic appearance and growth pattern, it may be clinically difficult or impossible to distinguish from other neoplastic or non-neoplastic lesions.

Bloch RS, Gartner S: The incidence of ocular metastatic carcinoma. Arch Ophthalmol *85*:673–675, 1971

Davis DL, Robertson DM: Fluorescein angiography of metastatic choroidal tumors. Arch Ophthalmol *89*:97–99, 1973

Ferry AP: The biological behavior and pathological features of carcinoma metastatic to the eye and orbit. Trans Am Ophthalmol Soc *71*:373–425, 1973

Ferry AP, Font RL: Carcinoma metastatic to the eye and orbit. A clinicopathologic study of 227 cases. Arch Ophthalmol *92*:276–286, 1974

Gass JDM: Differential Diagnosis of Intraocular Tumors. A Stereoscopic Presentation. St. Louis, CV Mosby, 1974, pp 140–158

Jaegar EA, Frayer WC, Southard ME, et al: Effect of radiation therapy on metastatic choroidal tumors. Trans Am Acad Ophthalmol Otolaryngol *75*:94–101, 1971

Reese AB: Tumors of the Eye. 3rd ed., Hagerstown, Md., Harper & Row, 1976, pp 424–431

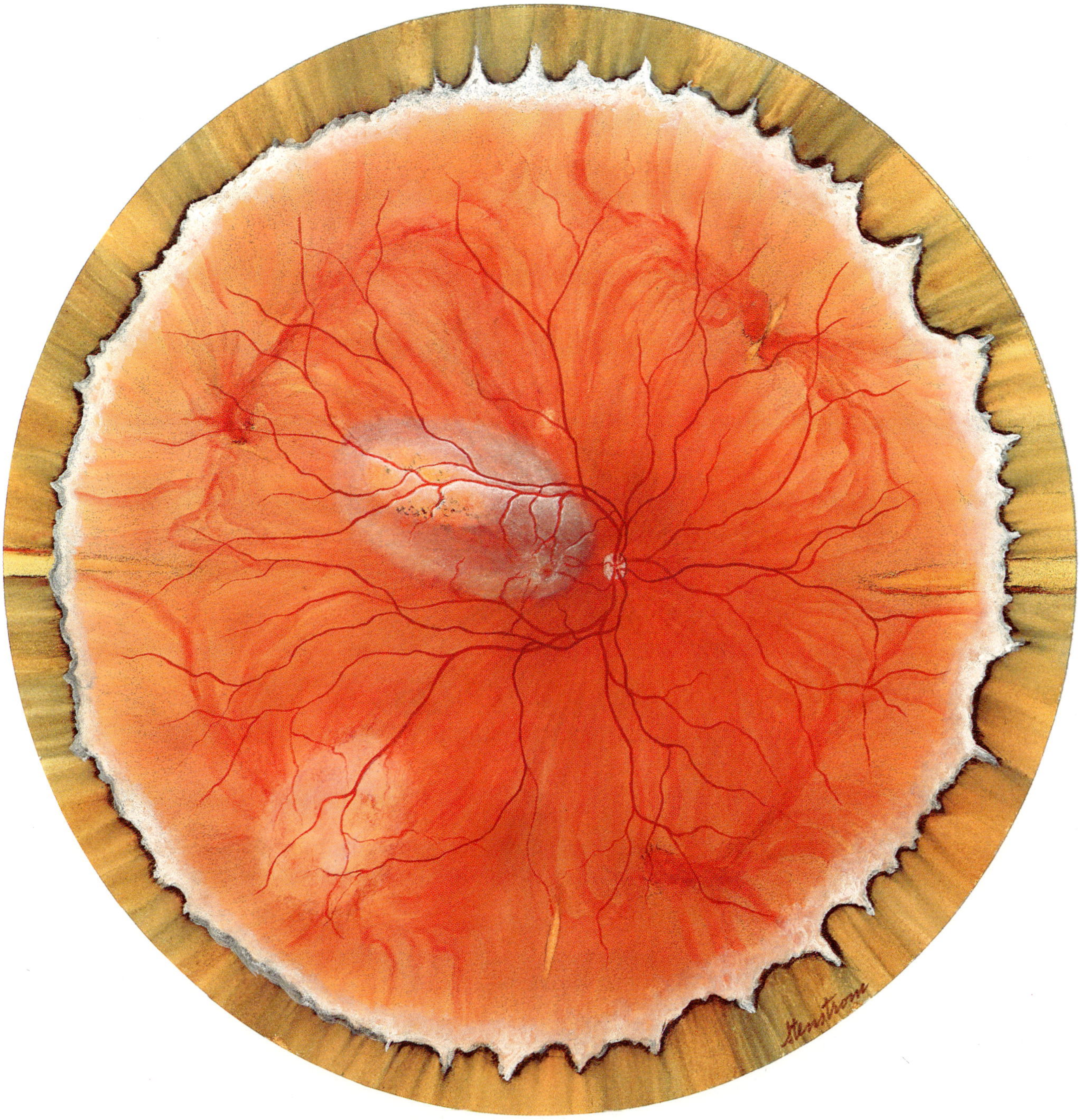

PLATE 47

METASTATIC CARCINOMA WITH SEROUS RETINAL DETACHMENT

The more advanced metastatic carcinoma lesions present with decreased vision due to a serous retinal detachment produced by the metastatic tumor, rather than with symptoms due to the mass lesion itself. Typical metastatic lesions appear in the posterior pole, usually temporal to the macula, where the blood supply is greatest because of the many short posterior ciliary arteries that supply the choroid in this region. Metastatic carcinoma appears as a flat white lesion with rather diffuse edges that is sometimes difficult to visualize beneath the detached retina. The subretinal fluid accumulates to produce a multilobed, bullous elevation of the retina dictated by the influence of gravity. There are no well defined margins to this serous exudative detachment as are present in a rhegmatogenous retinal detachment with an open retinal break. The subretinal fluid shifts readily with change in position, always assuming an inferior location. The serous exudative detachment does not extend to the ora serrata as does a rhegmatogenous detachment but extends only to the posterior vitreous base. Sometimes it is necessary to examine the eye in various positions to shift the subretinal fluid to another location so that the flat metastatic lesion becomes visible.

Metastatic carcinoma rarely erodes through Bruch's membrane to produce a collar-button subretinal lesion but may undergo necrosis, producing intraocular inflammatory signs and glaucoma. Rarely hemorrhage may be present. The most common origin of the primary tumor is in the breast and lung, with the kidneys, testicles, prostate, pancreas, colon, stomach, and thyroid also occurring rarely as primary sites. A most helpful diagnostic feature is a documented primary tumor outside the eye.

Albert DM, Rubenstein RA, Scheie HG: Tumor metastasis to the eye. Part I. Incidence in 213 adult patients with generalized malignancy. Am J Ophthalmol 63:723–726, 1967

Bloch RS, Gartner S: The incidence of ocular metastatic carcinoma. Arch Ophthalmol 85:673–675, 1971

Greear JN: Metastatic carcinoma of the eye. Am J Ophthalmol 33:1015–1025, 1950

Reese AB: Tumors of the Eye. 3rd ed., Hagerstown, Md, Harper & Row 1976, pp 424–428

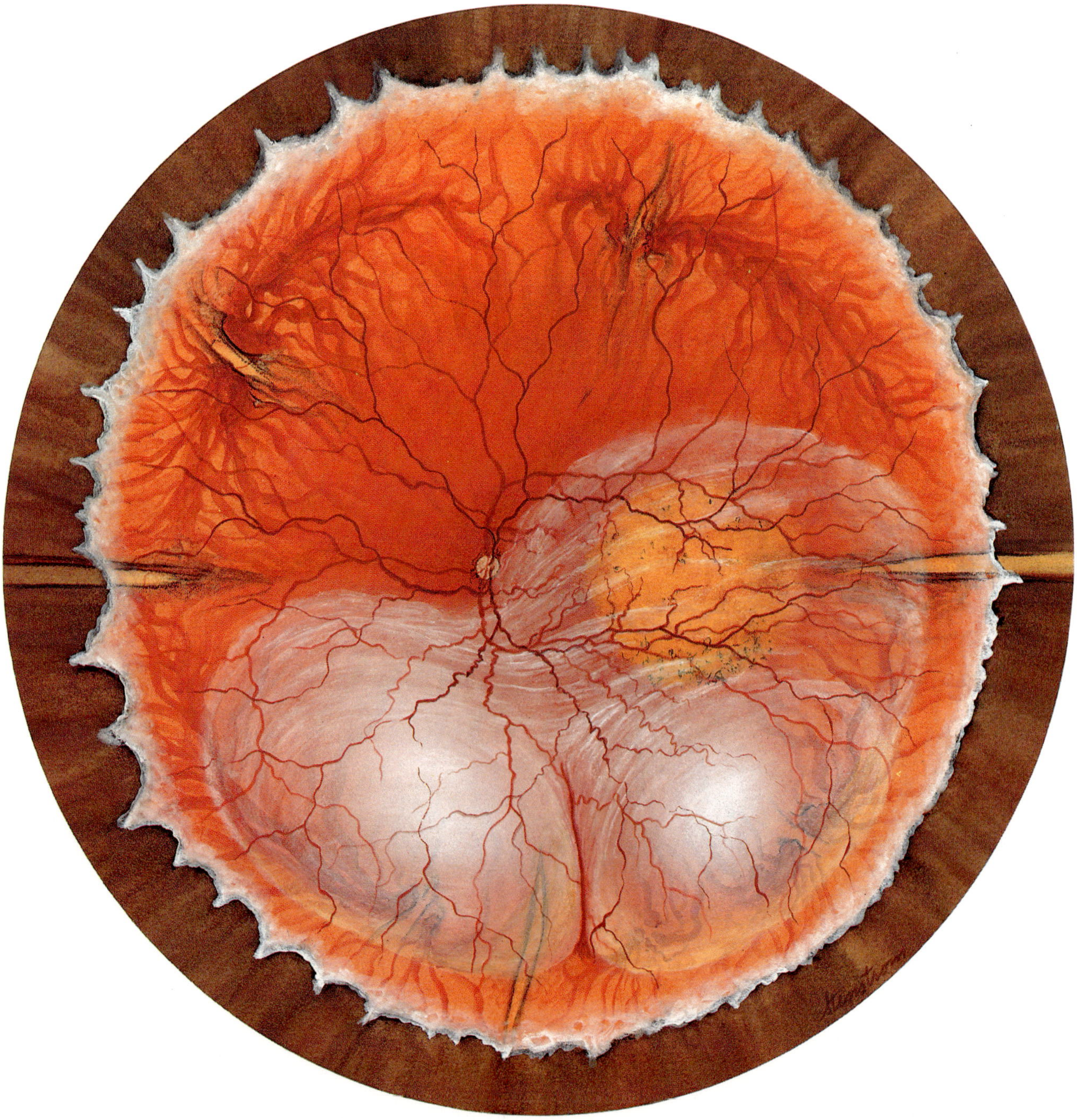

PLATE 48

CAVERNOUS HEMANGIOMA OF THE CHOROID

A cavernous hemangioma is a benign growth of choroidal vessels. It appears as a relatively flat, irregular mass of choroidal vessels beneath a serous retinal detachment. Usually, faint white strands of connective tissue can be seen within the pink to red hemangioma, which is usually from two to approximately eight disc diameters in size. Hemangiomas usually occur around the optic nerve or temporal arcades, especially temporal to the macula. They are usually asymptomatic until the serous detachment produced by the hemangioma extends into the foveal area, creating distortion and decreased acuity. The overlying retina is usually shallowly detached, but rarely very large serous detachments occur. The overlying retina has a cystic appearance, and varying degrees of subretinal pigment dispersion may be present. Yellow subretinal exudate may be present also in a carcinate pattern. In long-standing hemangiomas, bone formation has been found, which causes calcification that is visible clinically or by ancillary diagnostic studies.

Cavernous hemangiomas occur primarily in caucasians, with males outnumbering females. They may be observed from the third decade onward and show very little or no growth and may show spontaneous regression. Hemangiomas may blanch on compression of the eye and typically transilluminate easily, but caution is advised in the interpretation of these tests. The ultrasound examination, particularly the A scan, is more reliable. The fluorescein angiogram typically shows rapidly filling large vessels in the choroidal and early arterial phases. Patchy irregular areas of large vessels coalesce to produce intense staining. In the late phases there is the typical cystoid pattern of fluorescein accumulation in the overlying retina.

Gass JDM: Cavernous Hemangioma of the Choroid. *In* Differential Diagnosis of Intraocular Tumors. St. Louis, CV Mosby, 1974, pp 113–138

Jarrett WH, Hagler WS, LaRose JH, et al: Clinical experience with presumed hemangioma of the choroid: Radioactive phosphorus uptake studies as an aid in differential diagnosis. Trans Am Acad Ophthalmol Otolaryngol *81*:862–870, 1976

Jones IS, Cleasby GW: Hemangioma of the choroid: A clinico-pathologic analysis. Am J Ophthalmol *48*:612–628, 1958

MacLean AL, Maumanee AE: Hemangioma of the choroid. Am J Ophthalmol *50*:3–11, 1960

Norton EWD, Gutman F: Fluorescein angiography and hemangiomas of the choroid. Arch Ophthalmol *78*:121–125, 1967

Smith JL, David NJ, Hart LM, Levenson DS, Tillett CW: Hemangioma of the choroid. Fluorescein photography and photocoagulation. Arch Ophthalmol *69*:51–54, 1963

Witschel H, Font RL: Hemangioma of the choroid. A clinico-pathologic study of 71 cases and a review of the literature. Surv Ophthalmol *20*:415–431, 1976

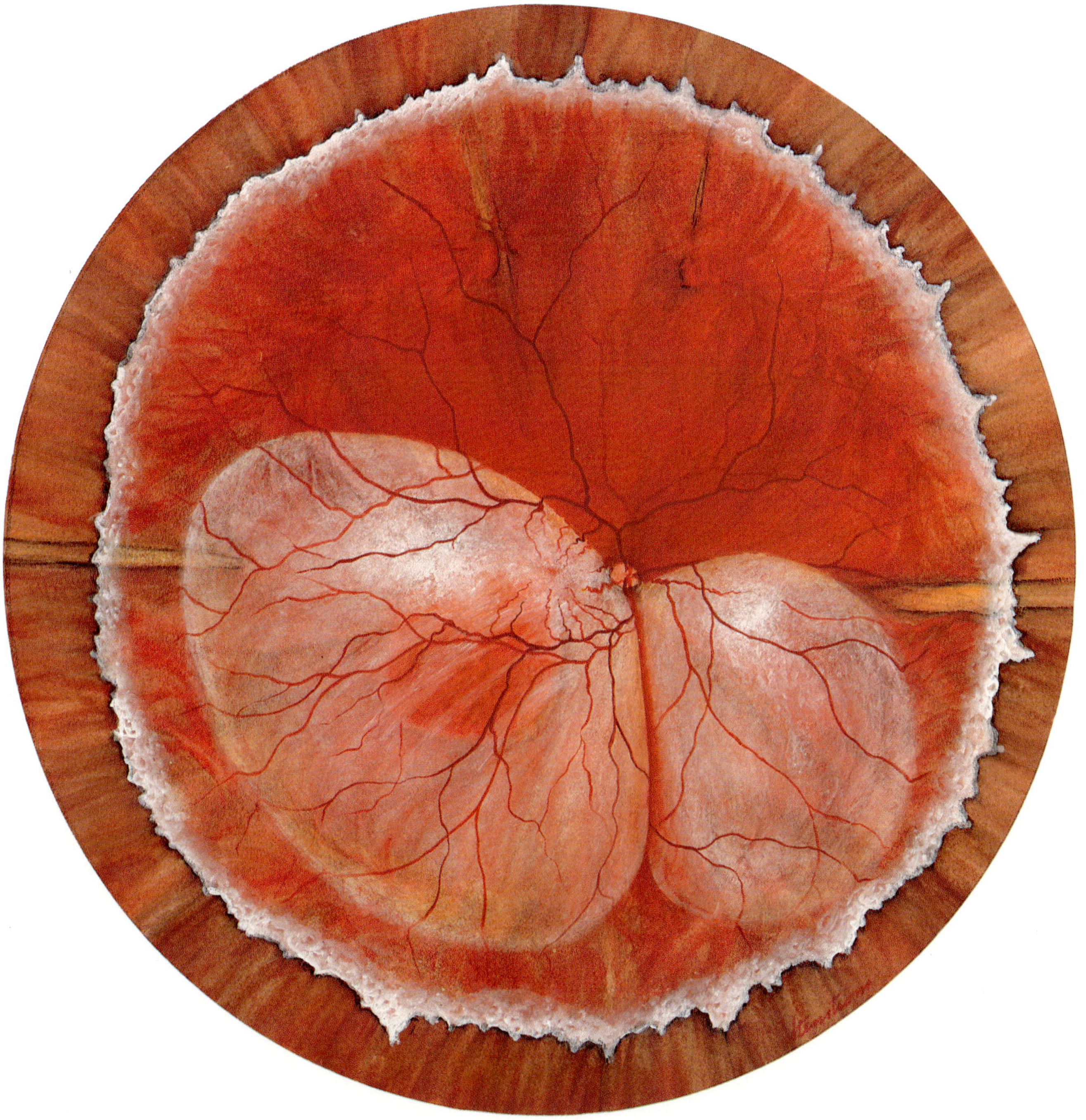

PLATE 49

CHOROIDAL DETACHMENT SIMULATING INTRAOCULAR TUMOR

A choroidal detachment is a highly elevated convex protrusion of the peripheral retina and choroid into the vitreous cavity. It is produced by serous or hemorrhagic fluid between the sclera and choroid. The solid appearance of a choroidal detachment, produced by the fact that the pigment epithelium is seen directly underneath the retina, is responsible for frequent confusion with tumors, particularly malignant melanomas of the peripheral fundus or ciliary body. The choroidal detachment is usually multilobed and frequently extends into several quadrants, although some portions may be much more highly elevated than others. The pars plana can usually be seen without scleral depression in the most highly elevated areas. Many eyes with choroidal detachments have been enucleated following a mistaken diagnosis of malignant melanoma.

There are many causes of choroidal detachment. A choroidal detachment may occur after almost any type of intraocular surgery, particularly when hypotony is present postoperatively. Scleritis, uveitis, or chorioretinitis may in certain instances produce a choroidal detachment. Uveal effusion and other rare entities may also be present with choroidal detachment. Choroidal detachment and retinal detachment may be combined, in which case the prognosis for successful repair is poor.

Aaberg TM: Experimental choroidal detachments. Mod Probl Ophthalmol *12*:167–172, 1974

Bard LA: Eyes with choroidal detachments removed for suspected melanoma. Arch Ophthalmol *73*:230–323, 1965

Ferry AP: Lesions mistaken for malignant melanoma of the posterior uvea. Arch. Ophthalmol *72*:463–469, 1964

Gottlieb F: Combined choroidal and retinal detachment. Arch Ophthalmol *88*:481–486, 1972

Hawkins WR, Schepens CL: Choroidal detachment and retinal surgery. Am J Ophthalmol *62*:813–819, 1966

McDonald PR, la Paz V, Sarin LK: Non-rhegmatogenous retinal separation associated with choroidal detachment. Trans Am Ophthalmol *62*:226–247, 1964

Schepens CL, Brockhurst RJ: Uveal effusion. Arch Ophthalmol *70*:189–201, 1963

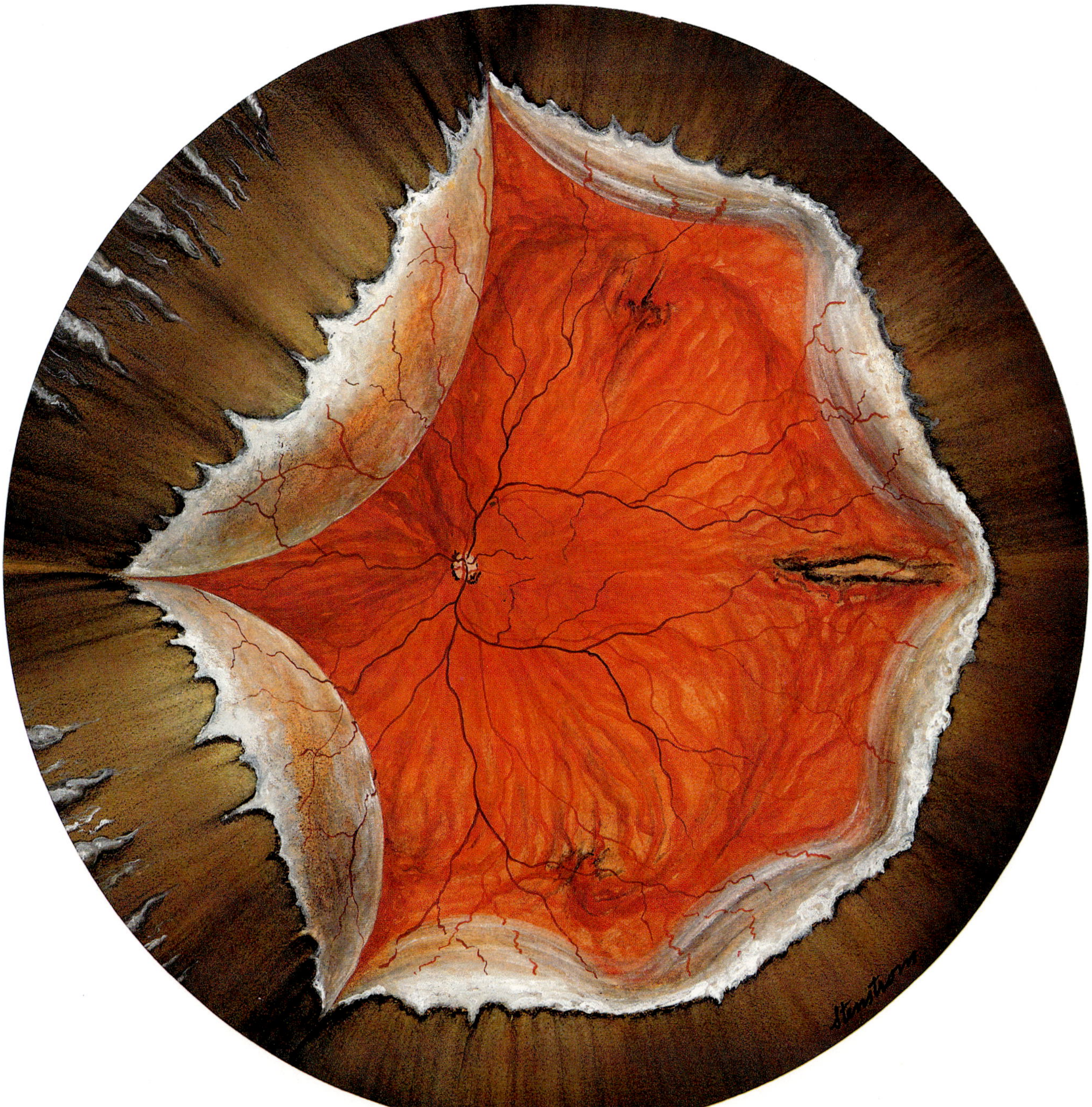

PLATE 50

RETINOBLASTOMA

Retinblastoma is the most common intraocular tumor in childhood. It is a malignant tumor that if undetected or misdiagnosed can metastasize and kill. It is a unique type of cancer, in that it is frequently genetically inherited, being transmitted as an autosomal dominant, and there may be a positive family history of similar tumors. Sporadic cases also occur. Retinoblastoma occurs in all races and has no sex predilection. Usually, the tumor presents during the first three years of life, although in neglected cases, it may present later, even in adulthood.

Retinoblastoma is usually discovered by observing a white reflex in a child's eye, but there are many less common presentations, such as intraocular inflammation or a presumed traumatic injury.

Retinoblastoma tumors may be single or multiple and as small as one disc diameter, or they may be large enough to fill the entire vitreous cavity. Individual tumors are usually white or creamy pink mounds with very fine blood vessels located on the surface or within the tumor substance. There may be a yellow exudate surrounding the tumor or rarely a pigmented annulus around the circumference of the tumor mass. A typical feature is calcification detectable by x-ray or ultrasound. A number of other intraocular diseases may mimic the lesions of retinoblastoma and may be difficult to differentiate from this neoplastic lesion. Particularly difficult to distinguish from retinoblastoma are some cases of Coats' disease, *Toxocara canis* granuloma, and tuberous sclerosis.

Chimonidou E, Palimeris G, Velissaropoulous P: Retinoblastoma: Some aspects concerning diagnosis, heredity and treatment. J Pediat Ophthalmol Strabismus *16*:101–104, 1979

Francois J, DeBie S, Matton-VanLeuven MT: The Costenbader Memorial Lecture. Genesis and genetics of retinoblastoma. J Pediat Ophthalmol Strabismus *16*:85–100, 1979

Reese AB: Tumors of the Eye. 3rd ed, Hagerstown, Md, Harper & Row, pp 90–132

Robertson DM, Campbell RJ: Analysis of misdiagnosed retinoblastoma in a series of 726 enucleated eyes. Mod Probl Ophthalmol *18*:156–159, 1977

Shields JA, Augsburger JJ: Current approaches to the diagnosis and management of retinoblastoma. Surv Ophthalmol *25*:347–372, 1981

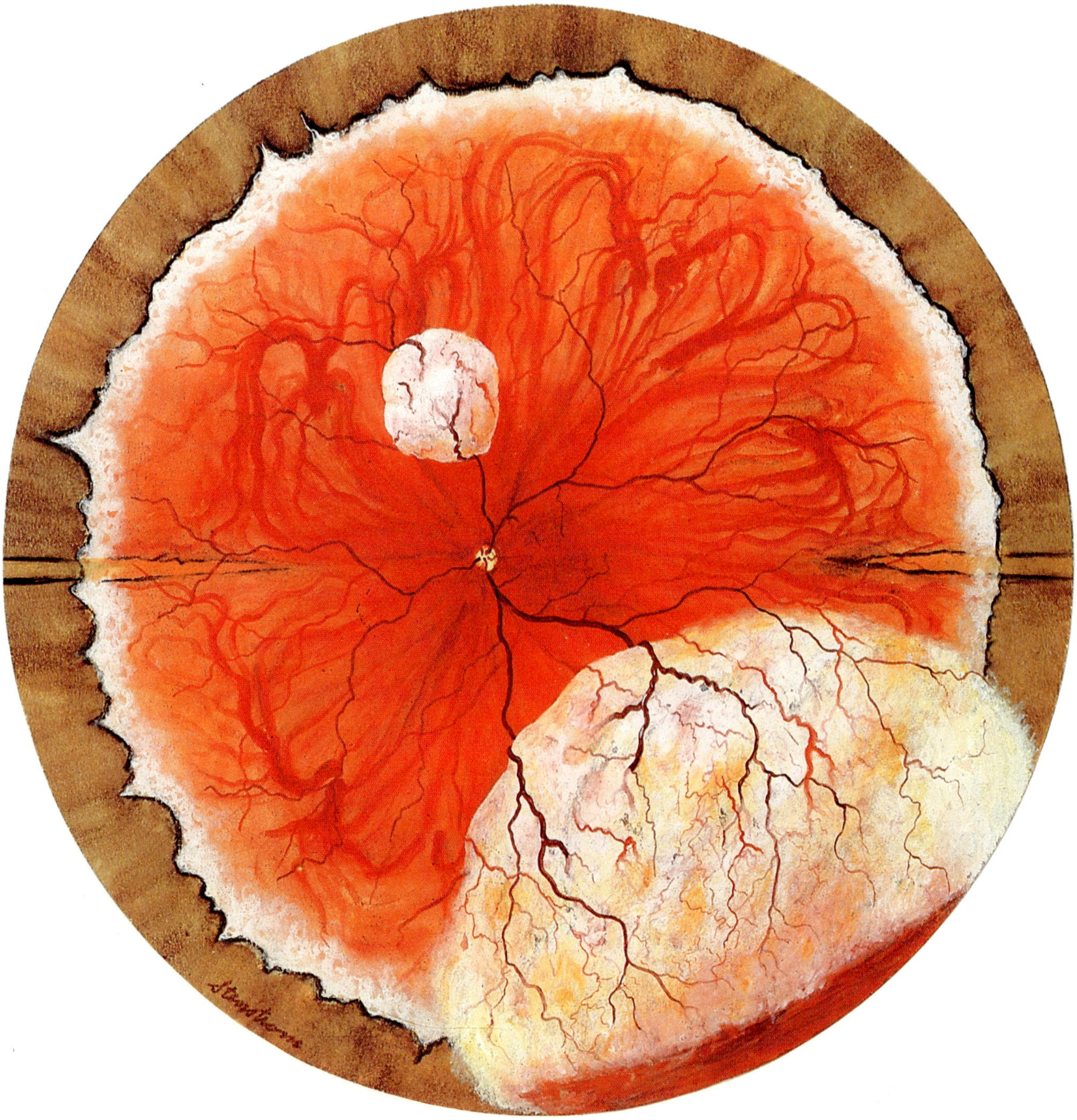

PLATE 51

EXOPHYTIC RETINOBLASTOMA

The exophytic growth pattern of retinoblastoma is less common but it causes more difficulty in diagnosis. The tumor grows outward toward the sclera in the subretinal space rather than inward toward the center of the vitreous cavity. Formation of subretinal fluid produces an initial impression of retinal detachment. On careful evaluation, however, no retinal break is discovered and the fluid shifts freely with no sharp demarcation line between attached and detached retina. The tumor requires detection through the overlying detached retina and may be very difficult to visualize. The view may be further compromised by subretinal hemorrhage or exudate. When subretinal white mounds are visualized in a young child, retinoblastoma should be suspected. It is important to distinguish this growth pattern from Coats' disease, which can be differentiated by the characteristic retinal vascular abnormalities.

Bedford MA, Bedotto, C, MacFaul PA: Retinoblastoma; a study of 139 cases. Br J Ophthalmol 55:19–27, 1971

Ellsworth RN: Retinoblastoma. *In* Duane TD: Clinical Ophthalmology. Hagerstown, Maryland, Harper & Row, 1979, Vol III, Chapter 35, pp 1–18

Gass JDM: Differential Diagnosis of Intraocular Tumors. A Stereoscopic Presentation. St. Louis, CV Mosby, 1974, pp 140–158

Jacobiec FAJ: Ocular and Adnexal tumors. Birmingham, Alabama, Aesculapius Publishing Co, 1978, pp 128–180

Sang DN, Albert DM: Recent advances in the study of retinoblastoma. *In* Peyman GA, et al: Intraocular Tumors. New York, Appleton-Century-Crofts, 1977, pp 285–329

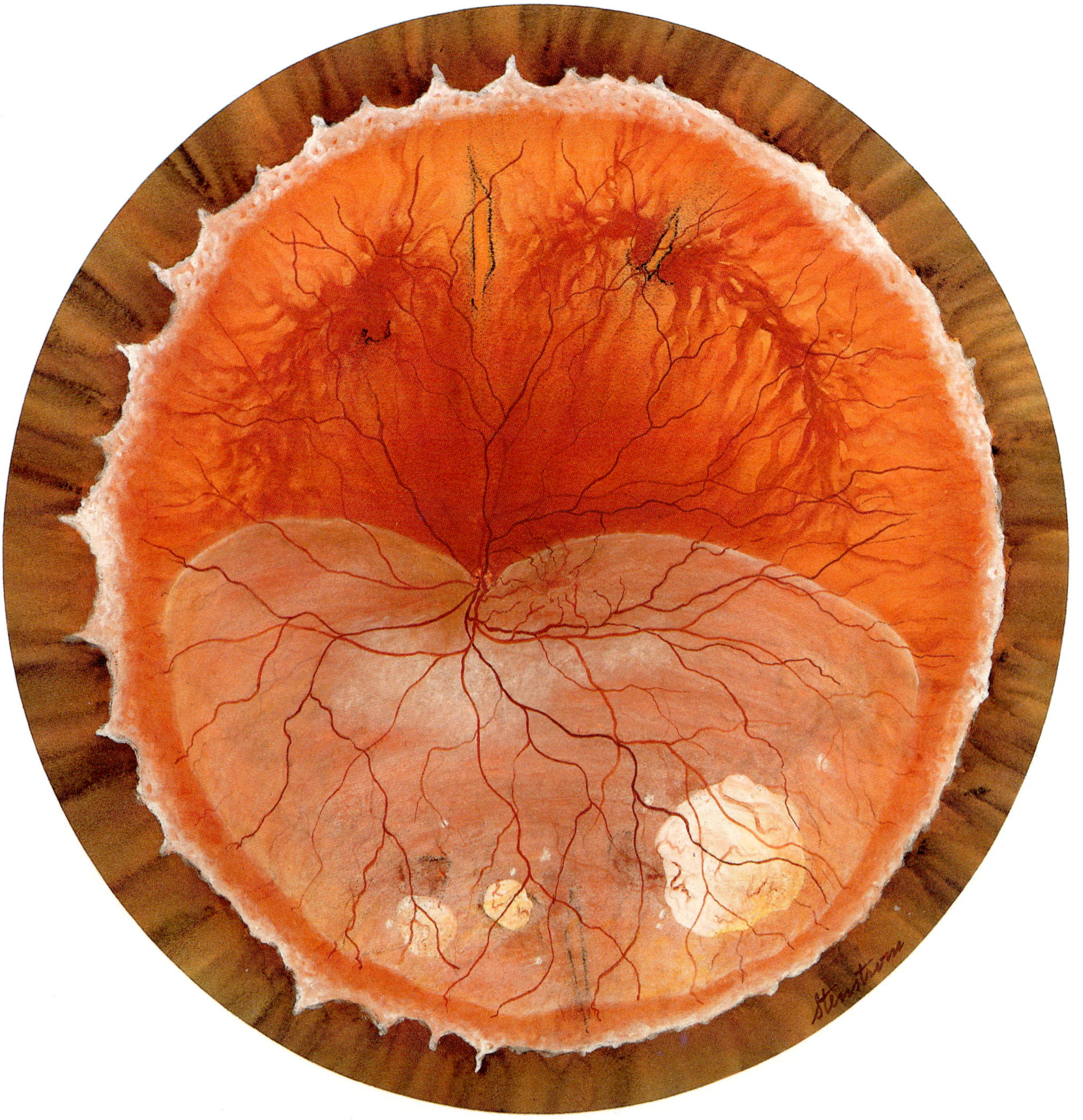

PLATE 52

RETINOBLASTOMA WITH VITREOUS SEEDING

Retinoblastomas may be unilateral or bilateral, and located anywhere in the fundus. Here, multiple tumors are located both in the posterior pole and in the far periphery. Notice especially the small tumors at the ora serrata, which may be found only by scleral depression. Of special note is the large tumor below, from which vitreous seeding has occurred. The cells of retinoblastomas are minimally cohesive and tend to slide over one another very easily and to become detached from the primary tumor. The cells tend to diffuse throughout the eye and may mimic uveitis. These cells may also accumulate in the anterior chamber and produce a clinical appearance of hypopyon. It is important to avoid a mistaken diagnosis of inflammatory disease; however, if vitreous seeding is recognized, it is a typical feature of retinoblastoma and will help in making a definitive diagnosis. Vitreous seeding also produces a white fundus reflex, which should not be misinterpreted as a cataract. As a rule, eyes containing retinoblastoma have clear lenses and are of normal size unless the tumor has developed in utero and there has been spontaneous necrosis of the tumor with phthisis soon after birth.

Andrew JM, Smith DR: Unsuspected retinoblastoma. Am J Ophthalmol *60*:536–540, 1965

Bishop JO, Madson EC: Retinoblastoma; review of the current status. Surv Ophthalmol *19*:324–366, 1975

Ellsworth RM: The practical management of retinoblastoma. Trans Am Ophthalmol Soc *67*:462–534, 1969

Howard GM, Ellsworth RM: Differential diagnosis of retinoblastomas. I. Relative frequency of the lesions which simulate retinoblastomas. Am J Ophthalmol *60*:610–618, 1965

Richards WW: Retinoblastoma simulating uveitis. Am J Ophthalmol *65*:427–431, 1968

Stafford WR, Yanoff M, Parnell BL: Retinoblastoma initially misdiagnosed as primary ocular inflammations. Arch Ophthalmol *82*:771–773, 1969

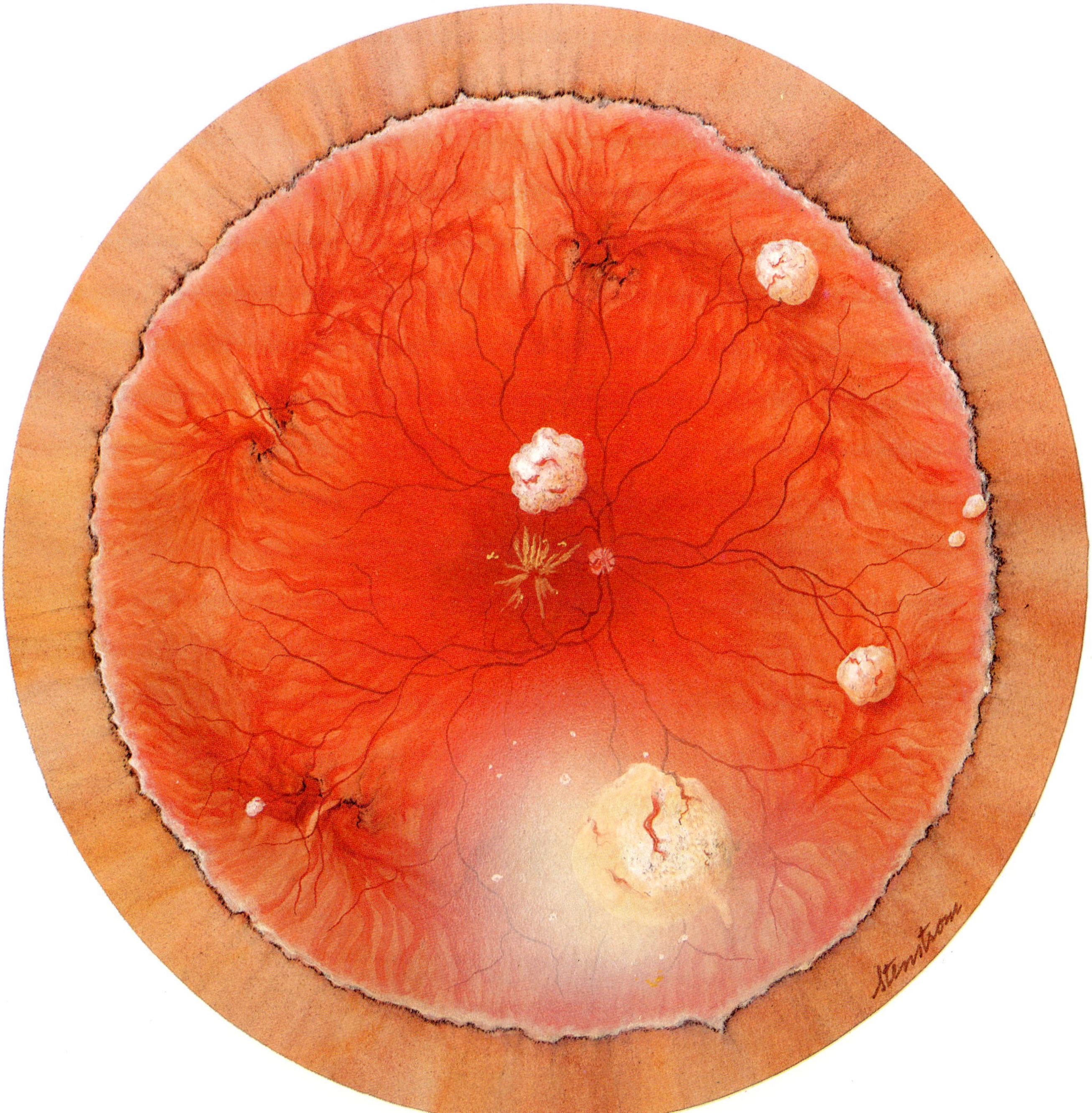

PLATE 53

Chapter Five

INFECTIOUS AND INFLAMMATORY RETINAL DISEASES

TOXOPLASMOSIS

Toxoplasmosis, caused by the organism *Toxoplasma gondii*, is an important and common infection of the retina. An active infection, seen here in the 7 o'clock meridian in the periphery, is characterized by a round to irregular white or yellow area of the retina with an overlying white haze, giving the appearance classically described as "a headlight in a fog." In this example, the area of retinal involvement is small and the symptoms produced by this infection include floating spots and a sensation of looking through a haze. If large areas of the retina are involved, the entire vitreous may be filled with a white, cloudlike cellular infiltrate.

Healed inactive lesions are shown in the posterior pole and mid-periphery above. A lesion in the macula is suggestive of congenital toxoplasmosis, although any part of the retina may be affected. Inactive lesions appear as rather sharply demarcated punched out areas of retinal and choroidal destruction surrounded by varying degrees of pigmentation at the margin of the lesion. A few large choroidal vessels may be observed in the base of these inactive lesions and there is no overlying white haze. Typically, there are recurrent episodes of activity, sometimes with years passing between active episodes. Reactivation frequently begins near the margin of a pre-existing inactive lesion. The clinical course can be quite variable depending on the area of retina involved and the location of the lesion. It is important to recognize toxoplasmosis clinically and confirm it serologically, for specific therapy is available.

Friedmann CT, Knox DL: Variations in recurrent active toxoplasmic retinochoroiditis. Arch Ophthalmol *81*:481–493, 1969

O'Connor GR: Manifestations and management of ocular toxoplasmosis. Bull NY Acad Med *50*:192–210, 1974

O'Connor GR, Frenkel JK: Dangers of steroid treatment in toxoplasmosis. Arch Ophthalmol *94*:213, 1976

Perkins ES: Ocular toxoplasmosis. Br J Ophthalmol *57*:1–17, 1973

Scott EH: New developments in toxoplasmosis. Surv Ophthalmol *18*:255–274, 1974

Spalter HF, Campbell CJ, Noyori KS, et al: Prophylactic photocoagulation of recurrent toxoplasmic retinochoroiditis. Arch Ophthalmol *75*:21–31, 1966

Tabbara KF, O'Connor GR: Treatment of ocular toxoplasmosis with clindamycin and sulfadiazine. Ophthalmol *87*:129–134, 1980

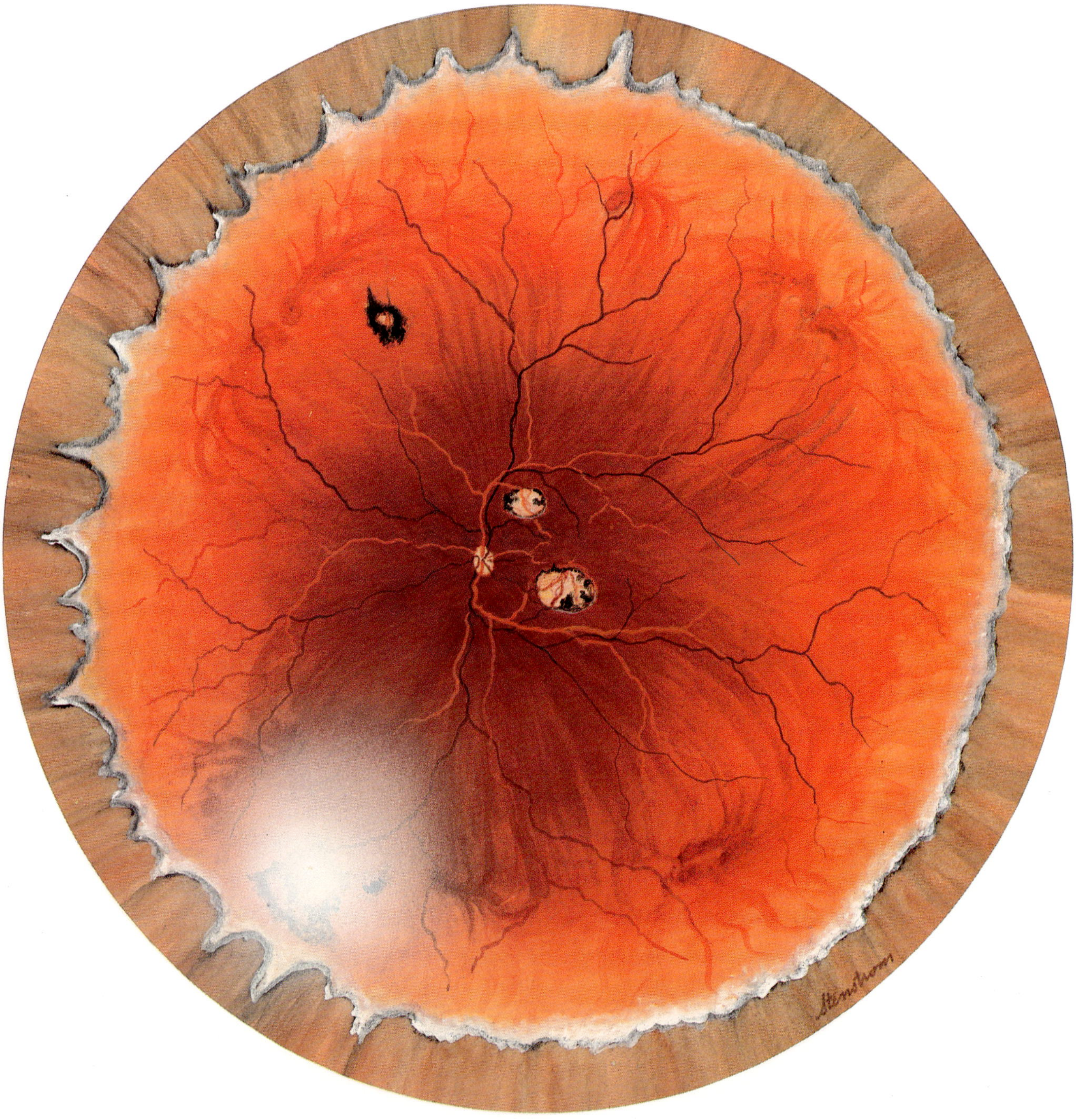

PLATE 54

HISTOPLASMOSIS

The presumed ocular histoplasmosis syndrome has a distinct retinal appearance characterized by small round atrophic areas in the midperipheral retina. These punched-out appearing spots may be surrounded by varying amounts of pigment. The optic nerve is typically surrounded by a ring of pigmented atrophic scarring, although the optic nerve itself is normal. The macula may be normal or affected by histoplasmosis spots. If present, histoplasmosis spots in the macula may lead to the development of subretinal neovascularization. Neovascularization may produce subretinal fluid and hemorrhage, culminating eventually in a fibrotic macular scar with permanent loss of central vision.

The peripheral spots first appear in young adulthood, while the macular involvement usually occurs in the second, third, or fourth decade. Even if histoplasmosis spots are not visible clinically in the macula, fluorescein angiography may show occult histoplasmosis spots that may later produce macular decompensation. Even when macular involvement occurs, the media typically remains crystal clear with no vitreous cellular infiltration.

The picture of presumed ocular histoplasmosis occurs most commonly in individuals who live for at least part of their life in an endemic area, which in the United States is along the Ohio and Mississippi River valleys. Ocular histoplasmosis is much more common in caucasian than in the more heavily pigmented races. The exact pathogenesis of ocular histoplasmosis is not fully known, but there appears to be some predilection for those with certain HLA antigens.

Braley RE, Meredith TA, Aaberg TN, et al: The prevalence of HLA-B7 in presumed ocular histoplasmosis. Am J Ophthalmol 85:859–861, 1978

Meredith TA, Smith RE, Duquesnoy RJ: Association of HLA-DR_w2 antigen with presumed ocular histoplasmosis. Am J Ophthalmol 89:70–76, 1980

Ryan SJ: De novo subretinal neovascularization in the histoplasmosis syndrome. Arch Ophthalmol 94:321–327, 1976

Schlaegel TF Jr: Ocular Histoplasmosis. New York, Grune & Stratton, 1977

Smith RE, Ganley JP: An epidemiologic study of presumed ocular histoplasmosis. Trans Am Acad Ophthalmol Otolaryngol 75:994–1005, 1971

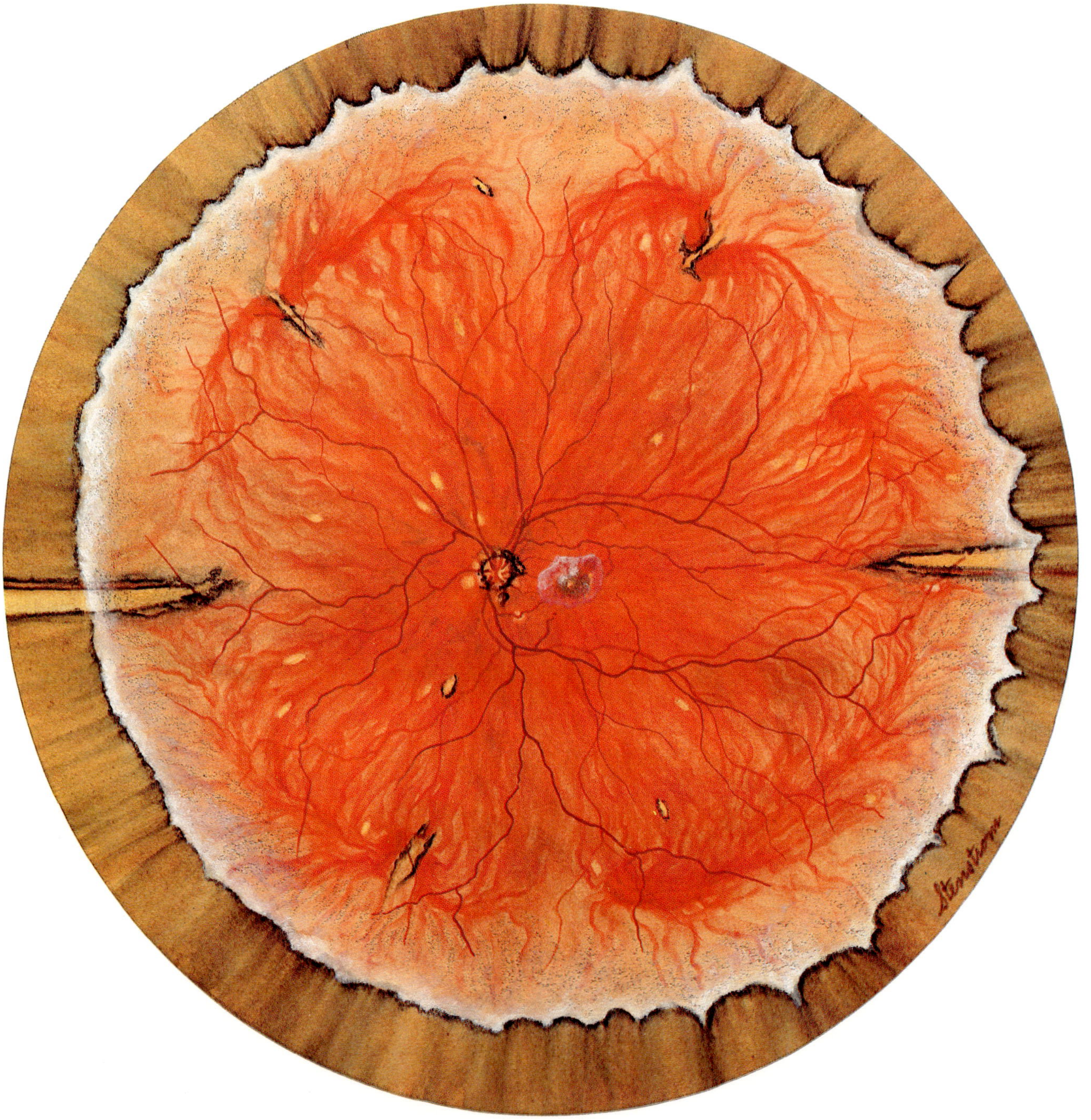

PLATE 55

SYPHILITIC CHORIORETINITIS

Syphilis remains the great mimic, producing a variety of clinical appearances in the fundus. Both congenital and acquired syphilis can produce retinal involvement and there may be little clinical difference in appearance between the two forms. In the acute stage of the infection there is vitreous haze with focal retinal exudates and splinter hemorrhages caused by involvement of the choriocapillaris. Clinically more common is the inactive stage, which produces three main clinical appearances. First there may be a minimal salt-and-pepper appearance to the entire fundus with a focal area of depigmentation and pigment clumping. Second, there may be multiple small focal areas of chorioretinal atrophy spread diffusely throughout the fundus. Third, there may be widespread involvement, with diffuse atrophy of the pigment epithelium and focal pigment clumping, producing a picture that resembles retinitis pigmentosa. Diffuse chorioretinal atrophy may occur, surrounding the optic nerve as shown here, but the same process may occur and be limited to the periphery. The retinal vessels frequently show white sheathing and vessel narrowing. Atrophy of the optic nerve may or may not be present, depending on the pattern of involvement. Visual function may be surprisingly well preserved, considering the dramatic retinal changes. The electroretinogram and electro-oculogram are usually normal. In rare instances neovascularization may develop from the optic nerve.

Blodi FC, Hervouet F: Syphilitic chorioretinitis. Arch Ophthalmol 79:294–296, 1968

Crouch ER, Goldberg MF: Retinal periarteritis secondary to syphilis. Arch Ophthalmol 93:384–387, 1975

Locker ES, Locker MJ, Rudolph AH: Syphilis and the eye. Perspect Ophthalmol 3:213–219, 1979

Savir H, Kurz O: Fluorescein angiography in syphilitic retinal vasculitis. Ann Ophthalmol 8:713–716, 1976

Schlaegel TF, Kao SF: A review of 28 presumptive cases of syphilitic uveitis. Am J Ophthalmol 93:412–414, 1982

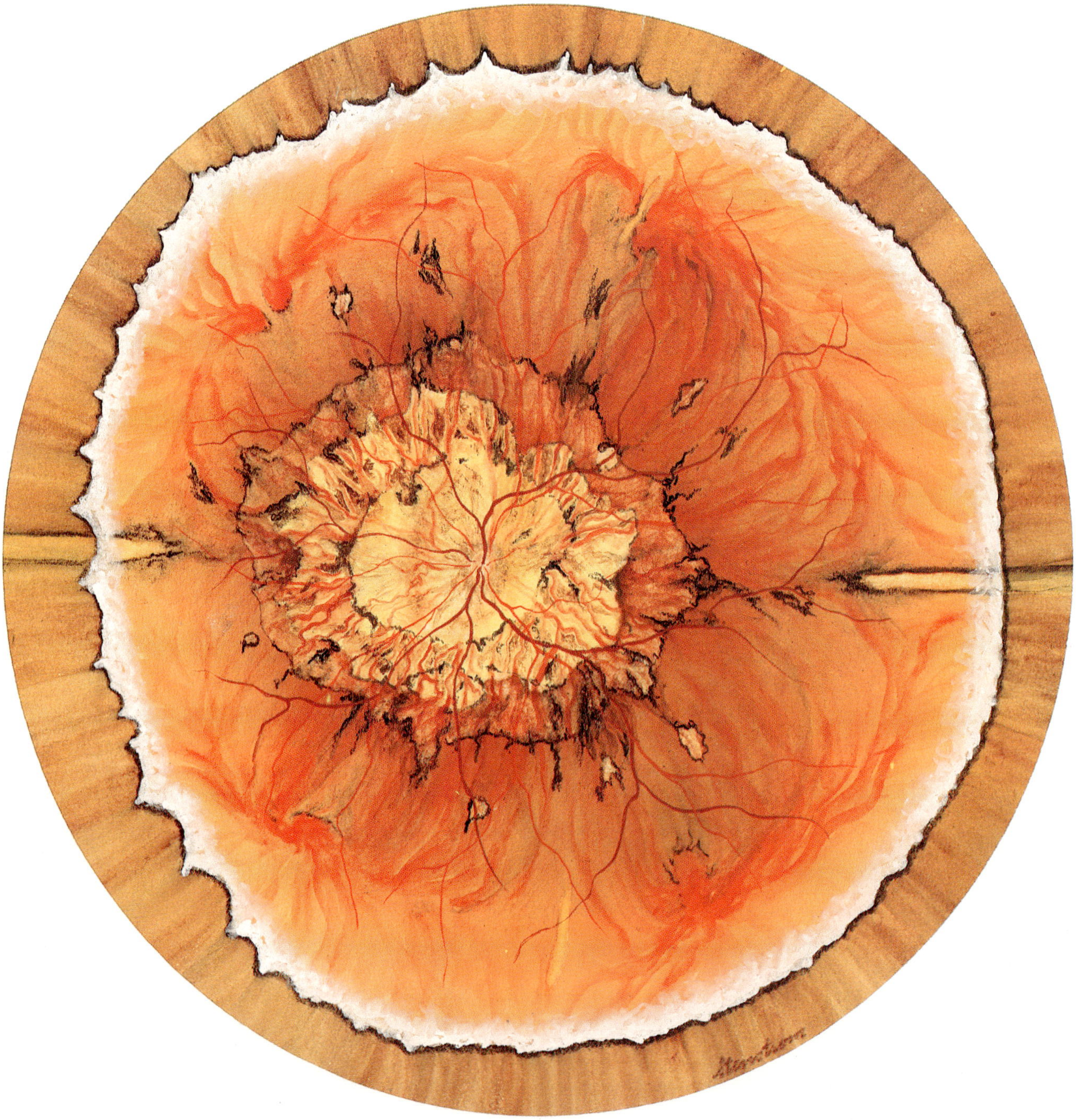

PLATE 56

TOXOCARA CANIS

Toxocara canis is the larval form of the intestinal parasite of dogs that infects humans through contaminated soil or food. Ova are ingested and develop into larvae in the human intestine. These larvae then penetrate the intestinal blood vessels and lymphatics and disseminate, eventually reaching the eye.

An overwhelming infection with *T. canis* results in the visceral larva migrans syndrome, but children affected with ocular *T. canis* rarely give a history of previous infection. The usual presentation is either the onset of strabismus or leukocoria in which the diagnosis of retinoblastoma is considered. In very young children the clinical picture is typically of a chronic unilateral uveitis with a cloudy vitreous and the development of a cyclitic membrane without specific localizing features. This picture may be very difficult to distinguish from that of retinoblastoma, but serological testing may be of value.

In the slightly older child in the early grade school years, the larval stage of *T. canis* typically wanders throughout the eye and finally dies, producing a localized granuloma. These granulomas may be anywhere in the eye, but are most common in the macula region. The granuloma appears intensely white and is usually subretinal, producing an elevated mass approximately two disc diameters in size. There is a surrounding serous detachment of the retina with subretinal pigment clumping and usually striae produced in a radiating pattern in the surrounding retina. Large granulomas may also occur in the retinal periphery in the vitreous cavity or beneath the retina. At this stage there is characteristically very little vitreous infiltrate, although localized vitreous abscess and iridocyclitis may occur.

Baldone JA, Clark WB, Jung RC: Nematode ophthalmitis. Am J. Ophthalmol 57:763–766, 1964

Brown DH: Ocular Toxocara canis. II. Clinical review. J Pediatr Ophthalmol 7:182–191, 1970

Byers B, Kimura SJ: Uveitis after death of larva in the vitreous cavity. Am J. Ophthalmol 77:63–66, 1974

Pollard ZF, Jarrett WH, Hagler WS, et al: ELISA for diagnosis of ocular toxocariasis. Ophthalmology 86:743–749, 1979

Wilder HC: Nematode endophthalmitis. Trans Am Acad Ophthalmol Otolaryngol 55:99–109, 1951

Wilkinson CP, Welch RB: Intraocular toxocara. Am J Ophthalmol 71:921–930, 1971

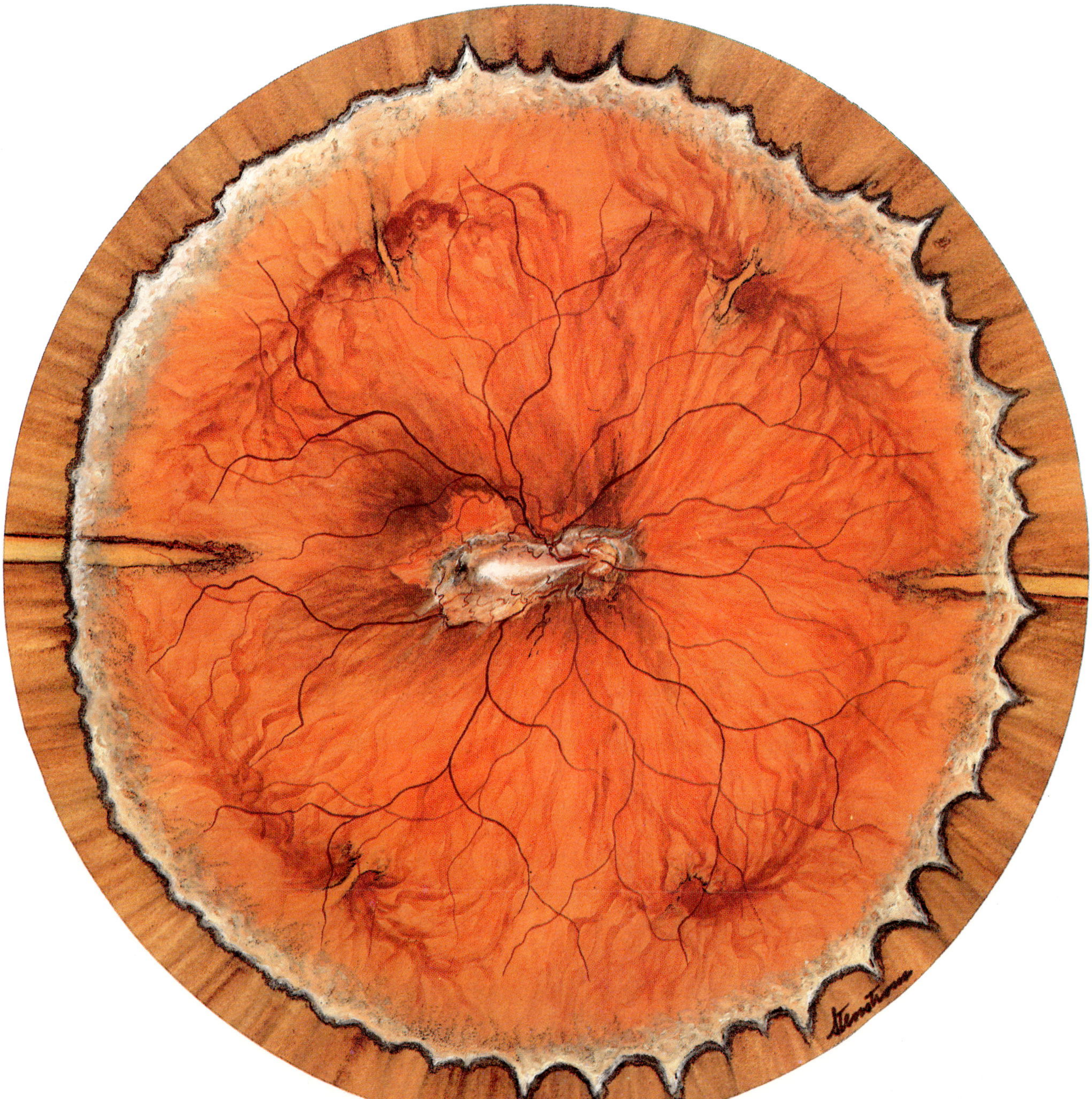

PLATE 57

TOXOCARA CANIS WITH TRACKS

The *Toxocara* larvae, it is believed, are capable of active motility while alive in the eye. They frequently migrate from one site to another inside the eye. The larvae are usually quite transparent and difficult to see by ophthalmoscopy. Also, they do not cause much inflammation in the living state and usually the eye is asymptomatic, so that the affected child does not complain. At a later stage it is possible to see larval tracks visible as a distinct pigmented line wandering in a random pattern throughout the fundus. Sometimes the pattern is so extensive that a diffuse pigment epithelial mottling is present. In either case, chorioretinal adhesions may be formed, as was described by Wilder in the original histologic description of ocular *T. canis*.

Eventually the parasite dies, producing the characteristic white granulomatous mound. Here it is shown at the equator with a surrounding subretinal hemorrhage. The tracks of its previous excursions are visible as a mottling of the pigment epithelium. There may be atrophy of the optic nerve in the later stages, resulting in rather profound visual loss even though the macula may appear intact.

Histological studies show many eosinophils surrounding the decomposed parasite, which may or may not be histologically identifiable. There are also numerous polymorphonuclear leukocytes, epithelioid cells, and giant cells present.

Ashton N: Larval granulomatosis of the retina due to toxocara. Br J Ophthalmol *44*:129–148, 1960

Biglan AW, Glickman LT, Lobes LA: Serum and vitreous toxocara antibody in nematode endophthalmitis. Am J Ophthalmol *88*:898–901, 1979

Bird AC, Smith JL, Curtin VT: Nematode optic neuritis. Am J Ophthalmol *69*:73–77, 1970

Gass JDM, Gilbert WR, Guerry RK, et al: Diffuse unilateral subacute neuroretinitis. Ophthalmology *85*:521–545, 1978

O'Connor PR: Visceral larva migrans of the eye. Subretinal tube formation. Arch Ophthalmol *88*:526–529, 1972

Wilder HC: Nematode endophthalmitis. Trans Am Acad Ophthalmol Otolaryngol *55*:99–109, 1951

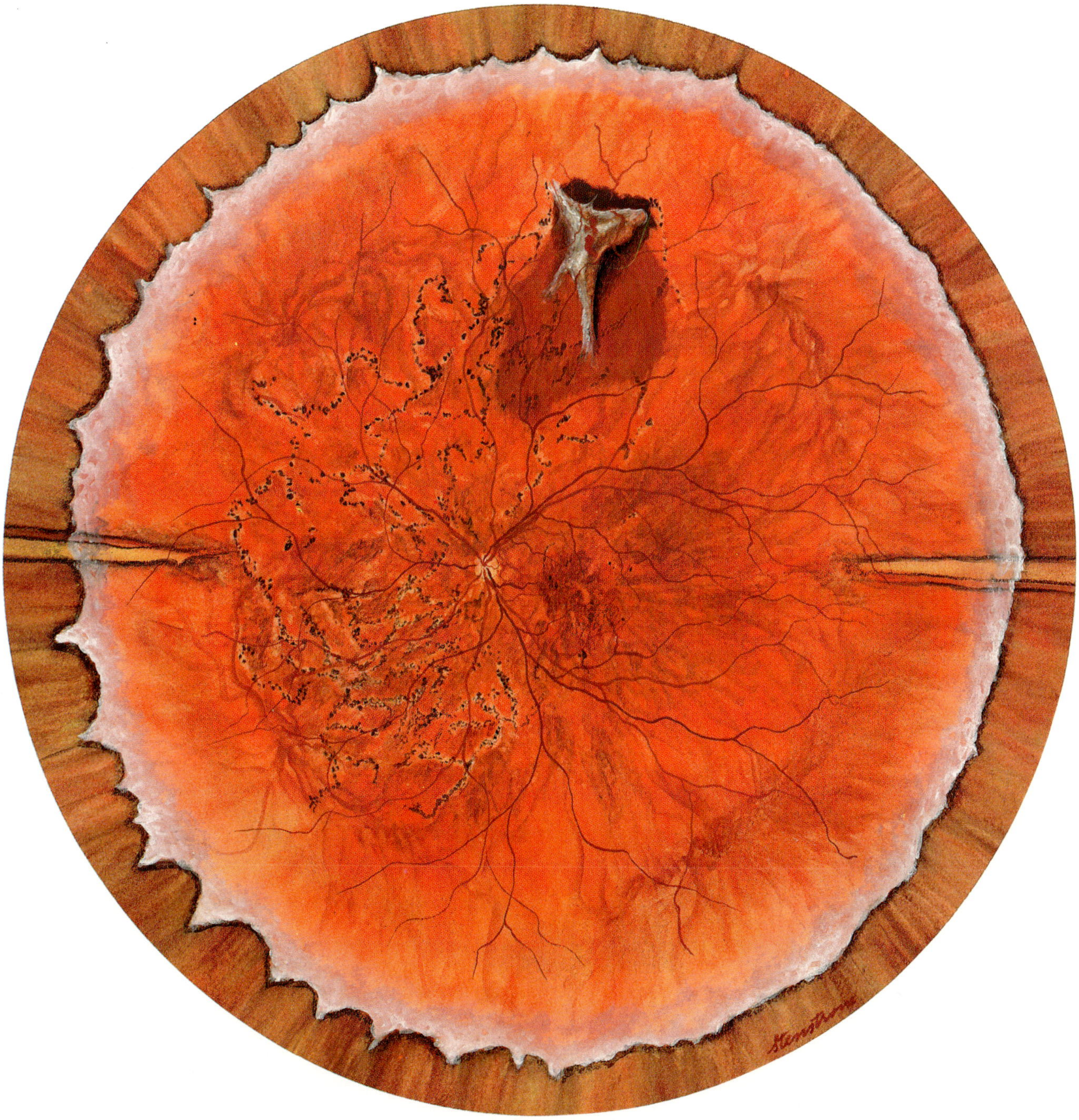

PLATE 58

TOXOCARA CANIS AT THE ORA SERRATA

Toxocara canis may present as a mass lesion at the ora serrata. Usually this clinical picture is found in older children in which a hemispheric, intensely white, elevated mass is present at the far periphery. There is a variable degree of vitreous inflammation surrounding the lesion. Fine lacy vascularization can usually be seen on the surface of the lesion. The appearance suggests the possibility of tumor, particularly retinoblastoma, or a parasitic lesion. It is a characteristic of peripheral *T. canis* lesions to develop dense connective tissue strands that extend posteriorly toward the disc and macula. Traction on these structures may produce retinal striae or traction detachment that will decrease central visual acuity. More peripherally, there usually are traction membranes and striae surrounding the elevated mass lesion.

There may be recurrent episodes of uveitis associated with these peripheral granulomas. Rarely retinal detachment may occur from such lesions. Vitrectomy has been proposed for selected cases of peripheral *T. canis*.

Hagler WS, Pollard ZF, Jarrett WH, et al: Results of surgery for ocular *Toxocara canis*. Ophthalmology *88*:1081–1086, 1981

Hogan MJ, Kimura SJ, Spencer WH: Visceral larva migrans and peripheral retinitis. JAMA *194*:1345–1347, 1965

Irvine WC, Irvine AR: Nematode endophthalmitis, *Toxocara canis*. Am J Ophthalmol *47*:185–191, 1959

Wilkinson CP, Welch RB: Intraocular toxocara. Am J Ophthalmol *71*:921–930, 1971

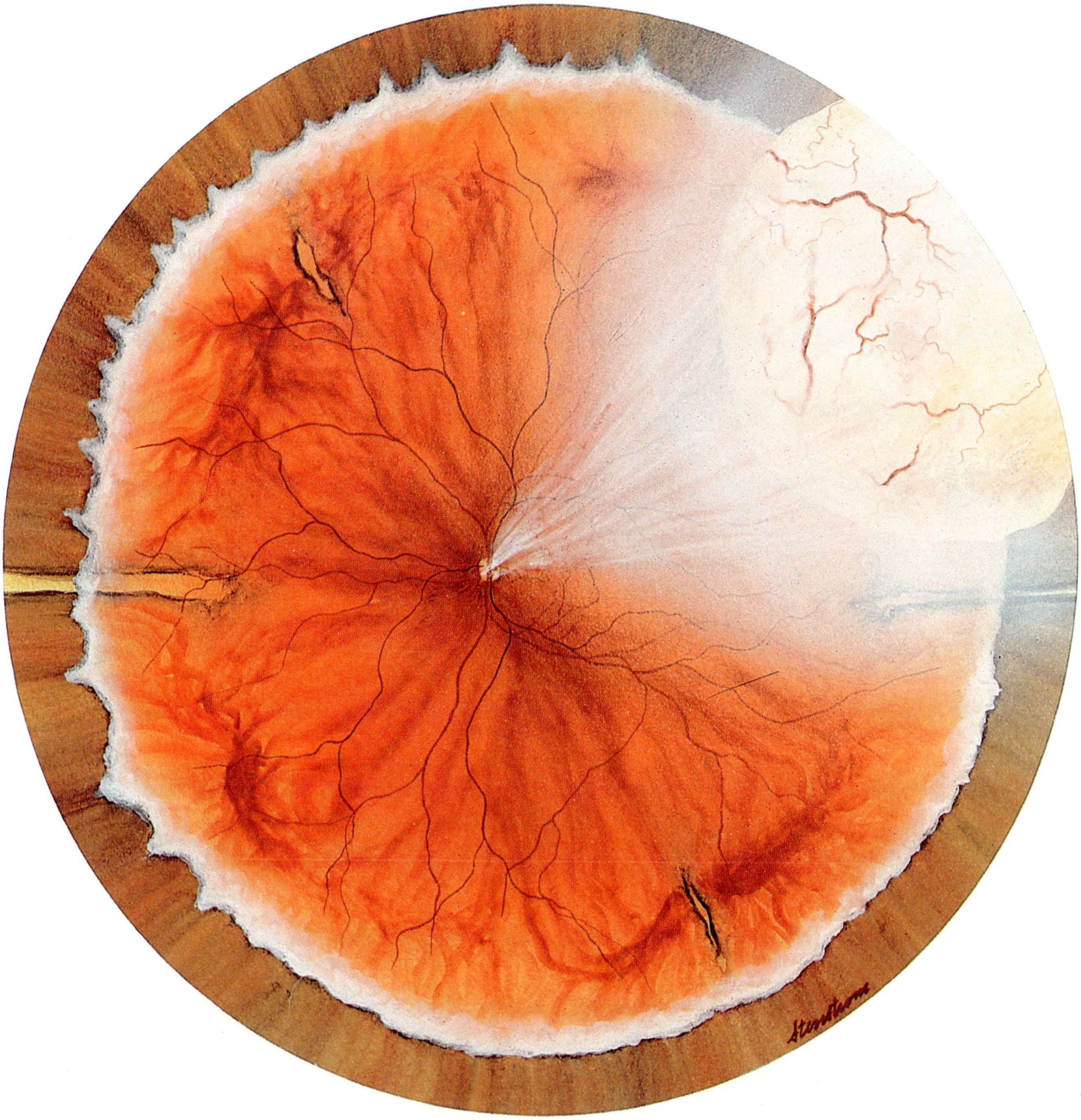

PLATE 59

CYTOMEGALOVIRUS

Cytomegalovirus infection of the retina occurs in two age groups, newborns and adults. The virus is opportunistic, infecting primarily those with diminished immunological defenses. In the newborn, cytomegalovirus occurs as an congenital infection transmitted through the placenta. The systemic infection of other major organ systems usually overshadows the eye findings. Retinal examination reveals large irregular areas of retinal necrosis with extensive retinal hemorrhages. In neonates the diagnosis is usually made by finding the typical inclusion bodies in cells in the urinary sediment.

The adult form, as pictured here, is usually found in adults with an underlying disorder of the immune system. This defect may be caused by a neoplastic disease such as leukemia, lymphoma, or multiple myeloma, or it may be medically induced by immunosuppression therapy in patients receiving organ transplantation. Very rarely cytomegalovirus infection occurs in an otherwise normal adult.

In the adult, the initial symptoms begin with decreased vision, photophobia, and intraocular inflammatory findings. Most cases are bilateral. The earliest retinal lesions are white punctate spots in the retinal periphery that represent areas of retinal necrosis. These spots enlarge and coalesce into large white areas of necrotic retina with superimposed retinal and preretinal hemorrhages. The posterior edge of the affected area contains the active leading edge of the infection, producing retinal edema and retinal hemorrhages as it marches relentlessly posteriorly toward the macula and optic nerve. Previously active areas in the periphery later show profound atrophy of the retina and pigment epithelium. Sometimes a retinal detachment occurs from large peripheral holes in necrotic retina. These detachments are very difficult to repair. Usually the disease process results in total blindness.

Hart WM, Reed CA, Freedman HL, et al: Cytomegalovirus in juvenile iridocyclitis. Am J Ophthalmol *86*:329–331, 1978

Meredith TA, Aaberg TM, Reeser FH: Rhegmatogenous retinal detachment complicating cytomegalovirus retinitis. Am J Ophthalmol *87*:793–796, 1979

Nicholson DH: Cytomegalovirus infection of the retina. Int Ophthalmol Clin *15*:151–162, 1975

Tarkkanen A, Merenmies L, Holmstrom T: Ocular involvement in congenital cytomegalic inclusion disease. J Pediatr Ophthalmol *9*:82–96, 1972

de Venecia G, Zu Rhein GM, Pratt MV, et al: Cytomegalic inclusion retinitis in an adult. Arch Ophthalmol *86*:44–57, 1971

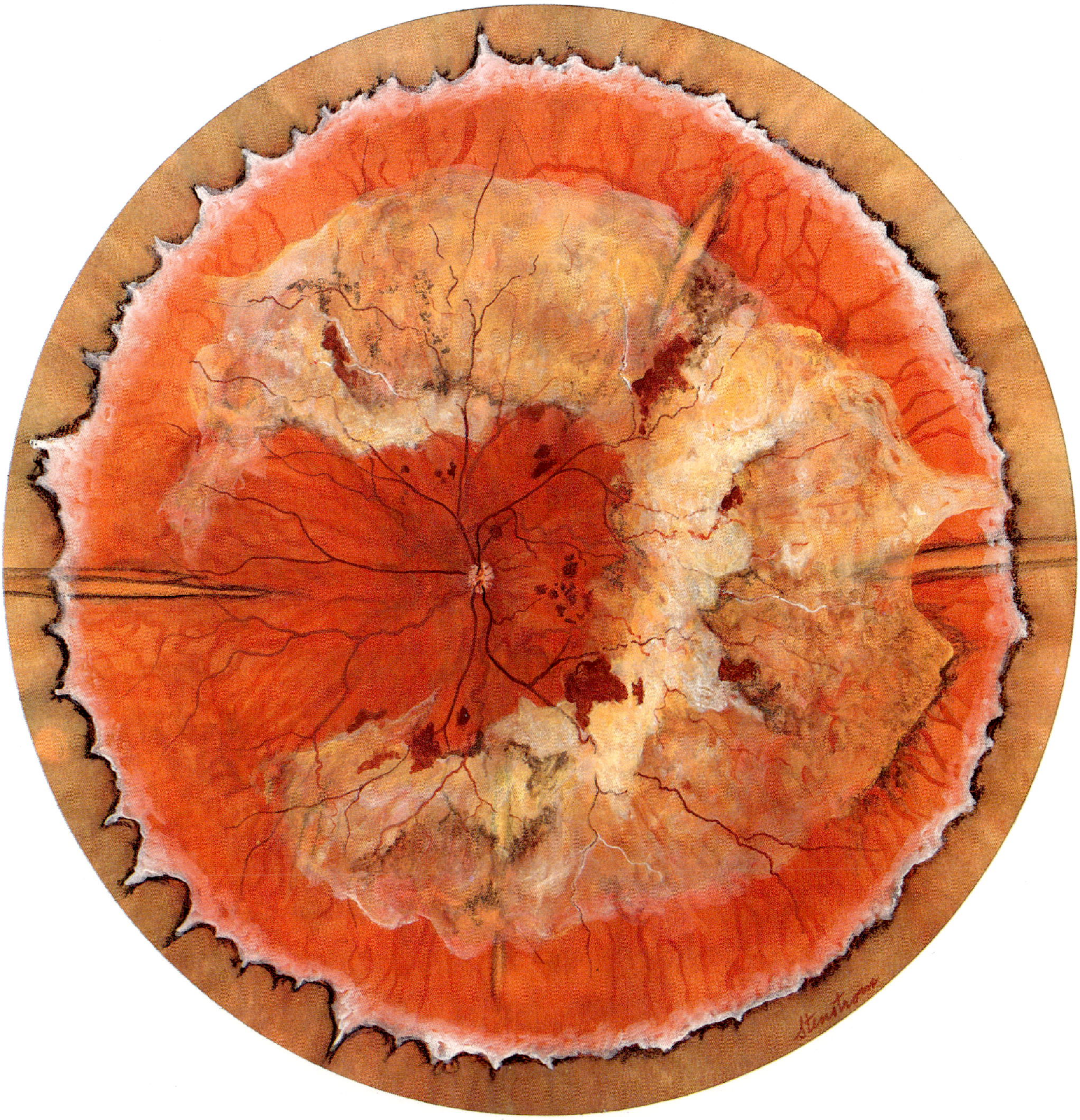

PLATE 60

FUNGAL ENDOPHTHALMITIS

Fungal endophthalmitis is either exogenous, coming from a source outside the body, or endogenous, coming from a source inside the body. Exogenous fungal endophthalmitis may occur after infection of the eye at cataract extraction or after a penetrating injury.

Most commonly, endogenous infection occurs by blood-borne spread of fungal infection elsewhere in the body. This is particularly likely to occur in patients with neoplastic or metabolic diseases, especially if they have been on chronic treatment with antibiotic, steroid, or cytotoxic drugs, or in patients with indwelling catheters. A longer interval occurs between inoculation and clinical onset of fungal endophthalmitis than with bacterial infections. The minimal interval is approximately eight days, and the interval may be as long as several months.

Initial symptoms begin to appear insidiously with blurred vision, pain, and minimal eye redness. The symptoms may be unilateral or bilateral. Purulent white accumulations may occur in the anterior or posterior vitreous, or particularly near the posterior pole. Initial lesions are white, circumscribed, and discrete, but quickly advance to appear as fluffy white infiltrates with a diffuse surrounding vitreous haze producing the "cotton balls in the vitreous" appearance. Progression from this stage may be slow or fulminant, with retinal hemorrhages and signs of anterior segment inflammation. Treatment is difficult at best and even after successful therapy, extensive scar tissue and vitrous traction may produce retinal detachment.

Axelrod AJ, Peyman GA: Intravitreal amphotericin B treatment of experimental fungal endophthalmitis. Am J Ophthalmol *76*:584–588, 1973

Clarkson JG, Green WR: Endogenous fungal endophthalmitis. *In* Duane TD, (ed): Clinical Ophthalmology, Hagerstown, Md, Harper & Row, 1981, Vol 3, Chapter 11, pp 1–44

Fine BS, Zimmerman LE: Exogenous intraocular fundus infections. Am J Ophthalmol *48*:151–165, 1959

Michelson PE, Stark WJ, Resser F, et al: Endogenous candida endophthalmitis. Int Ophthalmol Clin *3*:125–147, 1971

Peyman GA, Vastine DW, Diamond JG: Vitrectomy in endogenous candida endophthalmitis. Albrecht von Graefes Arch Klin Ophthalmol *197*:55–59, 1975

Sugar HS, Mandell GH, Shalev J: Metastatic endophthalmitis associated with injection of addictive drugs. Am J Ophthalmol *71*:1055–1058, 1971

Theodore FH, Littman ML, Almeda E: Endophthalmitis following cataract extraction. Am J Ophthalmol *53*:35–39, 1962

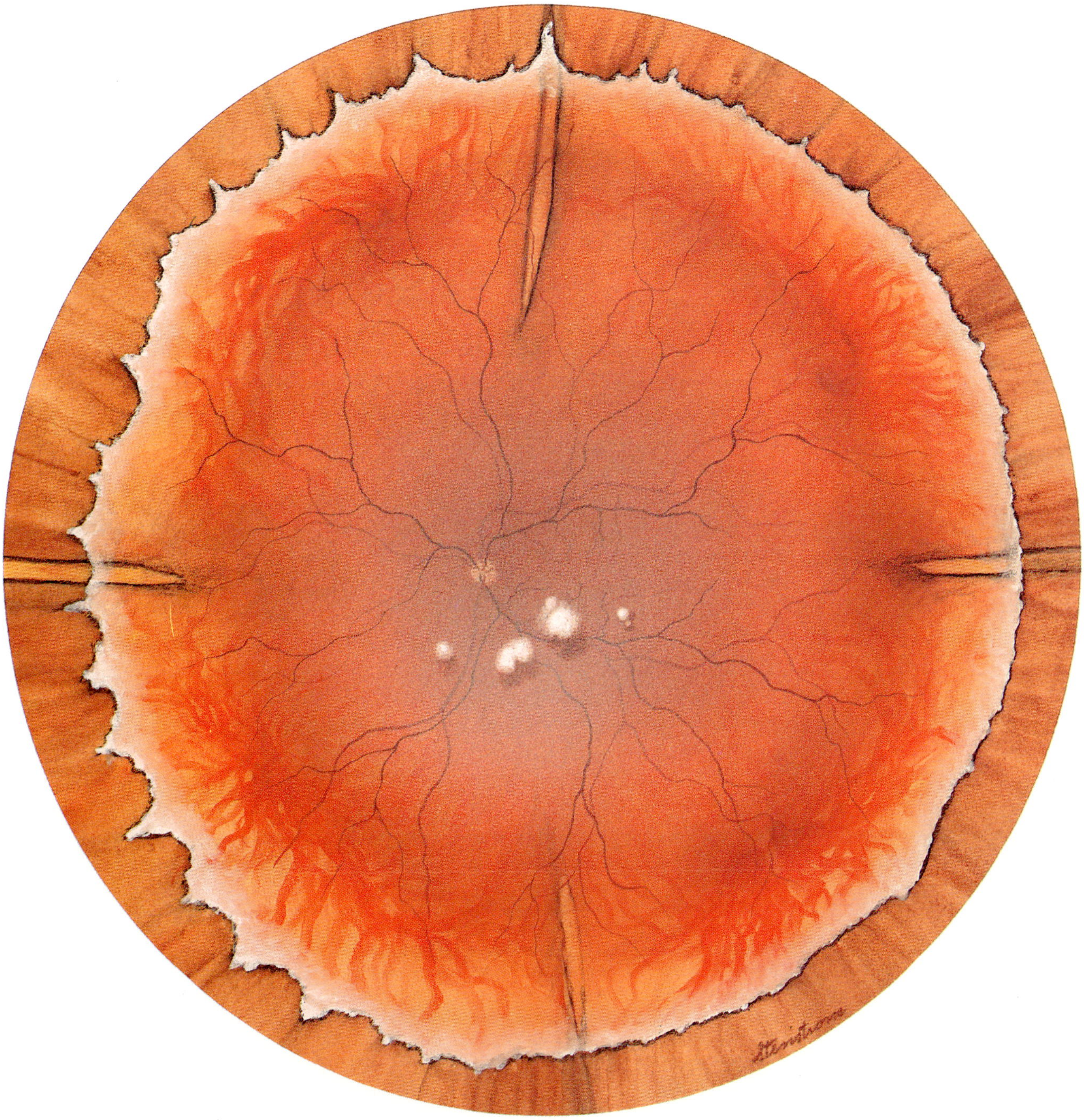

PLATE 61

BACTERIAL ENDOPHTHALMITIS

Bacterial endophthalmitis is an infection inside the eye that can rapidly lead to permanent destruction of all vision. It may be endogenous, resulting from a blood-borne infection caused by septic foci elsewhere in the body, especially in immunologically depressed patients, or it can be exogenous, having been directly inoculated into the eye during a surgical procedure or a perforating injury. The toxins and enzymes from the infecting bacteria and from degenerating tissues may produce irreversible damage to the eye. The prognosis depends on the virulence of the infecting organisms, the interval between onset of infection and the onset of treatment, and the effectiveness of the treatment.

The primary symptoms are severe pain and decreased vision in the eye. Lid and conjunctival edema, corneal haze, and hypopyon also appear early in the course. On fundus examination there is dense vitreous cellular infiltrate that produces a white reflex from the fundus. The vitreous infiltrate may be so dense that the retinal details may not be seen. In advanced infections, the retina itself may appear white and necrotic.

Bacterial endophthalmitis usually progresses rapidly, appearing clinically within 36 to 48 hours after the onset of bacterial infection. In the postoperative patient it is most important to distinguish bacterial endophthalmitis from noninfectious iridocyclitis, which typically occurs five to six days postoperatively.

The presence of retained lens material may be particularly irritating to the eye and cause an appearance that is clinically similar to early bacterial endophthalmitis. Fungal endophthalmitis usually is recognized clinically at a minimum of eight days, and usually appears several weeks later.

Allen HF, Mangiaracine AB: Bacterial endophthalmitis after cataract extraction: A study of 22 infections in 20,000 operations. Arch Ophthalmol *72*:454–462, 1964

Allen HF, Mangiaracine AB: Bacterial endophthalmitis after cataract extraction II. Incidence in 36,000 consecutive operations, with special references to preoperative topical antibiotics. Arch Ophthalmol *91*:3–7, 1974

Cottingham AJ, Forster RK: Vitrectomy in endophthalmitis. Arch Ophthalmol *94*:2078–2081, 1976

Forster RK: Endophthalmitis. Arch Ophthalmol *92*:387–392, 1974

Forster RK, Zachary IG, Cottingham AJ, et al: Further observations on the diagnosis, cause and treatment of endophthalmitis. Am J Ophthalmol *81*:52–56, 1976

Forster RK, Abbot RL, Gelender H: Management of infectious endophthalmitis. Ophthalmology *87*:313–319, 1980

Peyman GA, Sanders DR: Treatment of endophthalmitis. *In* Advances in Uveal Surgery, Vitreous Surgery and the Treatment of Endophthalmitis. New York, Appleton-Century-Crofts, 1975, pp 179–228

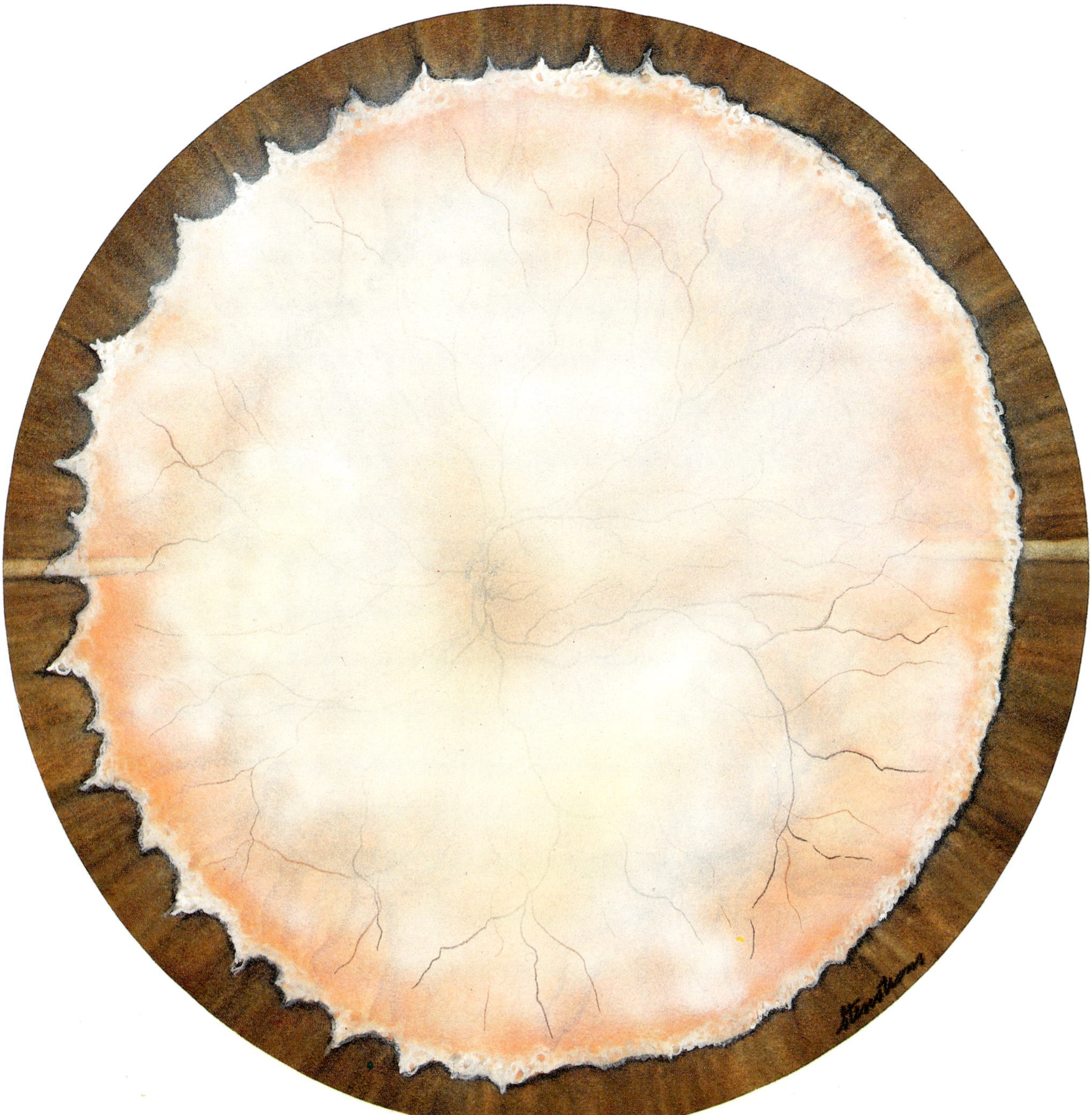

PLATE 62

ACUTE RETINAL NECROSIS

Acute retinal necrosis occurs in otherwise healthy individuals, presenting as a generally bilateral but asymmetrical uveitis of unknown cause. The anterior segment shows cells, flare, and mutton fat keratitic precipitates, but the major changes are in the posterior segment where there is a dense vitreous cellular infiltrate. In the early stages discrete opaque yellow-white lesions appear in the peripheral retina and may coalesce to become confluent. The process extends around the peripheral retina with relative sparing of the posterior pole. There is a well demarcated border between normal and abnormal retina. The choroidal pattern cannot be seen through the yellow-white necrotic retina, and fluorescein angiography shows that there is no capillary profusion in the affected areas. The major vessels are surrounded by perivascular hemorrhage and show staining of the vessel walls with fluorescein leakage. With the passage of time, affected areas of retina clear in a patchy manner, leaving a stippled pigment epithelium. The large vessels in the affected areas develop sheathing. At the same time the retina becomes less opaque and there is a sloughing of the necrotic retina into the vitreous, creating a marked increase in vitreous debris. There may be an exudative retinal detachment in the early stages of the process, and tractional and especially rhegmatogenous detachments in the later stages. Large retinal tears occur at the junction of the normal posterior retina and the affected anterior retina. Frequently these detachments are so complex as to be inoperable. The etiology of acute retinal necrosis is entirely unknown although the condition mimics certain features of Behçet's disease, cytomegalovirus infection, and herpes infection of the retina; however, the condition is generally considered to be a fulminant necrotizing retinal vasculitis of unknown etiology.

Aaberg TM, Cesarz TJ, Rytel MW: Correlation of virology and clinical course of cytomegalovirus retinitis. Am J Ophthalmol *74*:407–415, 1972

Minckler DS, McLean EB, Shaw CM, Hendrikson A: Herpesvirus hominis encephalitis and retinitis. Arch Ophthalmol *94*:89–95, 1976

Saari KM, Boke W, Manthey KF, et al: Bilateral acute retinal necrosis. Am J Ophthalmol *93*:403–411, 1982

de Venecia G, ZuRhein GM, Pratt MV et al: Cytomegalic inclusion retinitis. Arch Ophthalmol *86*:44–57, 1971

Willerson D, Aaberg TM, Reeser RH: Necrotizing vaso-occlusive retinitis, Am J Ophthalmol *84*:209–219, 1977

Young NJA, Bird AC: Bilateral acute retinal necrosis, Brit J Ophthalmol *62*:581–590, 1978

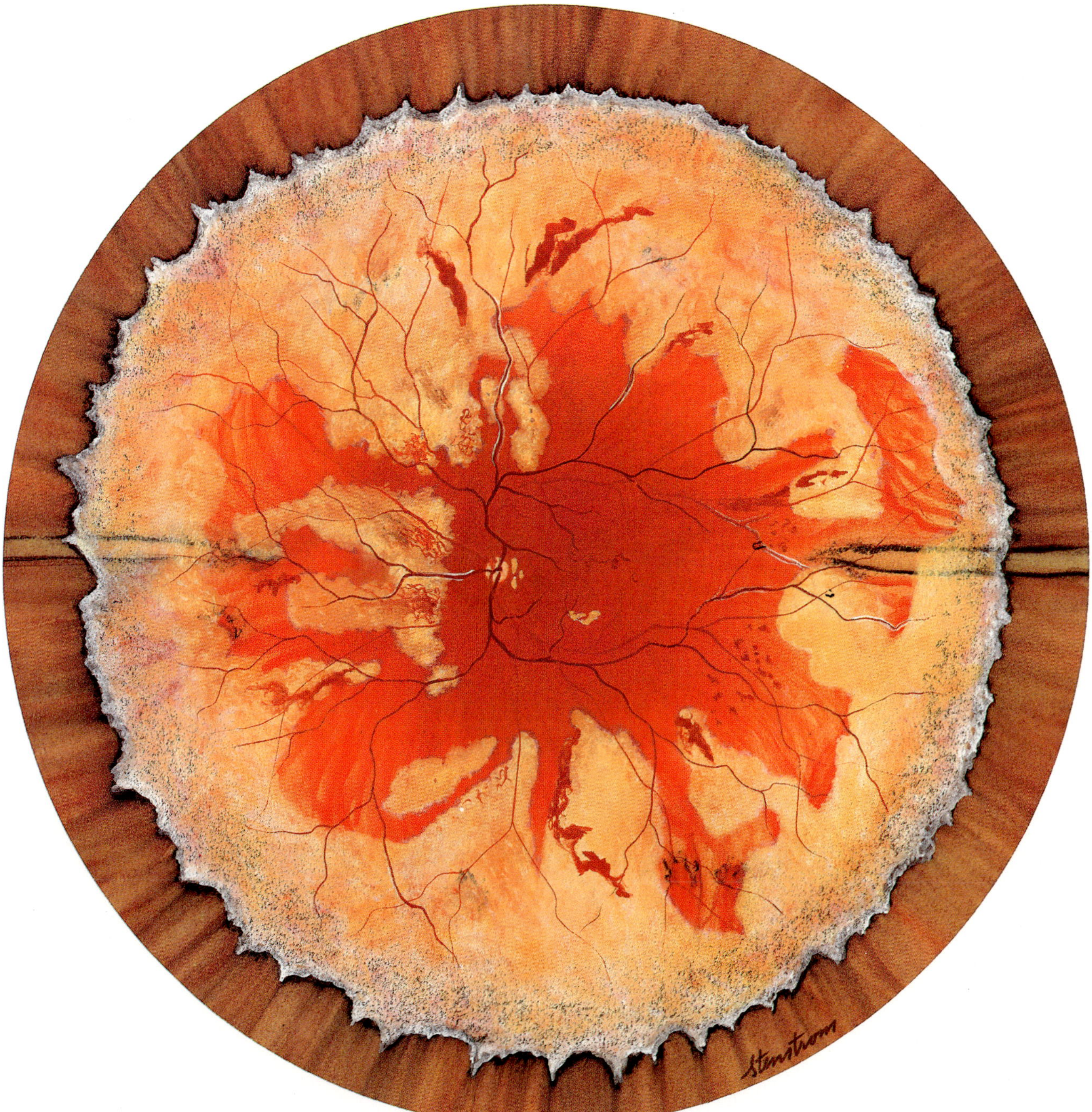

PLATE 63

PERIPHERAL UVEITIS

Peripheral uveitis, also called pars planitis, and chronic cyclitis, is a bilateral inflammatory disease affecting the vitreous and retinas of young adults. It is of completely unknown etiology. Initial symptoms include mild blurring of vision, floaters, and photophobia. Anterior segment findings include cells and aqueous flare, keratitic precipitates, posterior iris synechiae, and cataract formation.

Fundus examination reveals a vitreous cellular infiltrate primarily in the inferior vitreous cavity. The cellular infiltrate is concentrated particularly in the inferior vitreous base and accumulates along the inferior pars plana to produce a white covering resembling a snowbank. Peripheral uveitis is a chronic condition and with time, sheathing of the retinal vessels and cystoid macular edema develops. In severe cases there may be neovascularization of the optic nerve, and fine neovascular vessels may also be present over the snowbank in the periphery. Vitreous hemorrhage may occur from neovascularization, and phthisis bulbi may result. Typically, the inflammatory process waxes and wanes but may continue for years. Other causes of inflammatory ocular disease must be considered in the differential diagnosis, and in particular various tumors may masquerade as peripheral uveitis.

Aaberg TM, Cesarz TJ, Flinkinger RR: Treatment of peripheral uveoretinitis by cryotherapy. Am J Ophthalmol *73*:685–688, 1973

Brockhurst RJ, Schepens CL, Okamura ID: Uveitis II. Peripheral uveitis: Clinical description, complications and differential diagnosis. Am J Ophthalmol *49*:1257–1266, 1960

Brockhurst RJ, Schepens CL, Okamura ID: Uveitis III. Peripheral uveitis: Pathogenesis, etiology and treatment. Am J Ophthalmol *51*:19–26, 1961

Pruett RC, Brockhurst RJ, Letts N: Fluorescein angiography of peripheral uveitis. Am J Ophthalmol *77*:448–453, 1974

Schepens CL: L'inflammation de la région de l'"ora serrata" et ses séquelles. Bull Soc Ophthalmol Fr *63*:113–124, 1950

Smith RE, Godfrey SA, Kimura SJ: Chronic cyclitis I. Course and visual prognosis. Trans Am Acad Ophthalmol Otolaryngol *77*:760–768, 1973

Smith RE, Godfrey SA, Kumura SJ: Complications of chronic cyclitis. Am J Ophthalmol *82*:277–282, 1976

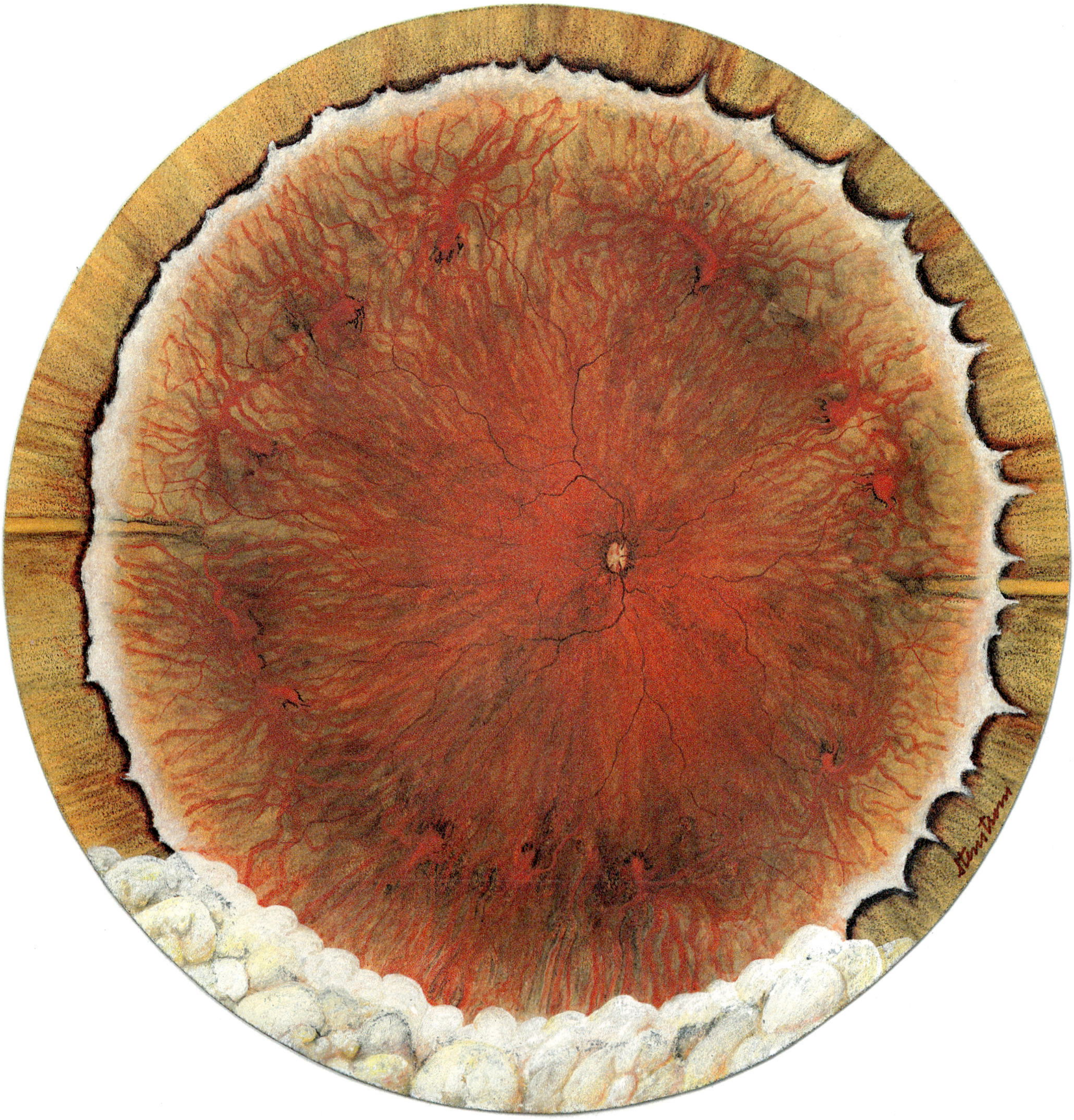

PLATE 64

Chapter Six

RETINAL VASCULAR DISEASES

CENTRAL RETINAL ARTERY OCCLUSION

Central retinal artery occlusion produces a sudden, profound loss of vision. The entire blood supply to the retina is obstructed, usually by atherosclerosis, embolism, or temporal arteritis. Within hours, the inner retinal layers supplied by the central retinal artery become milky white, representing ischemic edema. This milky appearance is more prominent in the posterior pole than in the far periphery. The foveal area stands out as a cherry red spot. The retina is anatomically thinner here; therefore, the normal red color of the choroid stands out in relief against the surrounding milky white retina. The retinal arteries and veins are not obscured by this milky white ischemic edema, and stand out prominently in relief. The arterioles are attenuated in size, and the veins may be either normal or slightly attenuated. Usually, the flow of blood is not completely obstructed, but, rather, there is a very slow flow, causing sludging of blood in the veins. With the direct ophthalmoscope, individual corpuscular flow can sometimes be observed.

After 7 to 10 days, the milky appearance of the retina gradually disappears as the inner retinal layers undergo atrophy and the retina becomes more transparent. By 6 weeks, optic atrophy is observed, and the retinal arteries become even smaller and show white sheathing. The veins are usually attenuated also, but the obstruction in the central retinal artery usually recanalizes and blood flow is re-established. Vision rarely returns, unless the macula is spared by the presence of a cilioretinal vessel supplied from the choroidal, rather than the retinal, circulation. Late complications include the development of rubeosis iridis and rarely neovascular glaucoma.

David NJ, Norton EWD, Gass JDM, et al: Fluorescein angiography in central retinal artery occlusion. Arch Opthalmol *77*:619–629, 1967

Karjalainen K: Occlusion of the central retinal artery and retinal branch arterioles. Acta Ophthalmol Suppl *109*:1–46, 1971

Kroll AJ: Experimental central retinal artery occlusion. Arch Ophthalmol *79*:453–469, 1968

Liversedge LA, Smith VH: Neuromedical and ophthalmic aspects of central retinal artery occlusion. Trans Ophthalmol Soc UK *82*:571–588, 1962

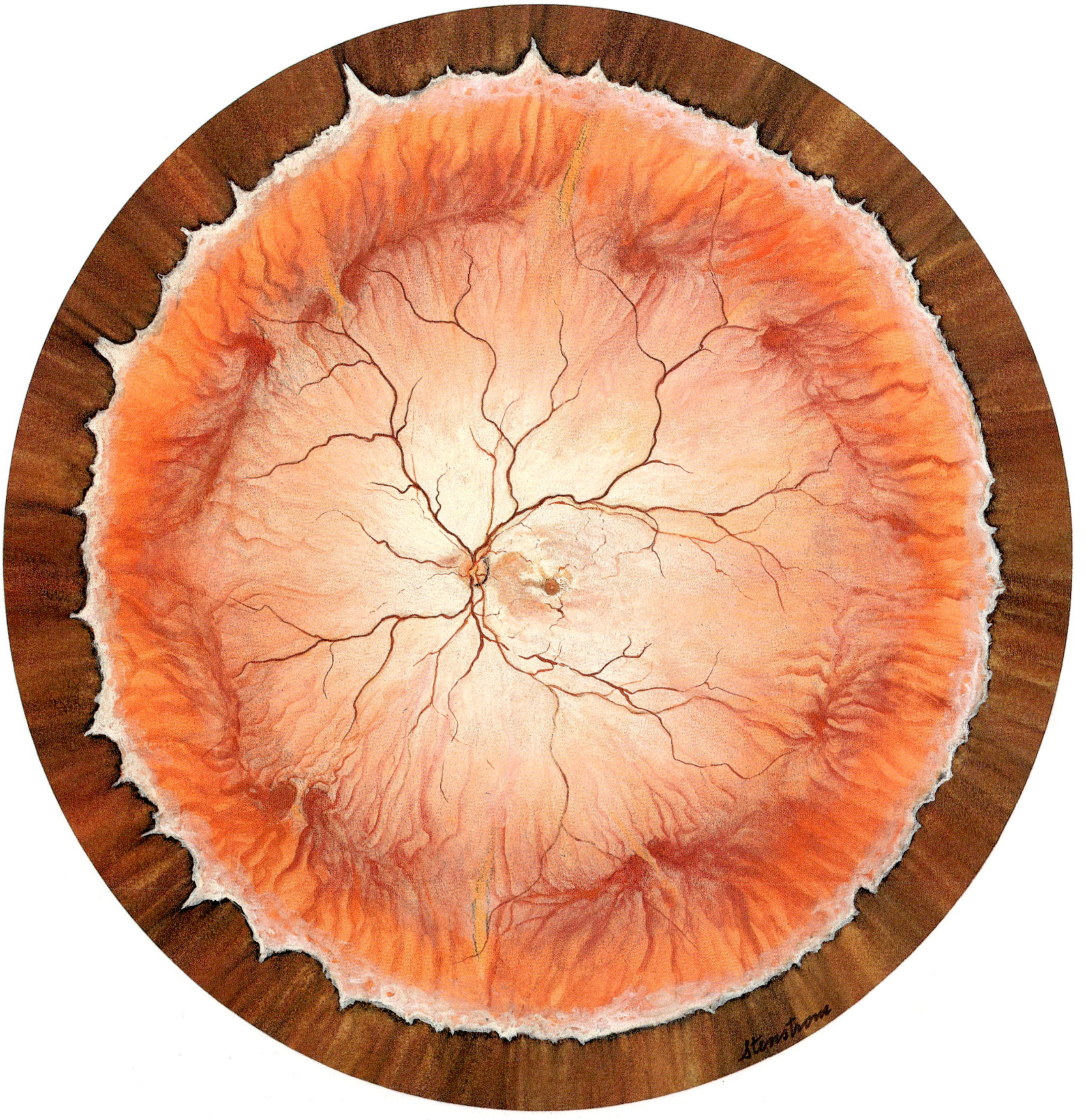

PLATE 65

BRANCH RETINAL VEIN OCCLUSION

Branch retinal vein occlusions of recent occurrence appear clinically as retinal hemorrhages and exudates in a distinctive pattern that corresponds to the drainage field of the occluded vein. The hemorrhages are either flame shaped and located in the nerve fiber layer, or dot hemorrhages located in the outer plexiform layer. Preretinal, or even vitreous hemorrhage may also occur. White exudates contrast sharply with the hemorrhage, and result from obstruction of axoplasmic flow in the retinal nerve fibers. The retina is diffusely thickened with florid edema. The obstructed vein itself appears engorged and tortuous, and the blood inside is dusky blue in color.

The pattern of hemorrhage and exudate is generally sector shaped, involving one full quadrant of the retina. The apex of the affected area, which is almost always where the vein is crossed by a retinal artery, is the site of the actual vein obstruction. The site of obstruction can generally be visialized ophthalmoscopically within several disc diameters of the disc. The superior temporal vein is most commonly affected, while the inferior temporal vein is next most common, and nasal branch retinal vein occlusions are relatively rare.

Occlusion of a branch retinal vein is most commonly associated with systemic hypertension. However, any systemic disease associated with hypercoagulability, slowing of blood flow, or any abnormality of erythrocytes or serum proteins may predispose to branch vein occlusion.

With the passage of months the hemorrhage, exudate, and edema may resolve somewhat. Chronic macular edema and preretinal membrane formation may develop, and neovascularization may lead to late vitreous hemorrhage. Anastomotic channels may form from dilated normal vessels to drain the obstructed vein, and such anastomotic channels must be differentiated from neovascularization.

Microaneurysms and white sheathing of both retinal arteries and retinal veins are seen in branch retinal vein occlusions of long standing. Visual field defects are demonstrable, corresponding to the area of affected retina.

Campbell CJ, Wise GN: Photocoagulation therapy of branch vein obstructions. Am J Ophthalmol *75*:28–31, 1973

Gutman FA: Macular edema in branch retinal vein occlusion: Prognosis and management. Trans Am Acad Ophalmol Otolaryngol *83*:488–493, 1977

Gutman FA, Zegarra H: The natural course of temporal retinal branch vein occlusion. Trans Am Acad Ophthalmol Otolaryngol *78*:178–192, 1974

Gutman FA, Zegarra H, Raver A, et al: Photocoagulation in retinal branch vein occlusion. Ann Ophthalmol *13*:1359–1363, 1981

Michels RG, Gass JDM: The natural course of retinal branch vein obstruction. Trans Am Acad Ophthalmol Otolaryngol *78*:166–177, 1974

Orth DH, Patz A: Retinal branch vein occlusion. Surv Ophthalmol *22*:357–376, 1978

Wetzig PC: The treatment of acute branch vein occlusion by photocoagulation. Am J Ophthalmol *87*:65–73, 1979

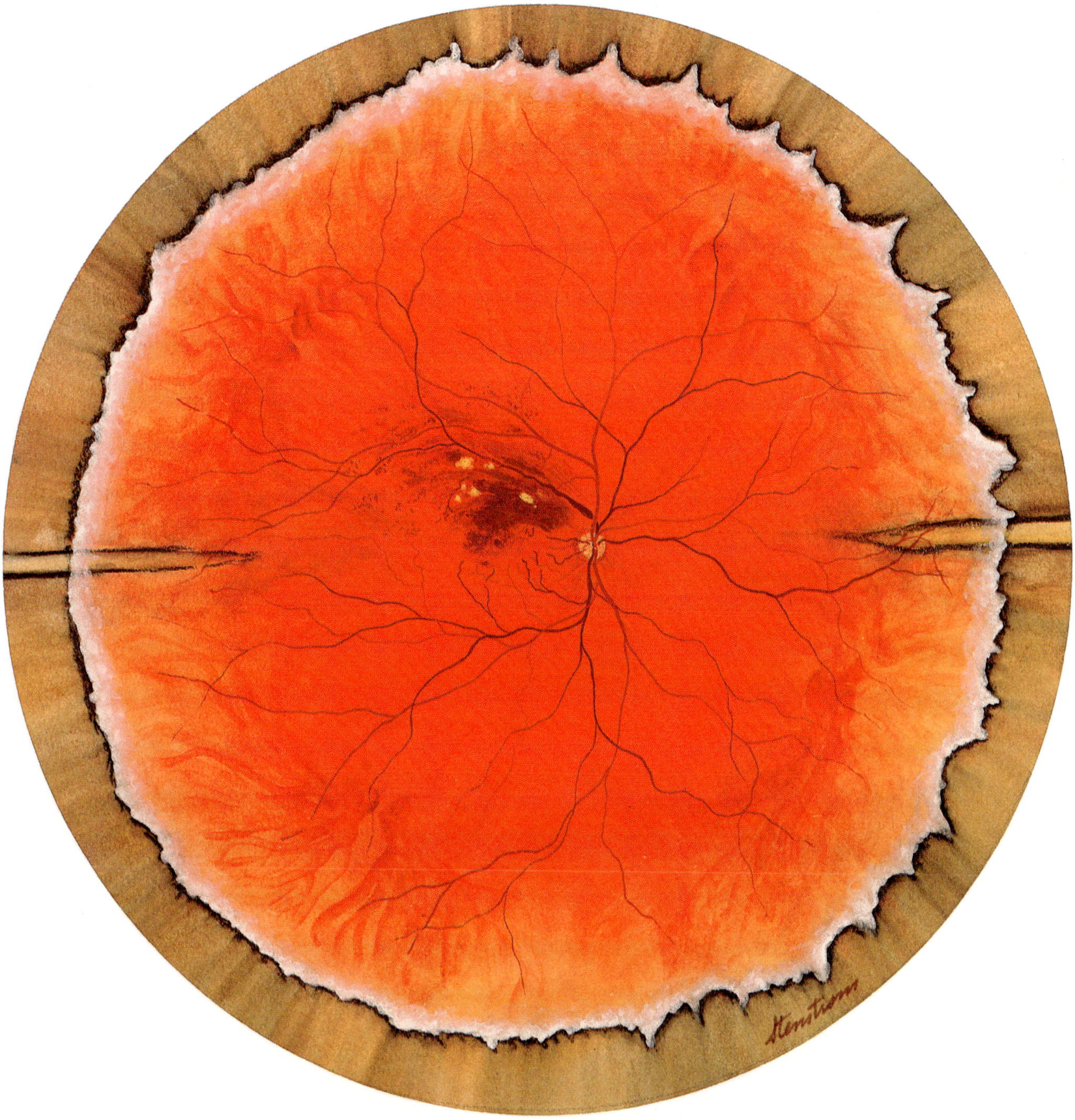

PLATE 66

CENTRAL RETINAL VEIN OCCLUSION

Central retinal vein occlusion produces the remarkable appearance of extensive retinal hemorrhages over the entire retina, described as the "blood and thunder" appearance. These hemorrhages are more dense surrounding the optic nerve, and are predominantly located in the nerve fiber layer, showing flame-shaped margins. Punctate hemorrhages are located deeper in the retina, and hemorrhage may break through the internal limiting membrane to become preretinal and extend into the vitreous. The nerve fiber layer frequently is markedly edematous, and yellow soft exudates (cotton wool spots) typically cluster around the disc. Microaneurysms may be present also, particularly in the macular area.

The optic disc is usually edematous, with blurred elevated margins, as in papilledema. Prominent capillaries are visible on the disc surface, along with small hemorrhages. In long-standing central retinal vein occlusions, enlarged vascular loops on the disc indicate venous shunting to the choroidal circulation.

The retinal veins are engorged and tortuous, and are a dusky, darker than normal color. With time, the veins become sheathed, with a white margin. The retinal arteries may be normal or may show generalized constriction.

The degree of macular edema determines the degree of visual decrease. With time, cystoid macular edema, lamellar macular hole, and preretinal membrane formation may occur.

Dreaded late complications include neovascular proliferation from the disc and rubeosis of the iris, which leads to hemorrhagic glaucoma.

Chester EM: Central retinal vein occlusion. *In* The Ocular Fundus In Systemic Disease. Chicago, Year Book Medical Publishers, 1973, pp 116–119

Hayreh SS: Occlusion of the central retinal vessels. Br J Ophthalmol 49:626–645, 1965

Jaeger EA: Venous obstructive disease of the retina. *In* Duane TD: Clinical Ophthalmology. Hagerstown, Maryland, Harper & Row, 1978, Vol 3, pp. 1–13

Wise GN, Dollery CT, Henkind P: Central vein occlusion. *In* The Retinal Circulation. New York, Harper & Row, 1971, pp 358–364

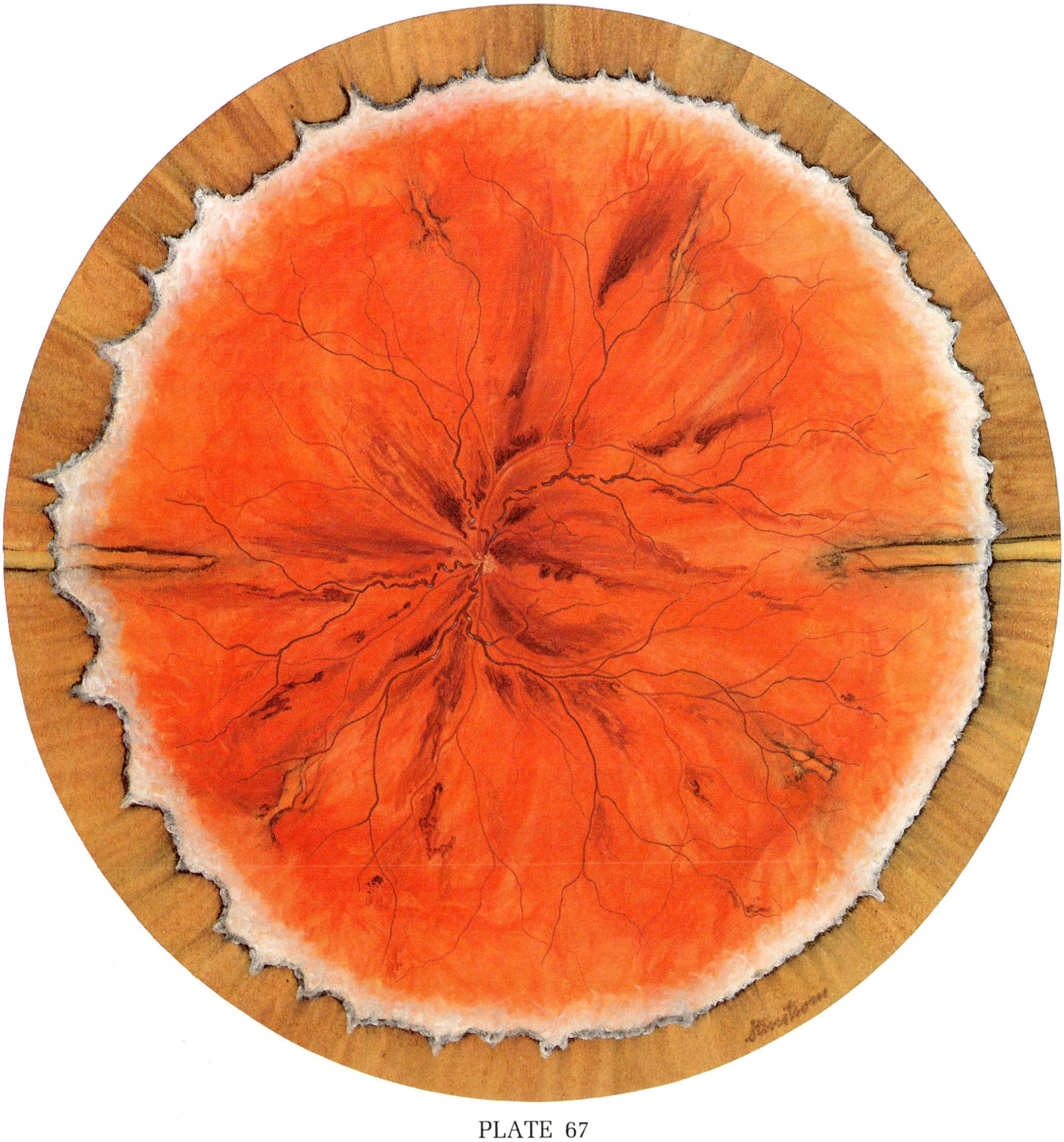

PLATE 67

CHOLESTEROL EMBOLI
(Hollenhorst Plaques)

Hollenhorst plaques are cholesterol emboli visible in retinal arteries. The source of these emboli is the heart or great vessels, most commonly the carotid arteries. Usually, emboli occur unilaterally in an elderly individual with advanced atherosclerosis. Typically, symptoms are fleeting alterations of vision (amaurosis fugax), but sometimes there are no symptoms at all.

Cholesterol emboli appear as highly refractile, glistening, white crystals that frequently lodge at arterial bifurcations. Sometimes they appear larger than the containing vessel because of their visibility. The entire column of blood is not usually occluded, and the cholesterol embolus frequently breaks up and travels further down the arterial tree, sometimes to disappear completely.

When complete occlusion of a retinal artery does occur, an ischemic infarct of the inner retinal layers is produced. Clinically, the affected retina appears milky white and thickened. Microscopically, there is ischemic edema of the inner retinal layers. With time, atrophy of the inner retinal layers develops and the retinal appearance returns to nearly normal. There is a permanent field defect in the involved area, even though the artery may recanalize.

Cholesterol emboli seen in the retina suggest that emboli may be traveling to the brain as well; therefore, a medical evaluation may be indicated. Studies show a decreased survival for individuals with cholesterol embolization to the retina.

Ball CJ: Atheromatous embolism to the brain, retina and choroid. Arch Ophthalmol *76*:690–695, 1966

David NJ, Klintworth GK, Friedberg SJ, et al: Fatal atheromatous cerebral embolism associated with bright plaques in the retinal arterioles. Neurology *13*:708–713, 1963

Hollenhorst RW: Significance of bright plaques in the retinal arterioles. JAMA *178*:23–29, 1961

Pfaffenbach DD, Hollenhorst RW: Morbidity and survivorship of patients with embolic cholesterol crystalization in the ocular fundus. Am J Ophthalmol *75*:66–72, 1973

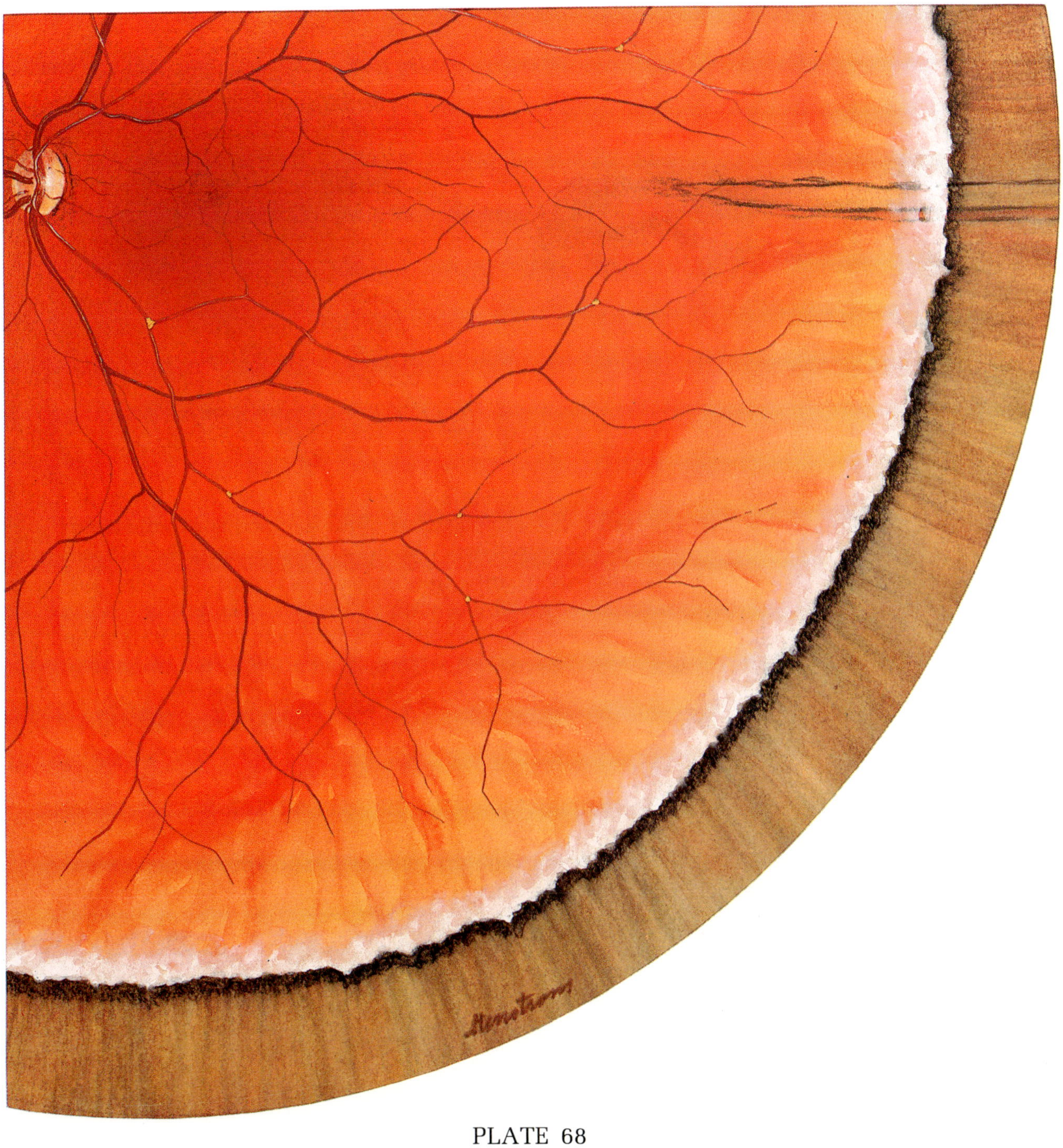

PLATE 68

FAT EMBOLI

Fat emboli appear in the fundus, usually as a result of crush injuries of the chest or long bones. The bone marrow contains fat, which is expressed into the blood stream and travels to the eye as microemboli. The visible lesion in the retina is the cotton wool spot. It is an ischemic infarct of the nerve fiber layer, the cause of which is obstruction of the small retinal arterioles by fat microemboli. The symptoms produced are entirely dependent on the pattern and degree of embolic occlusion. The patient frequently has many serious injuries which direct medical attention away from ocular findings. With the passage of time, the cotton wool spots disappear and the retina may become almost normal in appearance. The visual defects are usually permanent.

FIBRIN AND PLATELET EMBOLI

Fibrin and platelet emboli may occur together. They are usually the result of accumulations of these blood components on the surface of atherosclerotic plaques in the aorta or carotid arteries. Usually, there are symptoms of recurrent transient episodes of monocular blindness with recovery of vision (amaurosis fugax). Ophthalmoscopic examination frequently reveals that an arterial branch is plugged with a long length of dull white embolic material. If the amount of embolus is not too large, the embolus may break up and pass downstream to ultimately disappear. Blood flow in occluded vessels shows segmentation and marked slowing of flow, but usually obstruction is not complete. An ischemic infarct of the area supplied by the partially obstructed vessel appears white and thickened in the acute stages, but as time passes, the retinal transparency returns. Despite the normal retinal appearance, the visual loss is permanent and its degree depends upon the pattern and area of retina affected.

Cogan DG, Kuwabara T, Moser H: Fat emboli in the retina following angiography. Arch Ophthalmol 71:308–313, 1964

De Voe AG: Ocular fat embolism. Arch Ophthalmol 43:857–863, 1950

Henkind P, Dollery CT: Pathophysiology of the retinal vascular bed following acute embolization. Invest Ophthalmol 5:204–207, 1966

Kearns TP: Fat embolization of the retina. Am J Ophthalmol 41:1–2, 1956

Patterson JW, Dollery CT, Ramalho PS, et al: The effects of platelet aggregates on the retinal microcirculation. Bibl Anat 9:85–91, 1967

Wise GN, Dollery CT, Henkind P: The Retinal Circulation. New York, Harper & Row, 1971

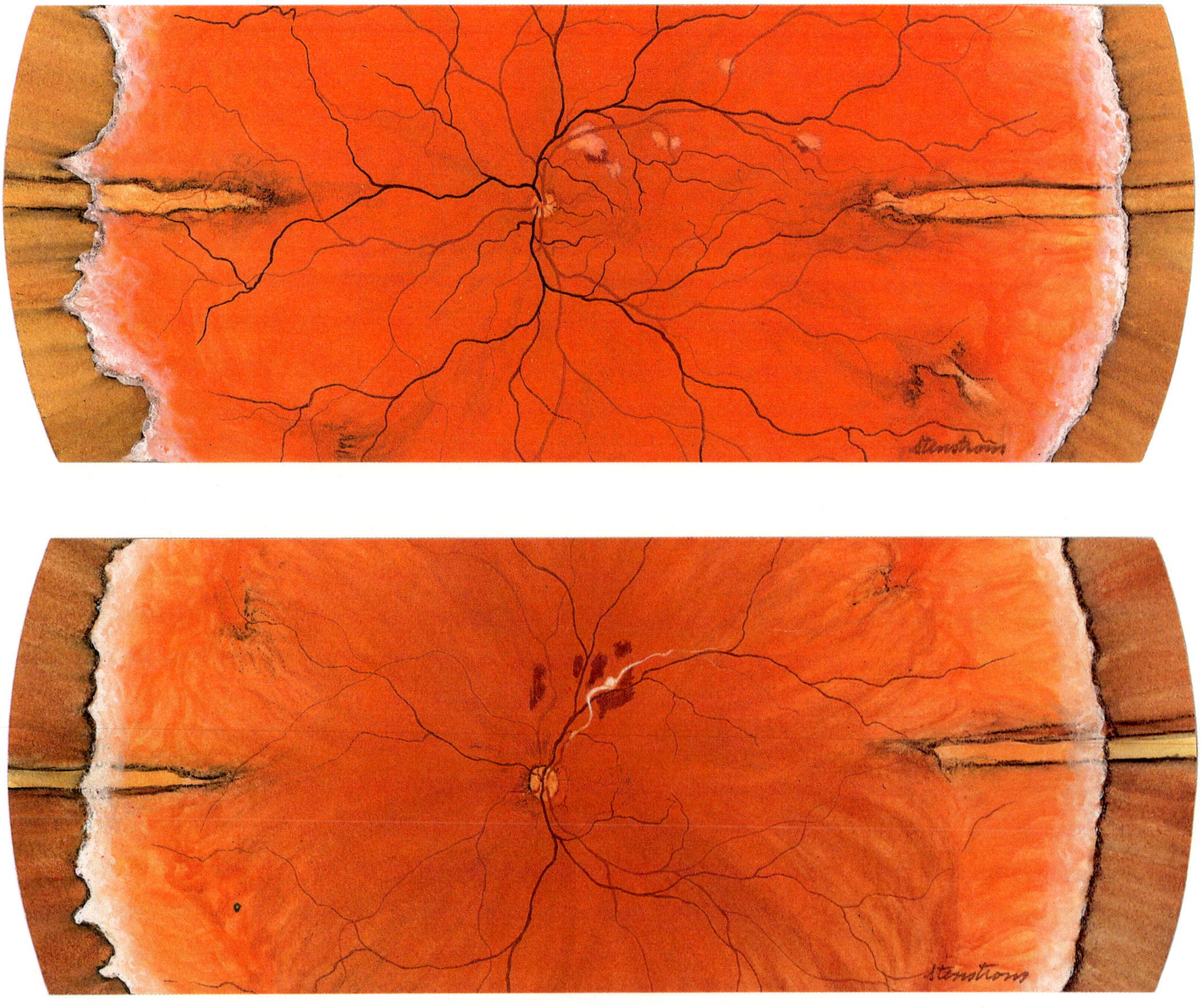

PLATE 69

COATS' DISEASE

Coats' disease is a disease of the retinal vasculature characterized by telangiectasis, large microaneurysms, and bizarre configurations of bulbous vascular dilatations. There are juvenile and adult forms of Coats' disease, which vary slightly in their clinical picture. In the juvenile form, shown in *A*, the irregular, dilated capillaries and convoluted, sausage-like vascular dilatations produce extensive vascular leakage and hemorrhage. The hemorrhage may be into the retina or vitreous, or typically beneath the retina, where old blood may give the fundus a peculiar green tint. Also characteristic of the juvenile form of Coats' disease is extensive subretinal, white to yellow exudate surrounding the vascular abnormalities. A circinate pattern may be present in the fovea, far removed from the vascular abnormalities in the retinal periphery. The vascular abnormalities, hemorrhage and exudate, may be much more extensive than shown here. In advanced cases there will be sheets of subretinal exudate, with embedded cholesterol crystals, and total serous detachment of the retina. The juvenile form of Coats' disease usually occurs in the first decade of life in a male patient, and is most commonly unilateral.

The adult form of Coats' disease, shown in *B*, typically has the vascular changes without extensive exudates or hemorrhage. Irregular dilatations and unusual vascular patterns of the retinal vessels are typical. There also may be marked sheathing and occlusion of the affected retinal vessels. The adult form usually presents in the second or third decade, and has a somewhat better prognosis than the juvenile form. The etiology of Coats' disease is entirely unknown.

Eger ERI, Tasman W, Tomer TL: Coats' disease. Arch Ophthalmol *92*:109–112, 1974

Fox KR: Coats' disease. Metab Pediat Ophthalmol 4:121–124, 1980

Harris GS: Coats' disease—diagnosis and treatment. Can J Ophthalmol 5:311–320, 1970

Tasman W: Coats' disease. *In* Tasman W (ed): Retinal Disease in Children. New York, Harper & Row, 1971, pp 59–69

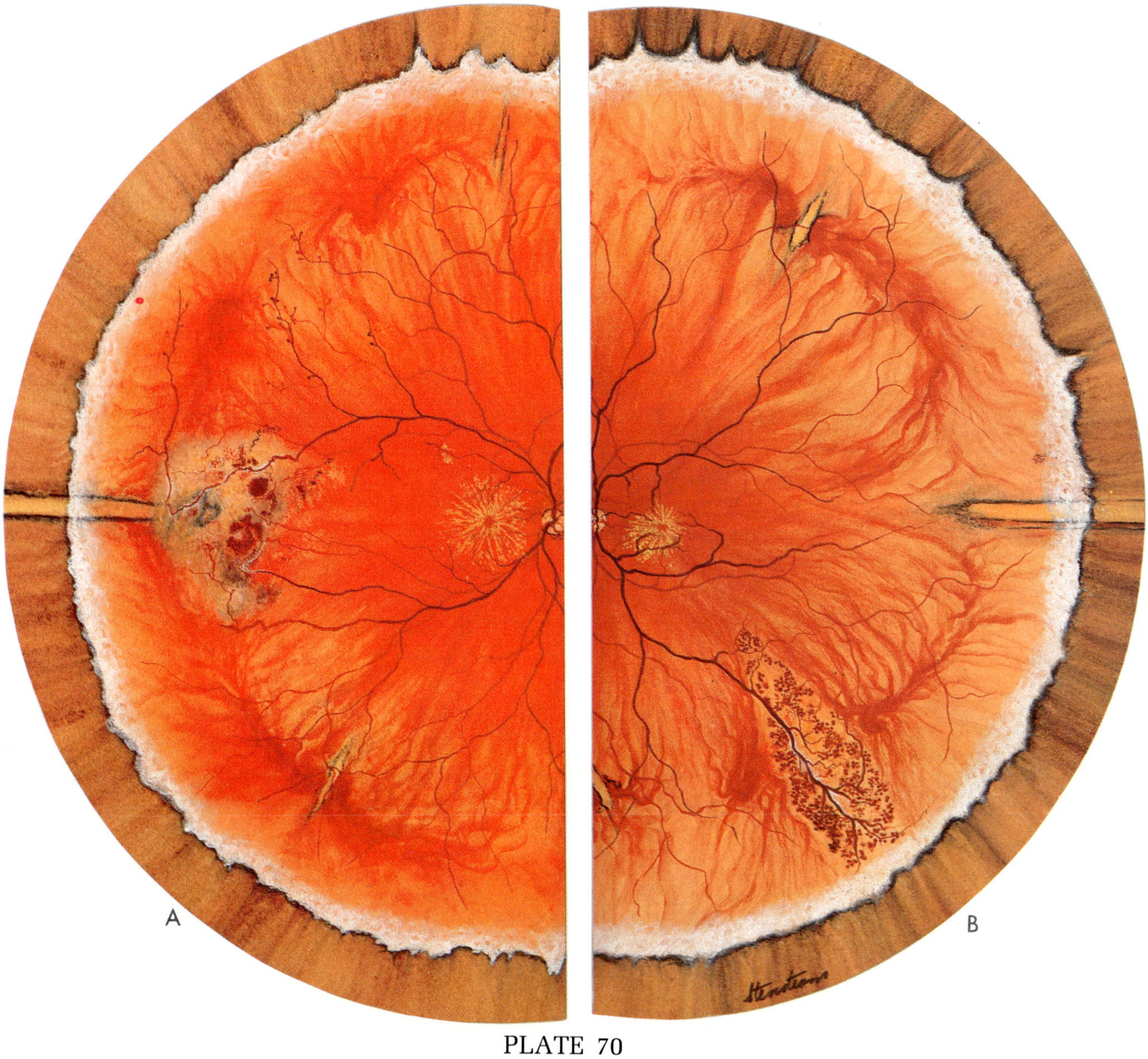

PLATE 70

RETROLENTAL FIBROPLASIA

Retrolental fibroplasia occurs most commonly in premature infants treated with supplemental oxygen for respiratory distress syndrome. It is known that retrolental fibroplasia may very rarely develop in full term infants who have had no exposure to oxygen.

In the premature infant, the peripheral retina is incompletely developed. The temporal retinal periphery appears gray and opaque, and lacks vascularization. It is thought that a high level of oxygen is toxic to the growing capillary endothelial cells. If oxygen toxicity obliterates the developing capillary bed, neovascular proliferative tissue develops leading to acute proliferative retrolental fibroplasia. In severe cases, there may be a massive overgrowth of vasoproliferative tissue into the vitreous, over the retinal surface, and onto the ciliary body and posterior lens surface. Fortunately, most cases are not so severe, and there is a high incidence of spontaneous regression of proliferative changes.

During the regression process, there is a contraction of the tissues, which may produce dragging of the retina, retinal folds, and traction retinal detachment. A typical appearance of cicatricial retrolental fibroplasia in a young adult is shown here many years after the acute proliferative stage. A retinal fold extends inferotemporally, obliterating macular architecture. In less severe cases, the macula may be dragged toward the temporal periphery. Perpheral retinal pigmentation is common, and lattice degeneration occurs more commonly than in the normal population. Retinal breaks may occur in this lattice, which may lead to rhegmatogenous retinal detachment. Vitreous traction on the peripheral retinal vessels may produce an exudative retinal detachment as well. A high degree of myopia is characteristic of eyes with retrolental fibroplasia, and associated findings of amblyopia, strabismus, and nystagmus also occur frequently.

Ashton N, Ward B, Serpell G: Effect of oxygen on developing retinal vessels with particular reference to the problem of retrolental fibroplasia. Br J Ophthalmol *38*:397–432, 1954

Faris BM, Brockhurst RJ: Retrolental fibroplasia in the cicatricial stage. Arch Ophthalmol *82*:60–65, 1969

Kingham JD: Acute retrolental fibroplasia. Arch Ophthalmol *95*:39–47, 1977

Patz A: Retrolental fibroplasia. Surv Ophthalmol *14*:1–29, 1969

Tasman W: Late complications of retrolental fibroplasia. Ophthalmology *86*:1724–1740, 1979

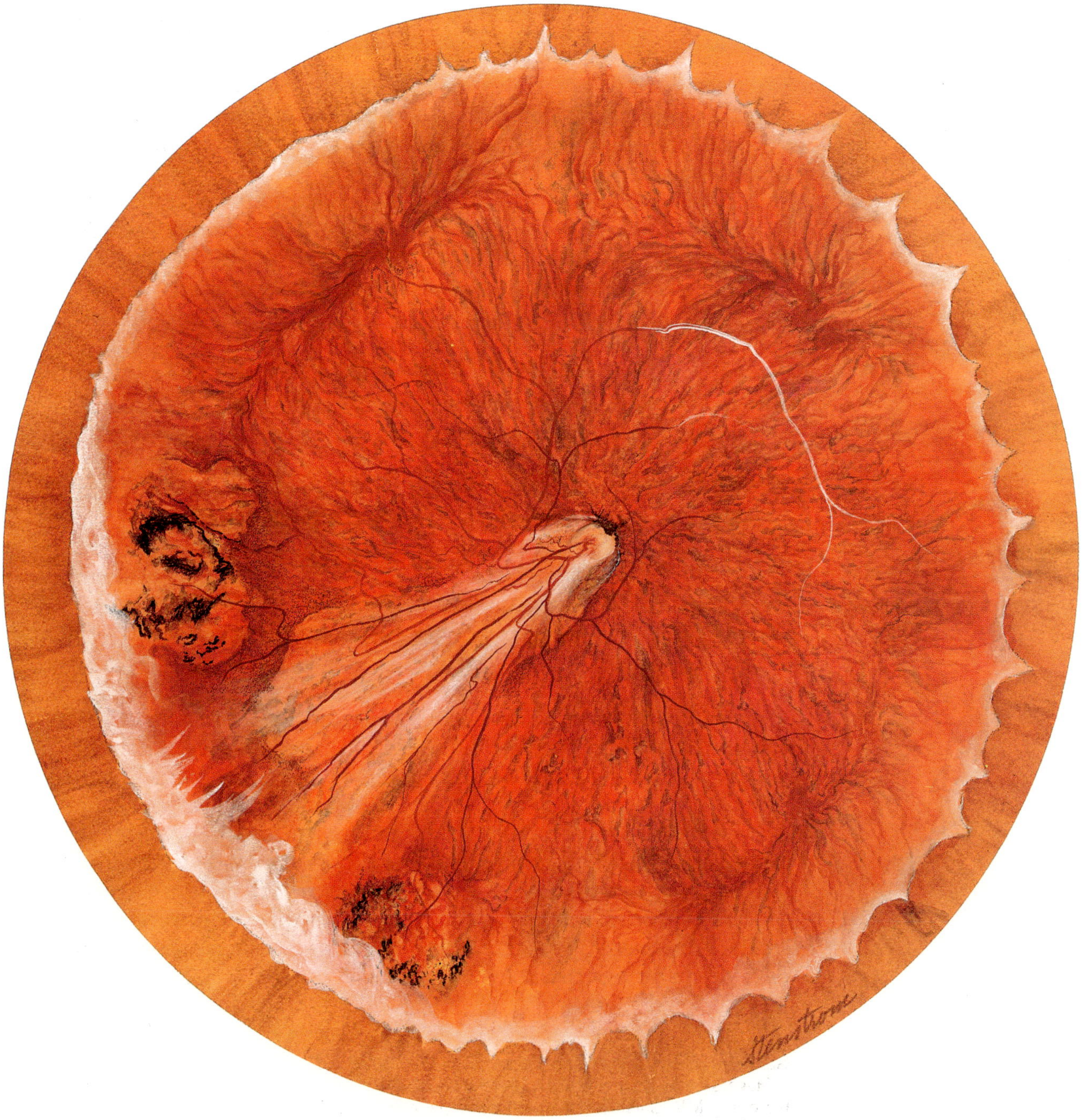

PLATE 71

SICKLE CELL RETINOPATHY

Sickle cell disease is caused by the inheritance of abnormal hemoglobin in the red blood cells. The abnormal hemoglobin produces vascular occlusions in the retinal blood vessels, leading to progressive fundus changes. Goldberg has carefully catalogued the ocular findings in the various combinations, hemoglobin S, C, D, and thalassemia.

Sickle cell retinopathy may be either nonproliferative or proliferative. Nonproliferative retinopathy appearances include venous tortuosity, in which the veins are engorged. Black sunburst spots typically occur in the temporal periphery as sharply demarcated round to ovoid lesions from one half disc diameter to two disc diameters in size. The pigment accumulates in a spicule pattern and may be present with refractile yellow granules. Intraretinal or preretinal hemorrhage, referred to as a salmon patch hemorrhage, occurs also in the midperiphery. Rarely, central retinal artery or vein occlusions, or branch vascular occlusions may occur. Occlusions of the choroidal vasculature and angioid streaks are described in sickle cell retinopathy.

Proliferative sickle cell retinopathy has been classified by Goldberg into five stages. In stage I, there are vascular occlusions, particularly in the temporal periphery. Fluorescein angiography shows a sharp demarcation between the avascular peripheral fundus and the normally vascularized posterior fundus. At this junction, arteriolar-venular connections arise, producing stage II. In stage III, neovascular capillary buds proliferate in a fan-shaped configuration, called "sea fans" because they resemble a marine organism with a similar radiating pattern. The sea fans are true neovascularization and leak fluorescein profusely. Sea fans may grow into huge neovascular proliferations that appear white, as there is a large fibrous component as well as new vessel formation. These lesions may undergo spontaneous involution or, more likely, produce vitreous hemorrhage, which is stage IV of proliferative sickle retinopathy. Progression of the vitreous hemorrhage and developing fibrous tissue leads to stage V, retinal detachment.

Goldberg MF: Sickle cell retinopathy. *In* Duane TD (ed.): Clinical Ophthalmology. Hagerstown, Harper & Row, 1976, Vol 3, pp 1–45

Goldberg MF: Classification and pathogenesis of proliferative sickle retinopathy. Ophthalmology 71:649–665, 1971

Goldberg MF: Natural history of untreated proliferative sickle retinopathy. Arch Ophthalmol 85:428–437, 1971

Goldberg MF: Treatment of proliferative sickle retinopathy. Trans Am Acad Ophthalmol Otolaryngol 75:532–556, 1971

Welch RB, Goldberg MF: Sickle cell hemoglobin and its relation to fundus abnormality. Arch Opthalmol 75:353–362, 1966

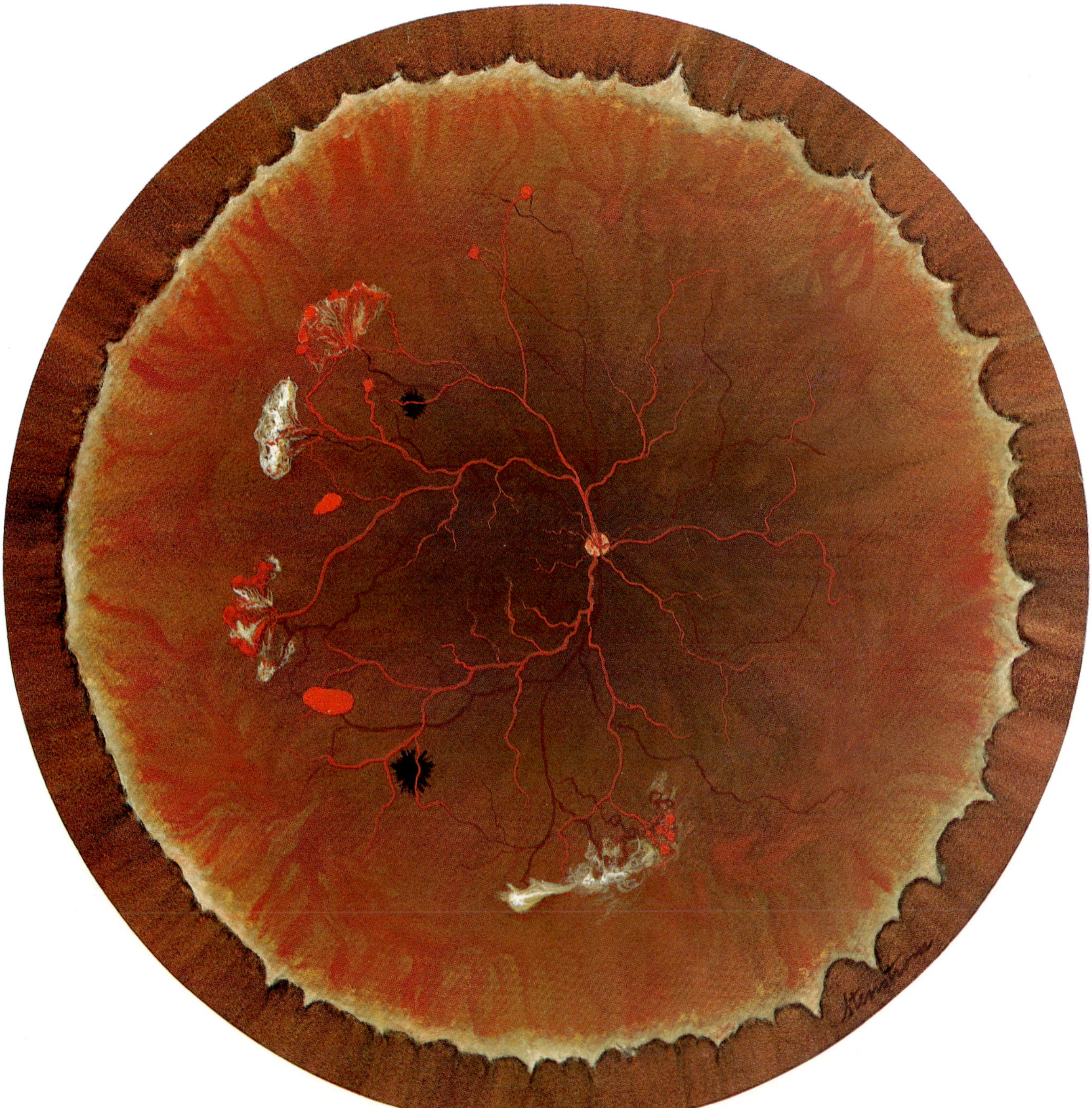

PLATE 72

Chapter Seven

DIABETIC RETINOPATHY

BACKGROUND DIABETIC RETINOPATHY

Background diabetic retinopathy is the first visible manifestation of diabetes in the eye. The initial onset of background diabetic retinopathy is related to the length of time that diabetes has been present. In juvenile diabetics, in whom the onset of diabetes is generally acute, almost three fourths of patients will show evidence of background diabetic retinopathy after 10 years of known disease. There may be few or no symptoms in the early stages.

Background diabetic changes develop first in the posterior pole of the eye, particularly the macula. Characteristic findings are punctate dot hemorrhages, which occur in the middle retinal layers, and microaneurysms, which also appear as red dots. It is frequently difficult to distinguish clinically between dot hemorrhages and microaneurysms. Superficial small hemorrhages in the nerve fiber layer are called blot hemorrhages because they have feathered edges, as observed with the direct ophthalmoscope. Exudates are also typical and initially appear as punctate yellow dots or blotches. Those exudates, which have diffuse margins, are called soft exudates and are thought to represent small ischemic infarcts in the nerve fiber layer. The retinal veins usually appear dark red and may be slightly engorged and tortuous in appearance. In advanced stages, the veins show irregular dilatations or beading. By definition, background diabetic retinopathy contains no new vessel growth or proliferative changes.

Blankenship GW, Skyler JS: Diabetic retinopathy: A general survey. Diabetes Care *I*:127–131, 1978

Burditt AF, Caird FI, Draper GJ: The natural history of diabetic retinopathy. Q J Med *37*:303–317, 1968

Kahn HA, Bradely RF: Prevalence of diabetic retinopathy. Br J Ophthalmol *59*:345–349, 1979

Keen H: The prevalence of blindness in diabetes. J R Coll Phys *7*:53–61, 1972

Kohner EM: The evolution and natural history of diabetic retinopathy. Int Ophthalmol Clin *18*:1–16, 1978

Knowler WC, Bennett PH, Ballintine EJ: Increased incidence of retinopathy in diabetics with elevated blood pressure. N Engl J Med *302*:645–650, 1980

White P: Childhood diabetes. Its course, and influence on the second and third generations. Diabetes 9:345–355, 1960

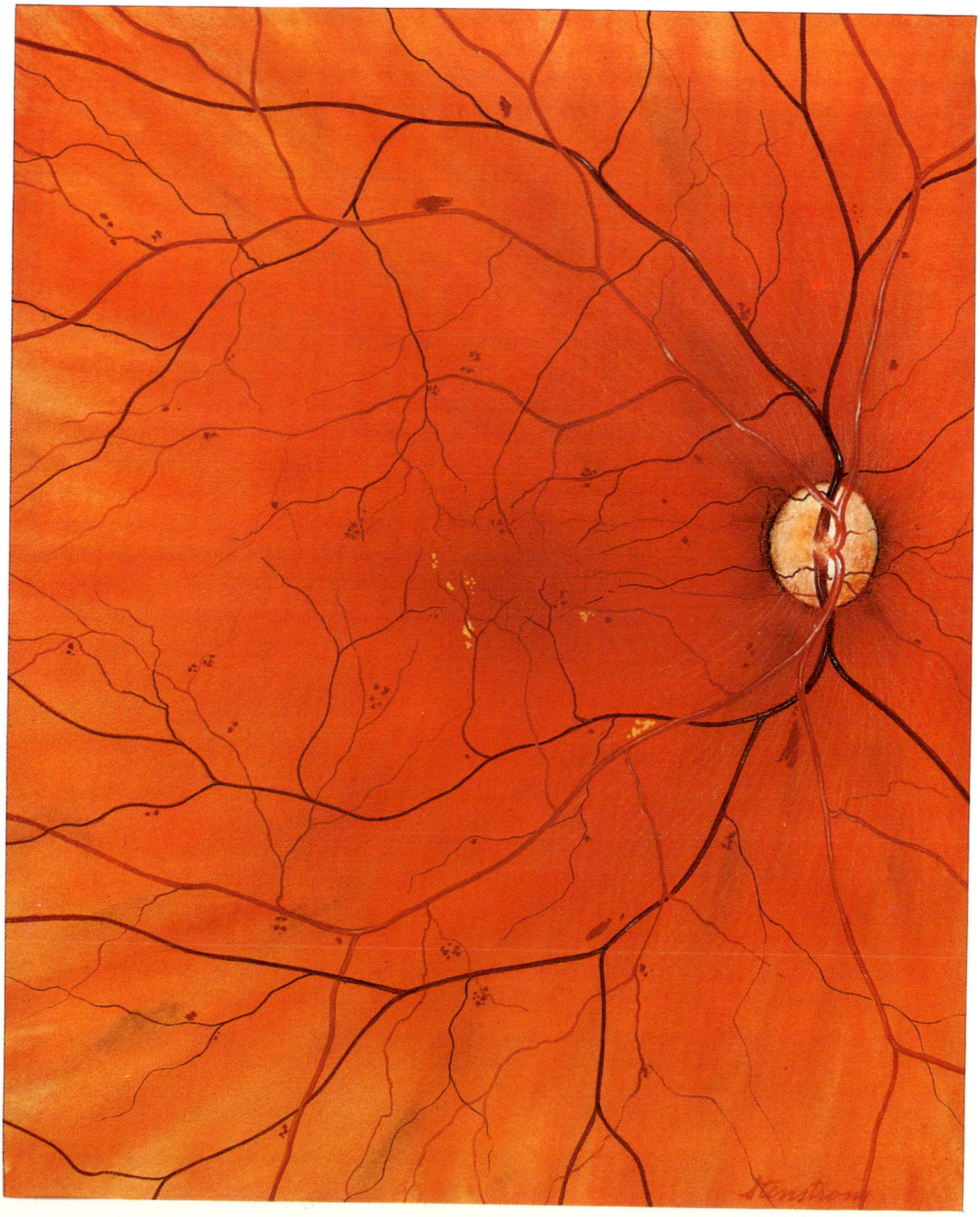

PLATE 73

STAGES OF DIABETIC RETINOPATHY

When background diabetic retinopathy progresses to the stage of severity as shown in *A*, vision generally is significantly decreased, and there is also decreased color discrimination. The dot and blot hemorrhages are more numerous and there is also generalized macular edema. No well defined foveal reflex is present as the macula is thickened by leakage of fluid into the retinal tissue, particularly the outer plexiform layer. When viewed with the higher magnification of the direct ophthalmoscope or fundus contact lens, discrete bubbles may be seen in the retina, producing the appearance called cystoid edema.

In *B*, a yellow ring of lipid exudate, called a circinate pattern, is shown. This is an example of a hard exudate, appearing as a well defined white or yellow accumulation of lipid in the outer plexiform layer of the retina. The circinate exudate is produced by leakage from microaneurysms in the center of the ring. When the fovea is touched by this ring, vision is significantly decreased. If photocoagulation treatment is given to the leaking microaneurysms, there may be resolution of the circinate pattern and improvement of vision, provided the process is not chronic.

Abnormal new blood vessels called neovascularization are produced as a later effect of diabetes on the retina. Commonly, neovascularization occurs along the vessels above and below the macula. In *C*, note the new vessels also have a white fibrous component and are elevated off the surface of the retina as a result of their attachment to the retracted vitreous. These new vessels will leak fluorescein profusely and are quite capable of producing a vitreous hemorrhage. In *D*, new vessels are seen as tortuous channels on the surface of the retina.

Bresnick GH, Davis MD, Myers FL, et al: Clinical pathologic correlations in diabetic retinopathy II. Clinical and histologic appearances of retinal capillary microaneurysms. Arch Ophthalmol 95:1215–1220, 1977

Dobree JH: Proliferative diabetic retinopathy. Evolution of the retinal lesions. Br J Ophthalmol 48:637–649, 1964

Patz A, Schatz H, Berkow JW, et al: Macular edema—an overlooked complication of diabetic retinopathy. Trans Am Acad Ophthalmol Otolaryngol 77:34–42, 1973

Schatz H, Patz A: Cystoid maculopathy in diabetics. Arch Ophthalmol 94:761–768, 1976

Ticho U, Patz A: The role of capillary perfusion in the management of diabetic macular edema. Am J Ophthalmol 76:880–886, 1973

Wiznia RA: Photocoagulation of nonproliferative exudative diabetic retinopathy. Am J Ophthalmol 88:22–27, 1979

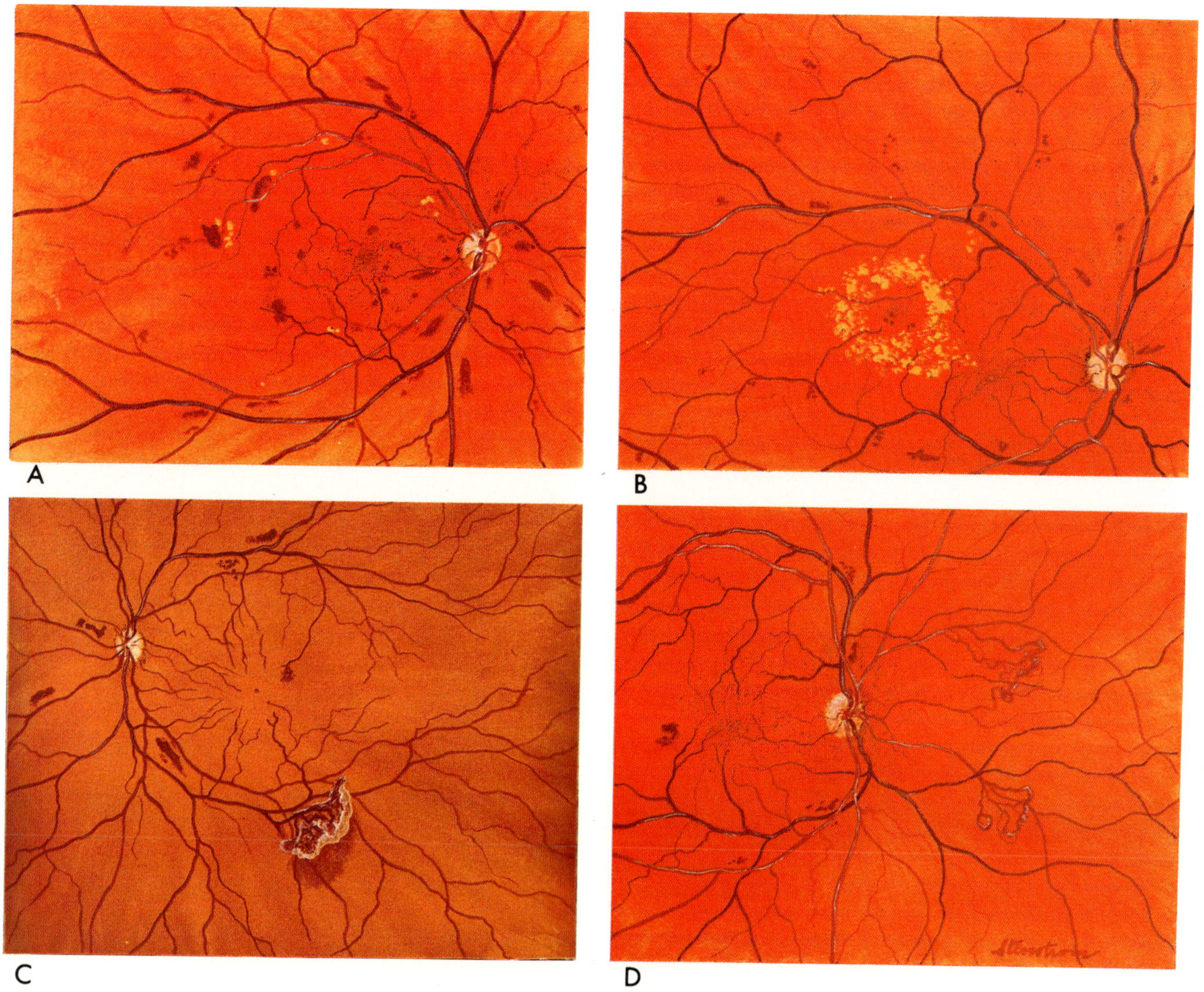

PLATE 74

DIABETIC RETINOPATHY WITH DISC NEOVASCULARIZATION

The optic nerve is a frequent site of new vessel formation, or neovascularization, in advanced diabetic retinopathy. In addition to the background diabetic retinopathy changes of dot and blot hemorrhages, exudates, including a circinate exudate, this eye contains florid neovascularization of the optic nerve. It is believed that retinal hypoxia is a precursor to the development of neovascularization. Important signs of hypoxia are cotton wool spots or soft exudates, irregular dilatations of the retinal veins, and small, dilated, intraretinal, anomalous vessels.

In reality, the neovascularization does not grow into the vitreous but, rather, is pulled forward by its attachment to the posterior surface of the slowly retracting vitreous. A neovascular frond growing from the disc contains not only fine blood vessels but also a fibrous component giving the frond a white appearance. The significance of these neovascular fronds growing from the optic nerve is that they have frequently been found to cause vitreous hemorrhage that may be extensive and cause a temporary or permanent loss of vision. Studies have shown the efficacy of photocoagulation treatment in reducing the incidence of blindness due to neovascular fronds on the disc. The neovascular frond is not treated directly; rather, the retina is treated with peripheral ablation photocoagulation treatments.

Davis MD; Vitreous contraction in proliferative diabetic retinopathy. Arch Ophthalmol *74*:741–751, 1965.

The Diabetic Retinopathy Study Group: Preliminary report on effects of photocoagulation therapy. Am J Ophthalmol *81*:383–386, 1976

The Diabetic Retinopathy Study Group: Photocoagulation treatment of proliferative diabetic retinopathy: The second report of diabetic retinopathy study findings. Ophthalmology *85*:82–105, 1978

Hercules BL, Gayed II, Lucas SB, et al: Peripheral retinal ablation in the treatment of proliferative diabetic retinopathy: A three-year interim report of a randomized, controlled study using the Argon laser. Br J Ophthalmol *61*:555–563, 1977

Tolentino FI, Lee PF, Schepens CL; Biomicroscopic study of vitreous cavity in diabetic retinopathy. Arch Ophthalmol *75*:238–246, 1966

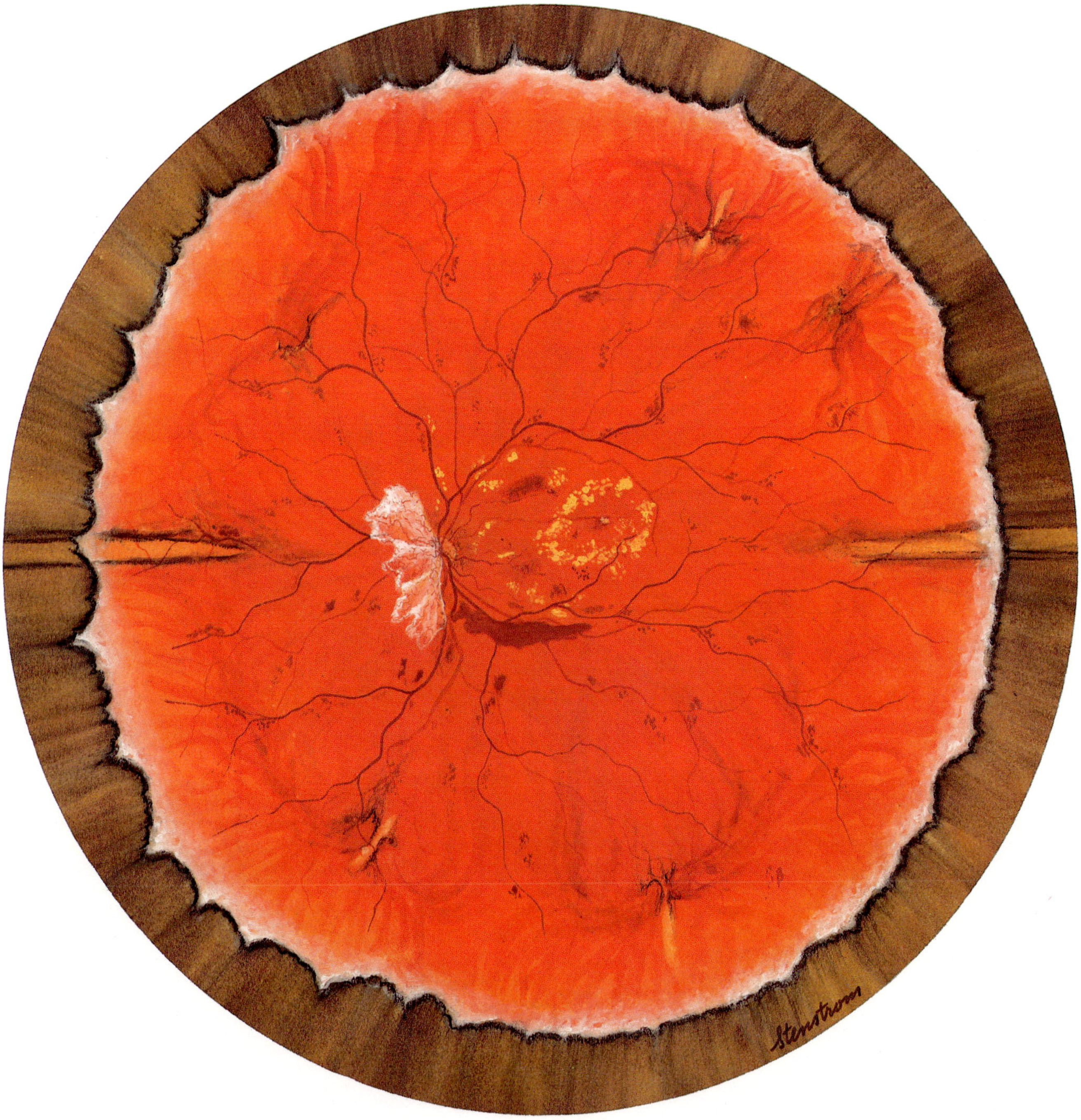

PLATE 75

DIABETIC RETINOPATHY WITH ACUTE VITREOUS HEMORRHAGE

An acute vitreous hemorrhage not uncommonly precipitates the initial eye care of a patient with known diabetes. The symptoms of dark floaters, a red haze, and profound loss of vision cause acute concern to the patient. This recent vitreous hemorrhage still has relatively well defined margins. As time passes, the vitreous hemorrhage will diffuse more completely throughout the eye and will obscure the entire retina. With further passage of time, the hemorrhage will eventually settle inferiorly and turn white in color.

No neovascularization is observed in this eye as a source of the vitreous hemorrhage. Only background diabetic retinopathy changes consisting of dot retinal hemorrhages and exudates can be directly visualized. It is quite likely, however, that neovascularization is present on or around the disc and is the cause of the vitreous hemorrhage. As the hemorrhage settles, the neovascularization may or may not become visible. If neovascularization is visible through a clear vitreous, photocoagulation may be performed, but if not, surgical removal of the vitreous hemorrhage with a vitrectomy may be indicated.

Benson WE, Spalter HF: Vitreous hemorrhage. A review of experimental and clinical investigations. Surv Ophthalmol *15*:297–311, 1971

Blankenship G: Pars plana vitrectomy for diabetic retinopathy. A report of eight years' experience. Mod Probl Ophthalmol *20*:376–386, 1979

Kupfer C: The diabetic retinopathy vitrectomy study. Am J Ophthalmol *81*:687–690, 1976

Mandelcorn MS, Blankenship G, Machemer R: Pars plana vitrectomy for the management of severe diabetic retinopathy. Am J Ophthalmol *81*:561–570, 1976

Michels RG: Vitrectomy for complications of diabetic retinopathy. Arch Ophthalmol *96*:237–246, 1978

Peyman GA, Raichand M, Huamonte FU, et al: Vitrectomy in 125 eyes with diabetic vitreous hemorrhage. Br J Ophthalmol *60*:752–755, 1976

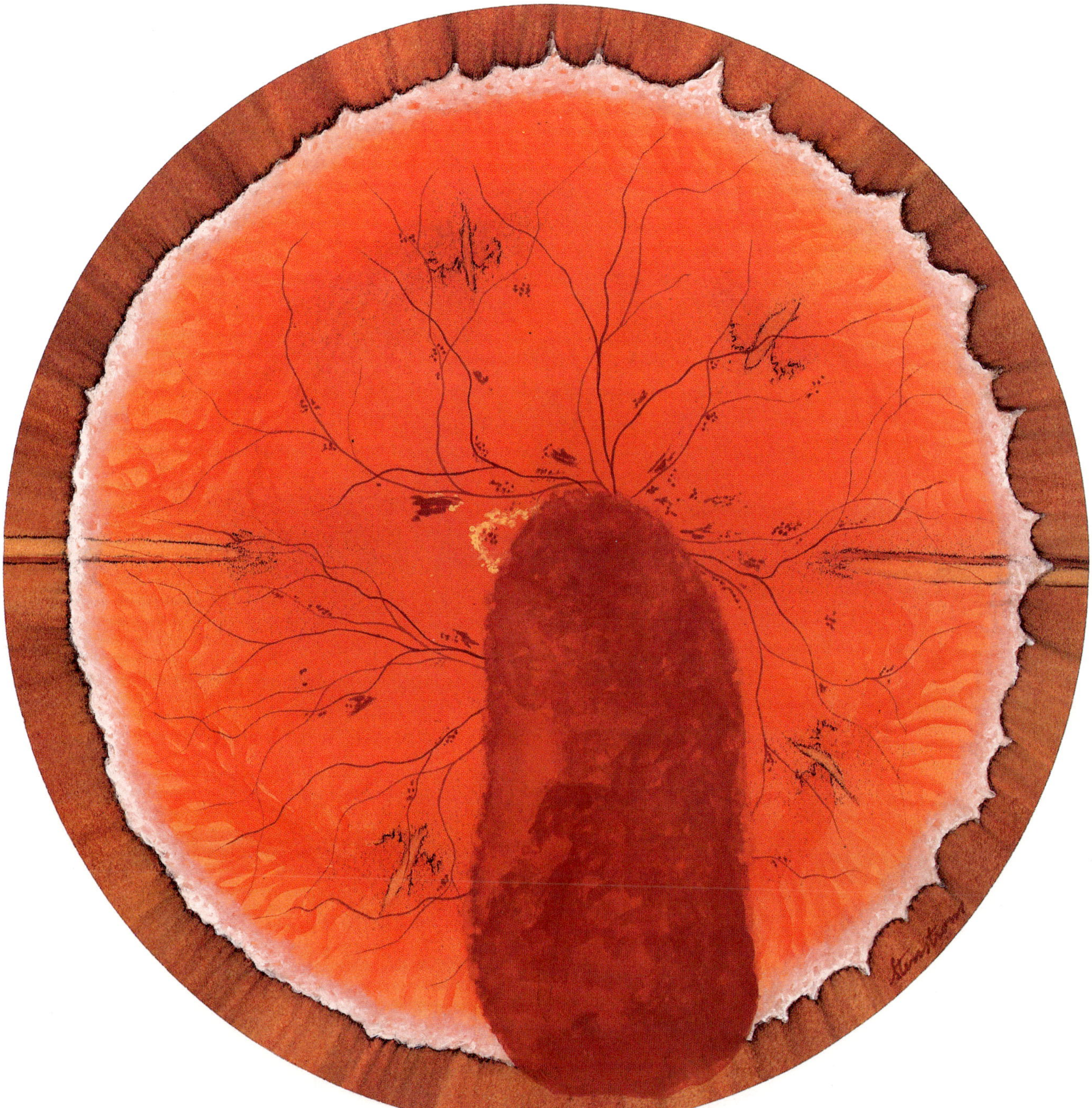

PLATE 76

DIABETIC RETINOPATHY WITH TRACTION RETINAL DETACHMENT

Traction retinal detachment is a complication of advanced proliferative diabetic retinopathy. Neovascularization initially develops on the surface of the retina, forming a strong adhesion between the retina and vitreous. The vitreous in advanced proliferative retinopathy contracts slowly, producing a pulling, or vitreous traction, on the retina. This vitreous traction pulls the retina into a tentlike, elevated, traction retinal detachment. These traction detachments typically occur along the temporal vascular arcades in the posterior pole and frequently involve the macula. The retina appears taut and shiny, and its surface is usually concave. Traction retinal detachments may enlarge leaving demarcation lines at the site of previous extension. In contrast to rhegmatogenous detachments, there is very little mobility of the retinal surface and no shifting fluid. Traction retinal detachments sometimes convert into rhegmatogenous detachments with the development of a full thickness retinal hole. These retinal holes usually occur near the posterior pole and may be quite difficult to visualize. When this occurs, the elevated retina changes in appearance from concave to bullous convex, and the inwardly scalloped edges at the margin of the detachment become bowed outward.

The inset shows a traction retinal detachment produced by a contracted vitreous and firm attachments between the vitreous and retina. Typically, these adhesions occur in a partial circle surrounding the optic nerve and macula in the posterior pole.

Aaberg TM: Clinical results in vitrectomy for diabetic traction retinal detachment. Am J Ophthalmol *88*:246–253, 1979

Blankenship G: Pars plana vitrectomy for diabetic retinopathy. A report of eight years' experience. Mod Probl Ophthalmol *20*:376–386, 1979

Mandelcorn MS, Blankenship G, Machemer R: Pars plana vitrectomy for the management of severe diabetic retinopathy. Am J Ophthalmol *81*:561–570, 1976

Michels RG: Vitrectomy for complications of diabetic retinopathy. Arch Ophthalmol *96*:237–246, 1978

Miller SA, Shafrin F, Bresnick GH, et al: Scleral buckling procedure for retinal detachments secondary to proliferative diabetic retinopathy. Am J Ophthalmol *89*:103–112, 1980

Tasman W: Retinal detachment secondary to proliferative diabetic retinopathy. Arch Ophthalmol *87*:286–289, 1972

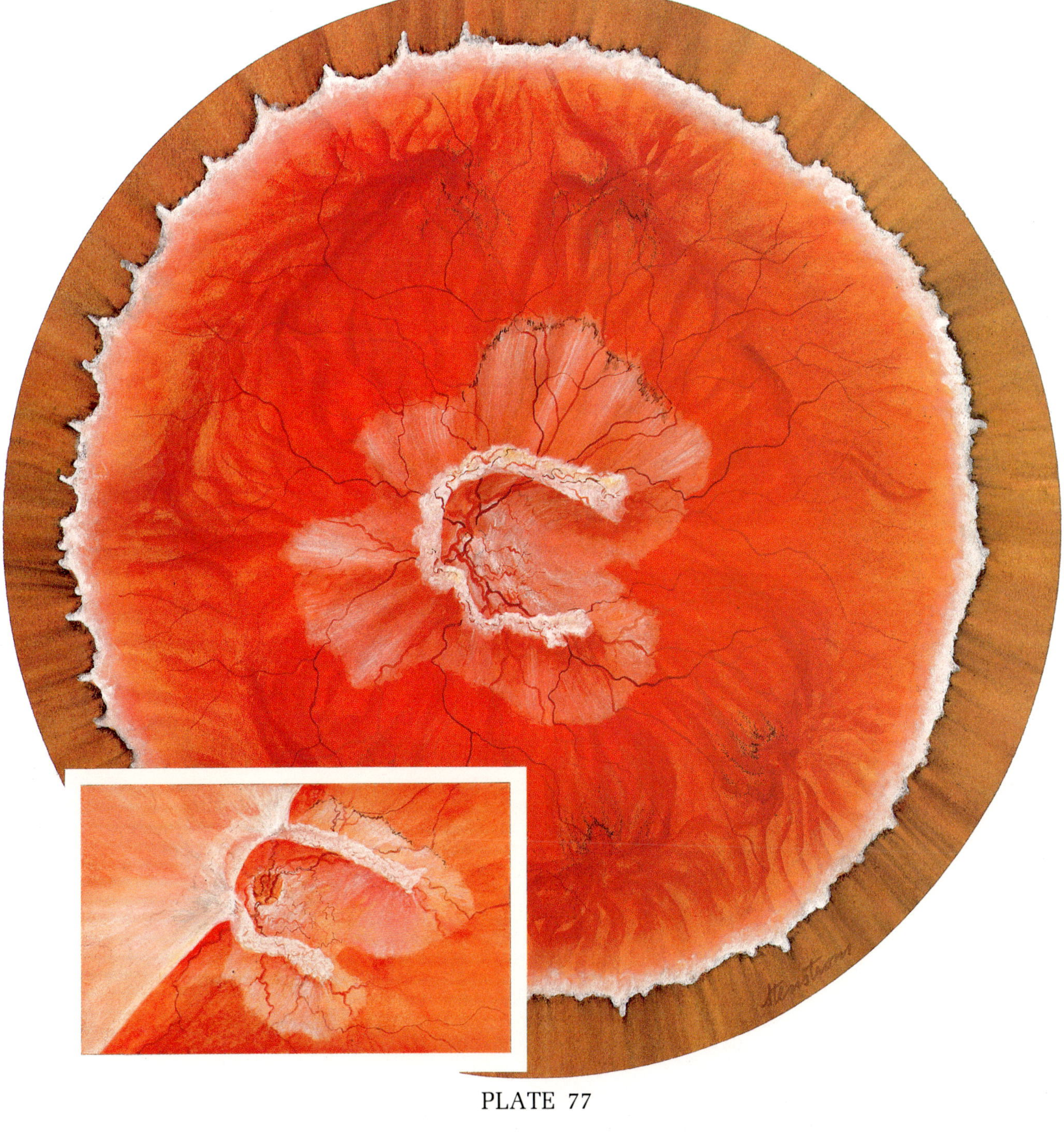

PLATE 77

LASER TREATMENT FOR PROLIFERATIVE DIABETIC RETINOPATHY

Proliferative diabetic retinopathy with neovascularization on the disc or elsewhere in the fundus is frequently treated with laser. The treated areas, multiple round discrete spots with pigmentation in the center or at the margins, should not be confused with an old chorioretinitis or other disease process. The areas treated with laser appear yellow to white immediately after treatment, but within several weeks pigmentation occurs, producing the fundus picture as shown. Note also that the neovascularization on the optic nerve has shown regression with an increase in fibrous tissue and a decrease in active vessels. There is no vitreous hemorrhage present, so this would be considered a successful treatment.

The pattern of treatment shown here is called a peripheral ablation. The neovascularization on the optic nerve is not treated directly; rather, extensive laser treatment is given throughout the periphery. It has been empirically determined that after such peripheral treatment, the disc neovascularization regresses, with a statistically proven decreased incidence of vitreous hemorrhage and blindness.

Apple DJ, Goldberg MF, Wyhinny G: Histopathology and ultrastructure of the argon laser lesion in human retinal and choroidal vasculatures. Am J Ophthalmol *75*:595–609, 1973

The Diabetic Retinopathy Study Research Group: Preliminary report on effects of photocoagulation therapy. Am J Ophthalmol *81*:383–386, 1976

The Diabetic Retinopathy Study Research Group: Photocoagulation treatment of diabetic retinopathy: The second report of diabetic retinopathy study findings. Ophalomology *85*:82–105, 1978

The Diabetic Retinopathy Study Research Group: Four risk factors for severe visual loss in diabetic retinopathy: The third report from the diabetic retinopathy study. Arch Ophthalmol *97*:654–655, 1979

The Diabetic Retinopathy Study Research Group: Protocoagulation of proliferative diabetic retinopathy: Clinical application of diabetic retinopathy study (DRS) findings. Ophalmology *88*:583–600, 1981

Little HL: Complications of Argon laser retinal photocoagulation. A five-year study. Int Ophthalmol *16*:145–159, 1976

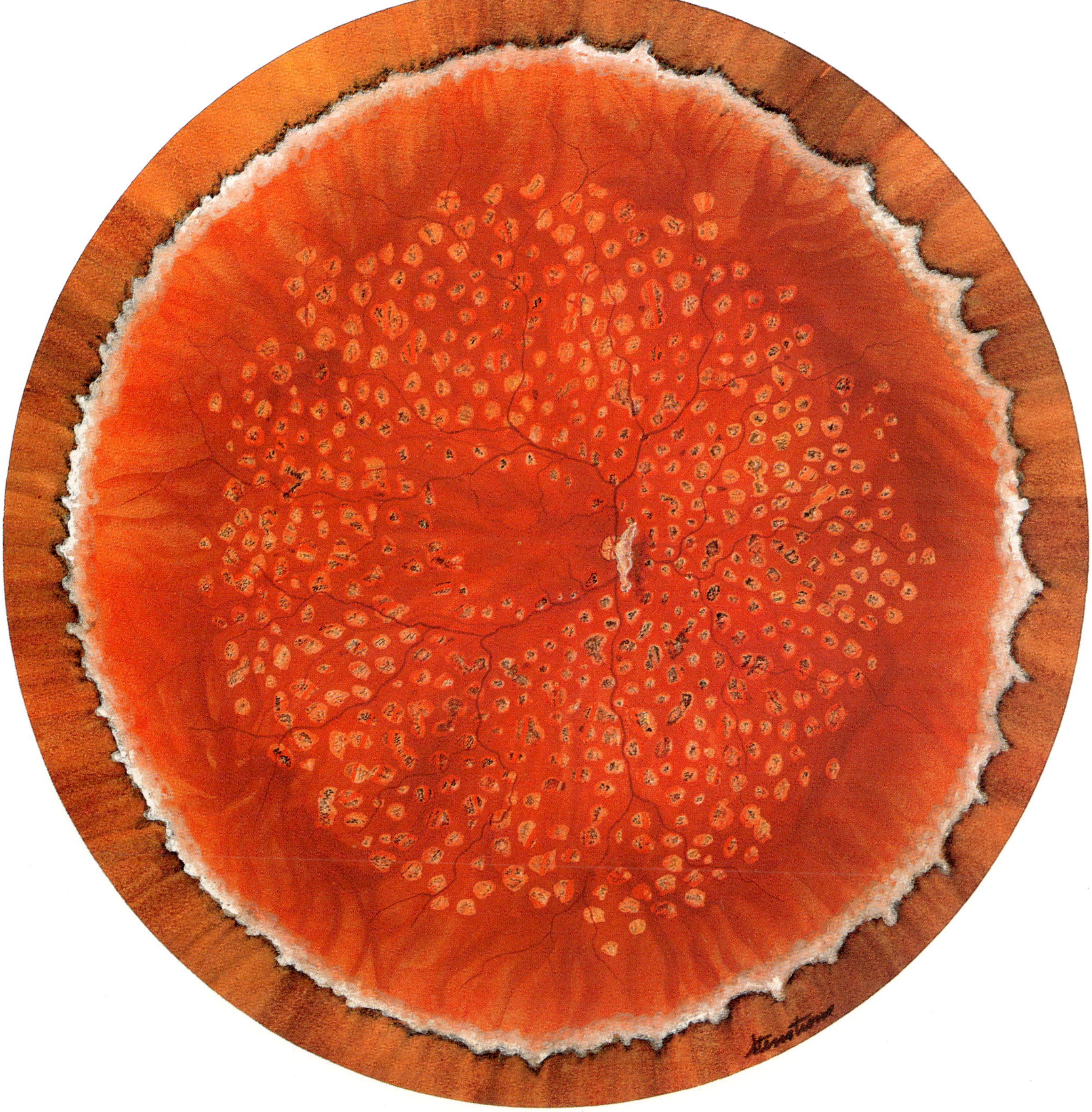

PLATE 78

Chapter Eight

THE PHAKOMATOSES

NEUROFIBROMATOSIS

Neurofibromatosis, or von Recklinghausen's disease, is a genetically inherited disease transmitted as an autosomal dominant with variable penetrance. Neurofibromatosis has many systemic manifestations, the most prominent of which are brown pigmented spots of the skin, called café-au-lait spots. Virtually every tissue of the eye, adnexa, and orbit may be involved, but fundus findings are relatively uncommon.

With the indirect ophthalmoscope, retinal, choroidal, and optic nerve changes have been described. The most common finding is a choroidal neurofibroma. Many times, these are not clinically visible and represent only a histological thickening of the choroid. Large choroidal nevi, as shown here, also occur in eyes of patients with neurofibromatosis. There is also a higher incidence of malignant melanomas in affected patients. Very rarely, small white retinal lesions have been noted that represent astrocytic hamartomas very much like those of tuberous sclerosis. Also, myelinated nerve fibers are commonly found in eyes affected with neurofibromatosis. Gliomas of the optic nerve present as an elevated white projection of the optic nerve into the vitreous cavity. The surface of this mass may be smooth or striated, and hemorrhage may occur on the surface of the lesion.

None of the fundus lesions that may occur in neurofibromatosis are pathognomonic, and specific diagnosis depends on finding characteristic lesions elsewhere in the orbit, or systemically.

Block FJ: Retinal tumor associated with neurofibromatosis (von Recklinghausen's disease). Report of a case. Arch Ophthalmol *40*:433–437, 1948

Cotlier E: Café-au-lait spots of the fundus in neurofibromatosis. Arch Ophthalmol *95*:1990–1992, 1977

Hales RH: Glioma of the optic disc. Arch Ophthalmol *70*:648–650, 1963

Hoyt WF, Baghdassarian SA: Optic glioma of childhood. Brit J Ophthalmol *53*:793–798, 1969

Van der Hoeve J: The Doyne memorial lecture: Eye symptoms in the phacomatoses. Trans Ophthalmol Soc UK *52*:380–401, 1932

Wolter JR, Gonzeles-Sirit R, Mankin WJ: Neurofibromatosis of the choroid. Amer J Ophthalmol *54*:217–225, 1962

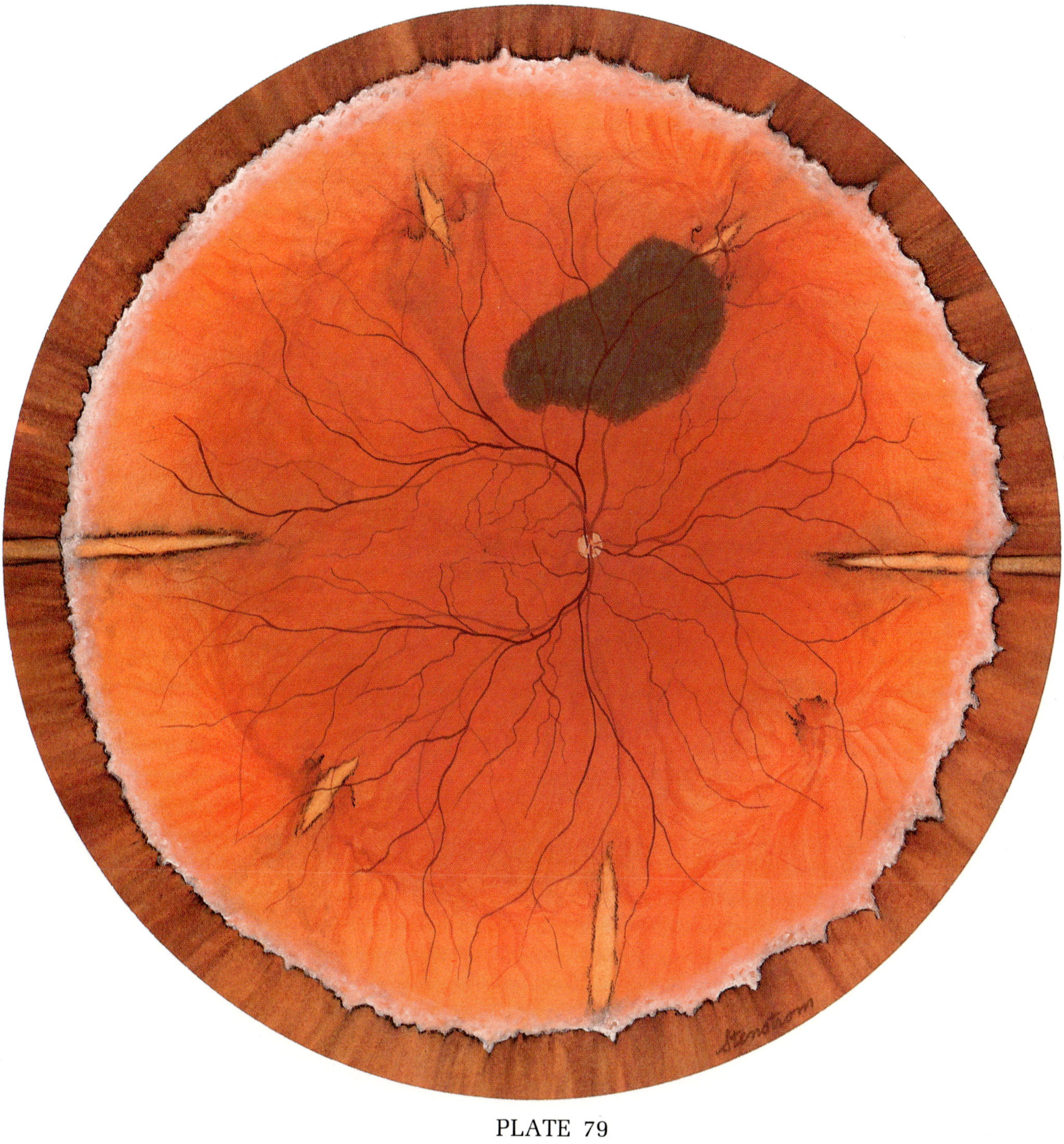

PLATE 79

STURGE-WEBER SYNDROME

Sturge-Weber syndrome is a congenital angiomatosis with skin, cerebral, and ocular manifestations. The typical skin involvement is a port wine hemangioma of the face that is usually unilateral. Similar vascular abnormalties occur in the central nervous system, with symptoms of epilepsy and x-ray findings of calcification occurring commonly. Ocular findings include buphthalmos, an enlargement of the globe due to congenital glaucoma as a result of choroidal hemangioma. Sturge-Weber syndrome is usually of sporadic occurrence, and no definite mode of genetic transmission is known.

The most typical fundus finding is hemangioma of the choroid. These may be small, diffuse, and flat, so that they are clinically inapparent, but more typically they are large and bright red in appearance, producing the typical "tomato-catsup" fundus. The deep red color of the choroidal markings is best appreciated after comparison with the fundus of the opposite eye, which is usually normal. The uniform, bright red fundus appearance obscures the underlying choroidal markings. The retina itself is generally normal, except that there may be some tortuosity of the retinal veins. Serous retinal detachment is known to occur rarely. Retinal pigment epithelial atrophy, drusen, and foci of calcification are rarely observed. The optic nerve is normal, unless buphthalmos produces glaucomatous cupping.

Alexander GL, Norman RM: The Sturge-Weber syndrome. Bristol, England, John Wright and Sons, Stonebridge Press, 1960

Jones IS, Cleasby GW: Hemangioma of the choroid: A clinicopathologic analysis. Am J Ophthalmol *48*:612–628, 1959

Stevenson RF, Morin JD: Ocular findings in nevus flammeus. Can J Ophthalmol *10*:136–139, 1975

Susac JO, Smith JL, Scelfo RJ: The "tomato-catsup" fundus in Sturge-Weber syndrome. Arch Ophthalmol *92*:69–70, 1974

Witschel H, Font R: Hemangioma of the choroid. A clinicopathologic study of 71 cases and review of the literature. Surv Ophthalmol *20*:415–431, 1976

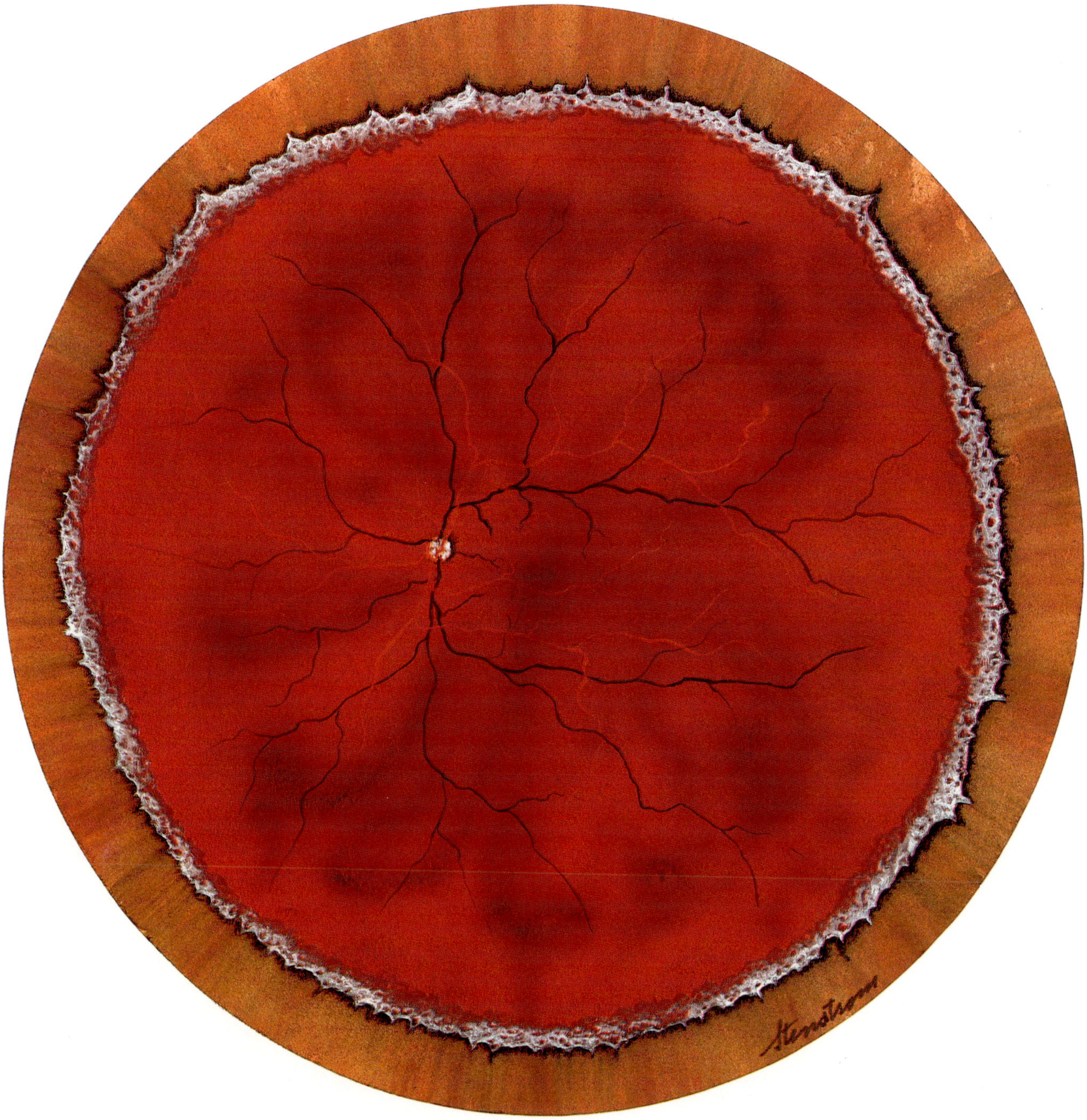

PLATE 80

TUBEROUS SCLEROSIS

Tuberous sclerosis is a hereditary disorder affecting the skin, brain, and eye. Skin manifestations include adenoma sebaceum, a brown nodular or papular rash over the face, and depigmented lesions on the extremities. Central nervous system glial proliferations occur, producing mental retardation and epilepsy in childhood. Fundus lesions may include giant drusen, which arise in superficial tissue of the optic nerve and which rarely interfere with optic nerve function. The most characteristic fundus finding is a small white lesion on the retinal surface that is slightly elevated and has poorly defined margins. *(A)* In very young children, these lesions may be confused with retinoblastoma. In young adults, these white lesions may become cystic, and on rare occasions the cyst may rupture, releasing granular material into the vitreous cavity. The classic mulberry phakoma has a multiple nodular collection of highly refractile drusenoid bodies, which gives the appearance of a berry. *(B)* Sometimes, very fine vascularization is present in these lesions and may rarely cause hemorrhages and exudates. Fluorescein angiography reveals that these vessels leak in the late stages and stain intensely. The retinal vessels are usually normal, and retinal function is undisturbed.

Tuberous sclerosis is inherited as an autosomal dominant with low penetrance, and many cases appear to be sporadic. All ethnic groups are affected, and there is an equal sex incidence.

Harley RD, Grover WD: Tuberous sclerosis—description and report of 12 cases. Ann Ophthalmol 1:477–481, 1970

Kinder RSL: The ocular pathology of tuberous sclerosis. J Pediat Ophthalmol 9:106–107, 1972

Loewenstein A, Steel J: Retinal tuberous sclerosis (Bourneville's disease). Am J Ophthalmol *24*:731–741, 1941

Pagenstecher WJ: Tuberous sclerosis. Historical review and report of two cases. Am J Ophthalmol *39*:663–676, 1955

Schwab F: Die Augenhintergrundveränderungen bei tuberöser Hirnsklerose. Klin Mbl Augenheilkd *128*:257–297, 1956

Van der Hoeve J: Eye symptoms in tuberous sclerosis of the brain. Trans Ophthalmol Soc UK *40*:329–334, 1920

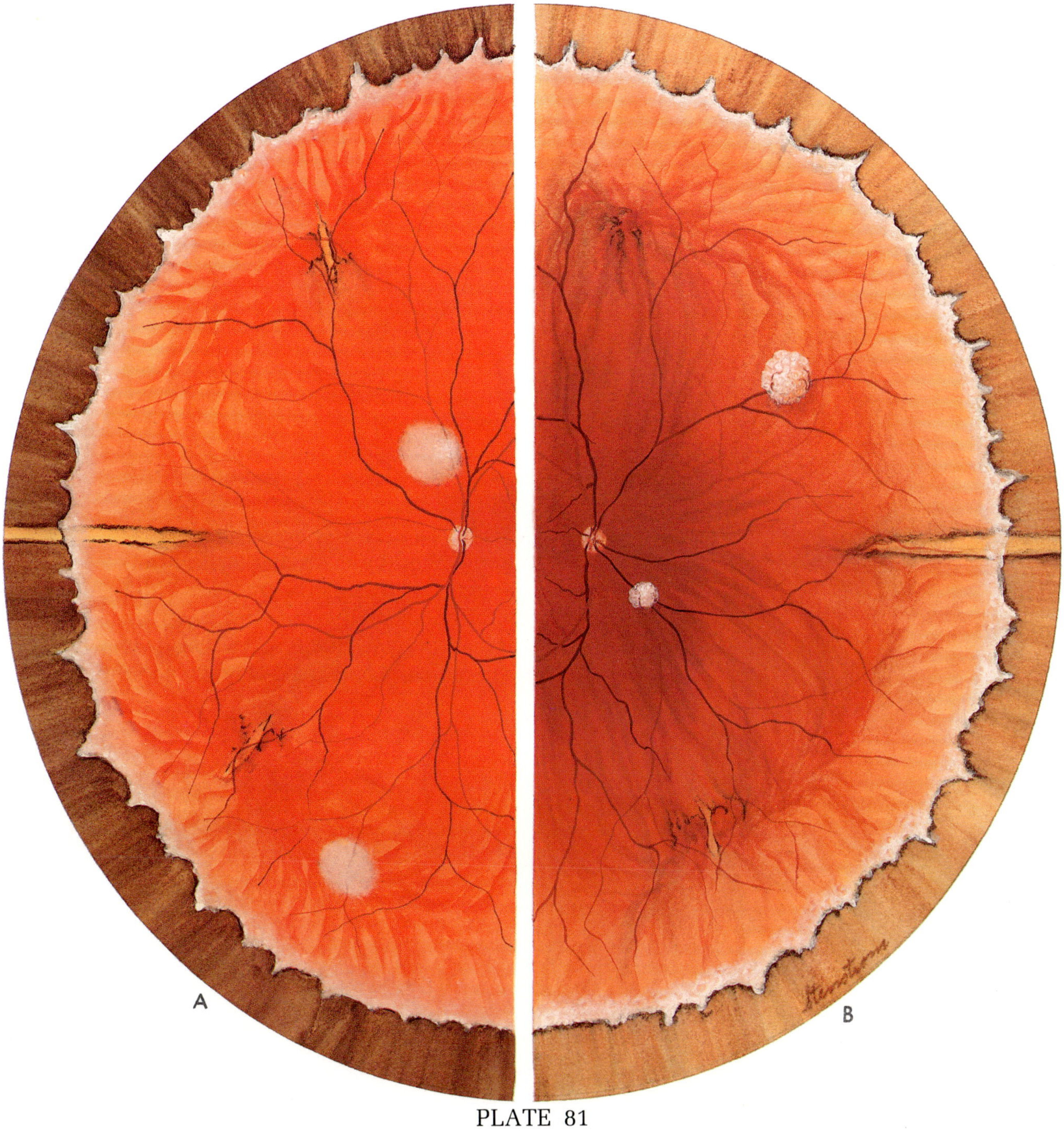

PLATE 81

WYBURN-MASON SYNDROME

Wyburn-Mason syndrome is characterized by arteriovenous malformations in the brain and dramatic retinal vessel changes. Markedly engorged and tortuous retinal blood vessels emanate from the optic nerve and may project forward from the surface of the retina. The vessels are so numerous and convoluted that it is difficult to distinguish retinal arteries from retinal veins.

The Wyburn-Mason syndrome is a congenital malformation of blood vessels, and is considered by many authorities not to be a true phakomatosis, although it is frequently grouped with them. The condition is congenital and usually does not progress. The vision is not affected unless the macula is involved. Wyburn-Mason syndrome occurs sporadically and has no known hereditary tendency.

Bech K, Jensen OA: On the frequency of coexisting racemose haemangiomata of the retina and brain. Acta Psychiatr Scand *36*:47–56, 1961

Wyburn-Mason R: Arteriovenous aneurysm of mid-brain and retina, facial naevi and mental changes. Brain *66*:163–203, 1943

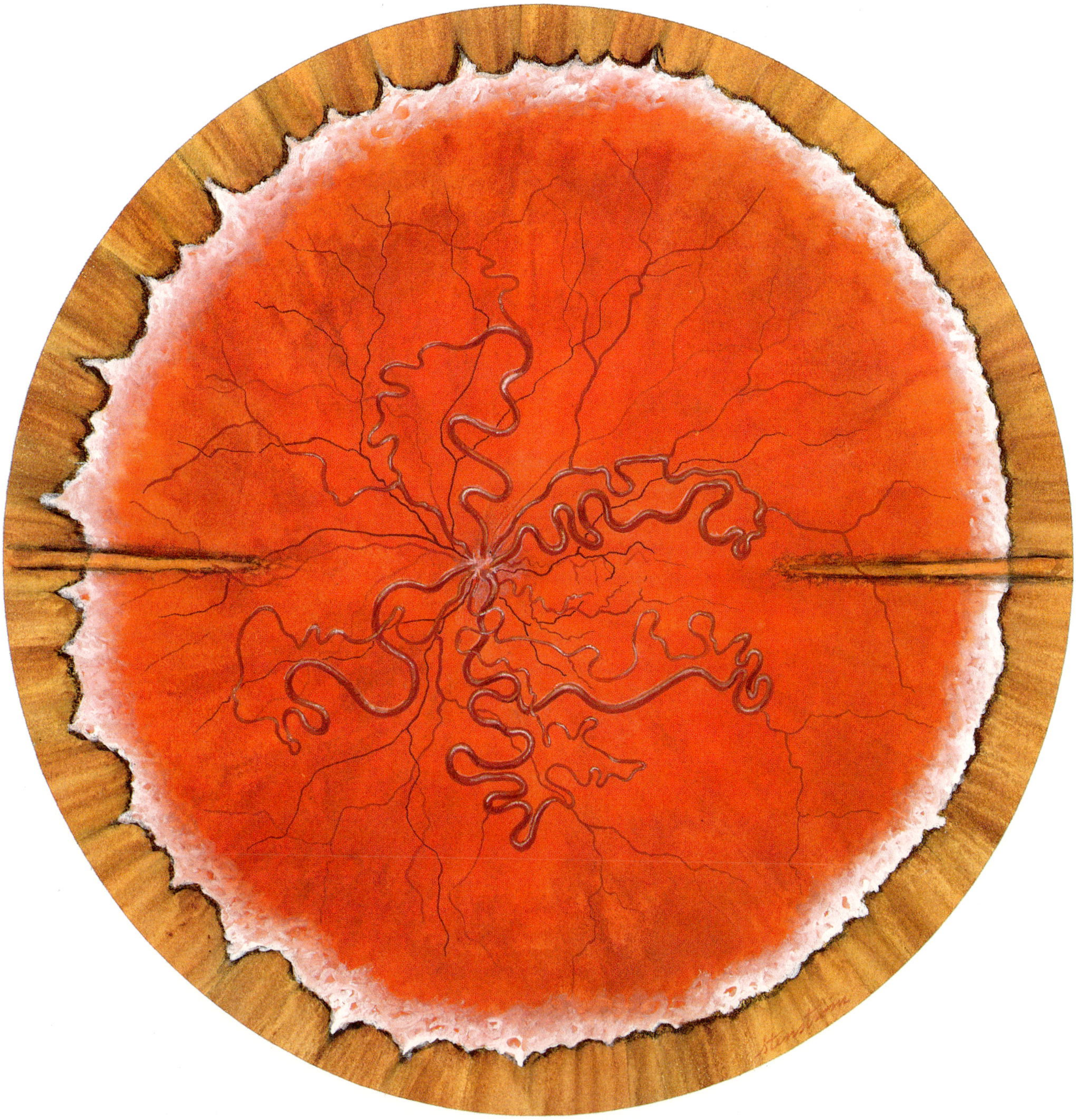

PLATE 82

VON HIPPEL-LINDAU ANGIOMATOSIS

Angiomatosis retinae of von Hippel-Lindau is a systemic disease that affects the viscera and central nervous system as well as the eye. The typical retinal appearance is a red nodule or globular balloon on the surface of the mid-peripheral retina. These lesions are, in reality, arteriovenous fistulas and are fed by dramatically engorged and tortuous retinal arterioles and venules. Yellow exudate may surround these angiomas, and advanced lesions may produce localized or even total serous retinal detachment.

The earliest visible lesions are a fan-shaped set of fine capillary-like vessels between arterioles and venules. Fluorescein angiography demonstrates leakage of dye from these vessels. Blood may leak also, producing a retinal or vitreous hemorrhage.

The posterior pole may be involved when an angioma is present in or on the optic nerve. Frequently, hard exudates produced by peripheral angiomas are visible in the macula. The macular exudate may be so dense that a solid yellow to white mound, which may be confused with retinoblastoma, is found in the macula.

Angiomatosis of von Hippel-Lindau is transmitted as an autosomal dominant, without sex predilection. Usually, lesions are found bilaterally and can develop from infancy to the sixth or seventh decade.

Blodi FC: Angiomatosis retinae. *In* Duane TD (ed): Clinical Ophthalmology. Hagerstown, Maryland, Harper & Row, 1978, Vol. 3, pp 4–8

Horowitz P: von Hippel-Lindau disease. *In* Tasman W (ed): Retinal Diseases in Children. New York, Harper & Row, 1971, pp 78–91

Watzke RC, Weingeist TA, Constantine JB: Diagnosis and management of von Hippel-Lindau disease. *In* Peyman GA, Apple DJ, Saunders DR: Intraocular Tumors, New York, Appleton-Century-Crofts, 1977, pp 199–217

Wing GL, Weiter JJ, Kelly PJ, et al: von Hippel-Lindau disease. Ophthalmology *88*:1311–1314, 1981

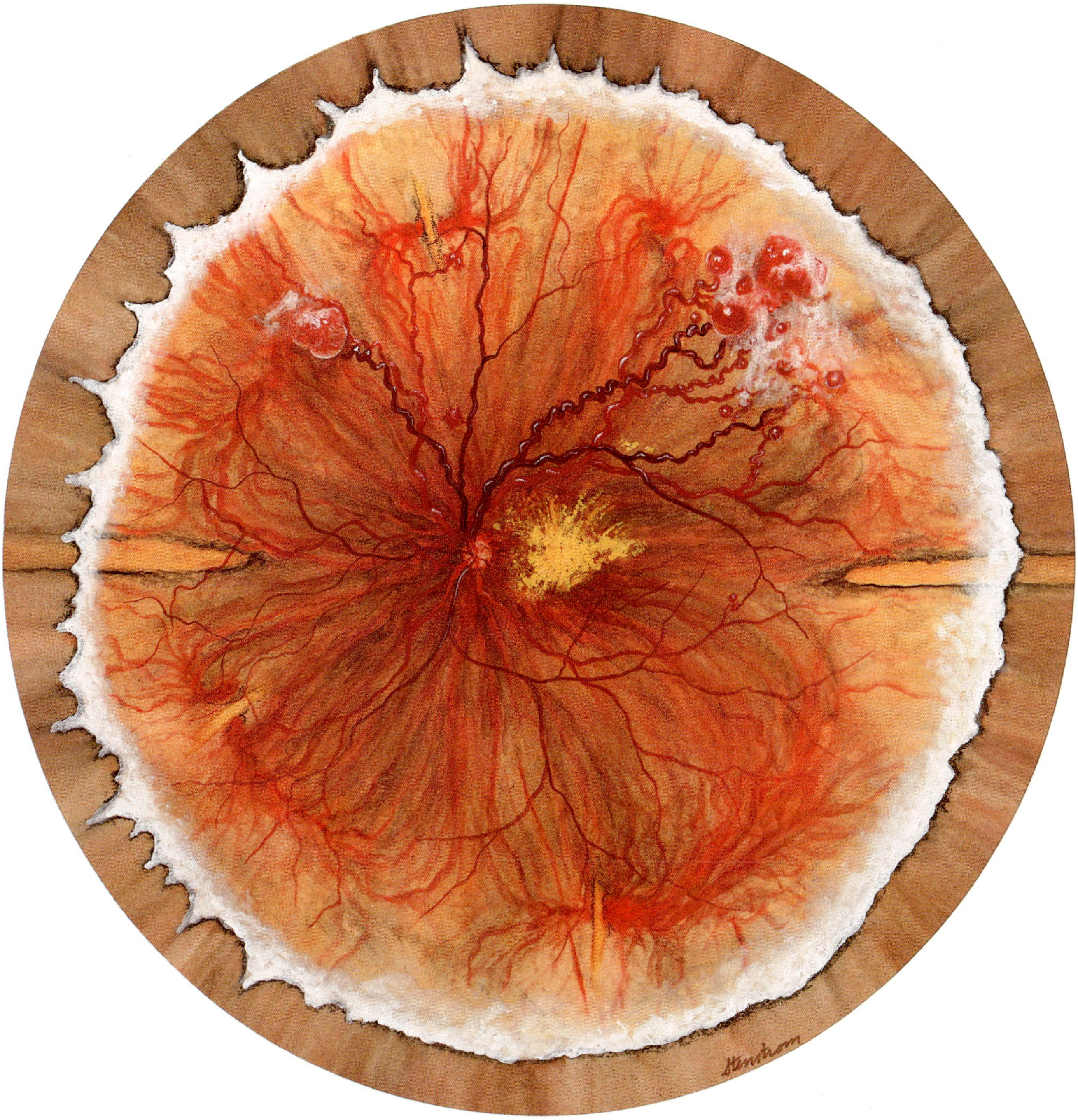

PLATE 83

Chapter Nine

MEDICAL RETINAL DISEASES

RETINITIS PIGMENTOSA

Retinitis pigmentosa is a genetically inherited, slowly progressive retinal degeneration characterized by bone spicule pigmentation in the retinal periphery and constricted retinal arterioles. Inheritance by autosomal recessive, autosomal dominant, and X-linked inheritance is known, but many sporadic cases also occur. The most common clinical picture is of a dramatic pigmentation in the mid-periphery, surrounding the retinal vessels in a bone spicule pattern. However, some cases show only salt and pepper diffuse pigmentation, and some cases totally lack pigmentation. Many variations have been described affecting only one quadrant of the fundus, and even unilateral cases have been reported. The retinal arterioles are markedly constricted, although the veins appear normal. The macula appears normal in the early stages, but later cystoid macular edema and macular atrophy may occur. The disc is normal in many cases, but as the condition progresses the disc may become pale and atrophic.

The initial symptom of retinitis pigmentosa is night blindness, usually presenting in the first or second decade of life. Later, there are visual field defects, with peripheral scotomas coalescing into a ring scotoma, and eventually markedly constricted peripheral visual fields. Central visual acuity is usually good for many years; only the progressive visual field constriction obliterates all vision from the eye.

The most helpful laboratory test in making the diagnosis is the electroretinogram. It may be diminished, even in the early stages, before the retinal picture becomes recognizable. In the late stages, the electroretinogram and electrooculogram are both extinguished.

There are many syndromes associated with retinitis pigmentosa. There are also many causes of pseudo-retinitis pigmentosa, such as inflammatory disease, infection, certain drugs, metabolic diseases, and a number of ocular and systemic syndromes of unknown etiology.

Carr RE: Primary retinal degenerations. *In* Duane TD (ed): Clinical Ophthalmology. New York, Harper & Row, 1981, Vol 3, pp 1–10

Dewar AJ, Reading HW: The biochemical aspects of retinitis pigmentosa. Int J Biochem 6:615–641, 1975

Lucas DR: Retinitis pigmentosa. Br J Ophthalmol *40*:14–23, 1956

Merin S, Auerbach A: Retinitis pigmentosa. Surv Ophthalmol *20*:303–346, 1976

Szamier RB, Berson DL: Retinal ultrastructure in advanced retinitis pigmentosa. Invest Ophthalmol *16*:947–962, 1977

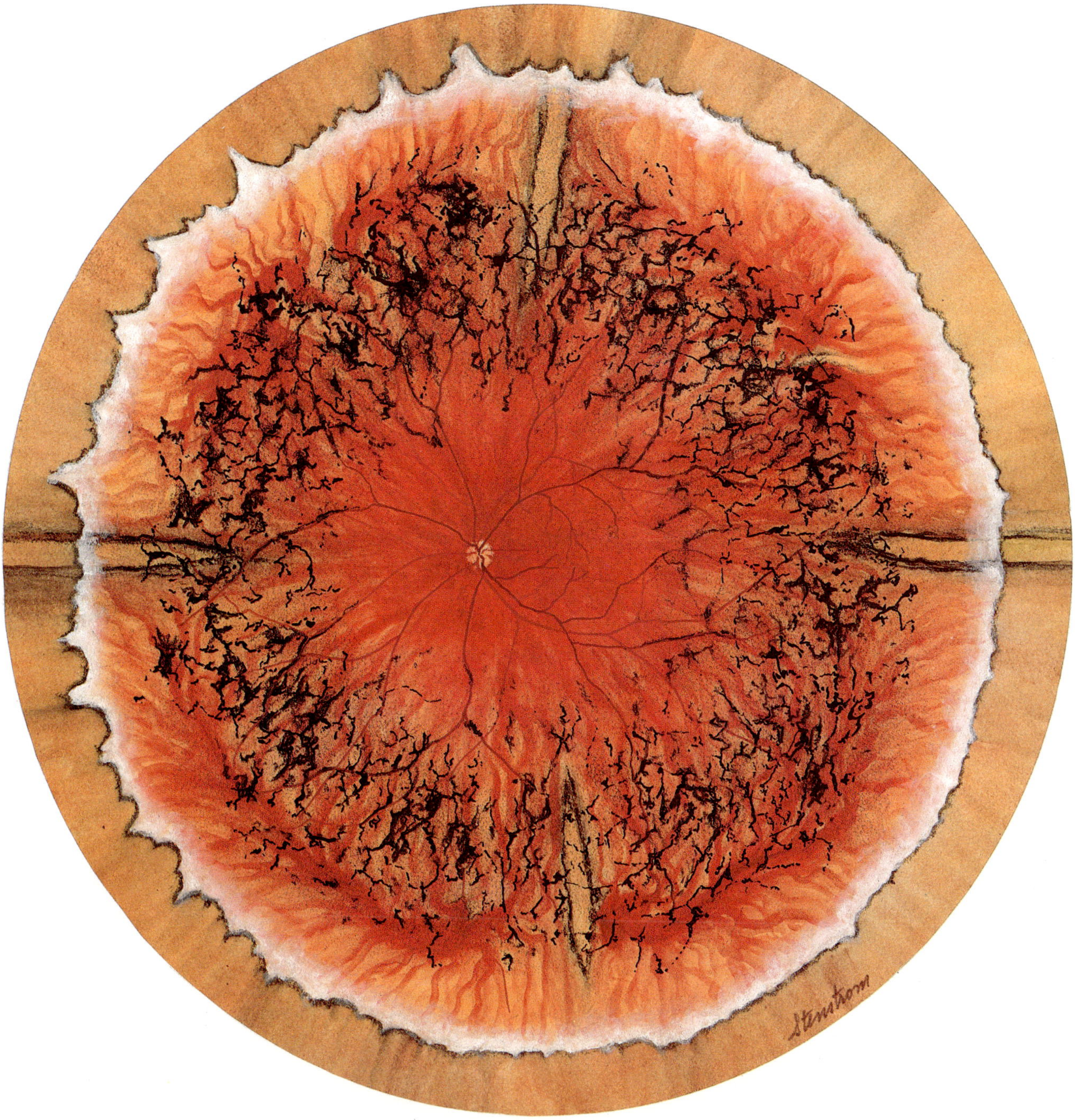

PLATE 84

MYELINATED NERVE FIBERS

Myelination of the optic nerve normally ends behind the lamina cribrosa of the optic nerve and does not extend into the disc or retina. In 0.3 to 0.4 per cent of patients, myelination does extend as a developmental defect so that it is ophthalmoscopically visible. When present, these myelinated nerve fibers are larger than the normal fibers, so that the nerve bulges from the added bulk, and the surrounding area appears thickened. Myelinated nerve fibers occur more often in males than in females, and are bilateral in about 20 per cent of affected patients.

Areas of myelination appear intensely white or light gray, and may partially or completely obscure the retinal vessels and choroidal markings. On careful observation with the direct ophthalmoscope, the margins of the individual myelinated fibers can be seen to extend to varying degrees into normal retina, producing a feathered edge appearance to the margin of the lesion.

Isolated patches of myelinated nerve fibers may be present in the mid periphery entirely separated from the disc. These myelinated patches may have punctate spots of microscystic degeneration within them. Such areas of myelination produce corresponding visual field defects that do not change with time. Myelinated nerve fibers may also be associated with high myopia, amblyopia, and strabismus.

Levy NS, Ernest JT: Retinal medulated nerve fibers. Arch Ophthalmol *91*:330–331, 1974

Merritt JC: Myelinated nerve fibers associated with afferent pupillary defect and amblyopia. J Pediatr Ophthalmol *14*:139–140, 1977

Straatsma BR, Foos RY, Hecklenlively JR, Taylor GN: Myelinated retinal nerve fibers. Amer J Ophthalmol *91*:25–38, 1981

Straatsma BR, Heckenlively JR, Foos RY, Shahinian J: Myelinated retinal nerve fibers associated with ipsilateral myopia, amblyopia and strabismus. Amer J Ophthalmol *88*:506–510, 1979

Walsh FB, Hoyt WF: Clinical Neuro-ophthalmology. 3rd ed., Baltimore, Williams & Wilkins, 1969, pp 665–668

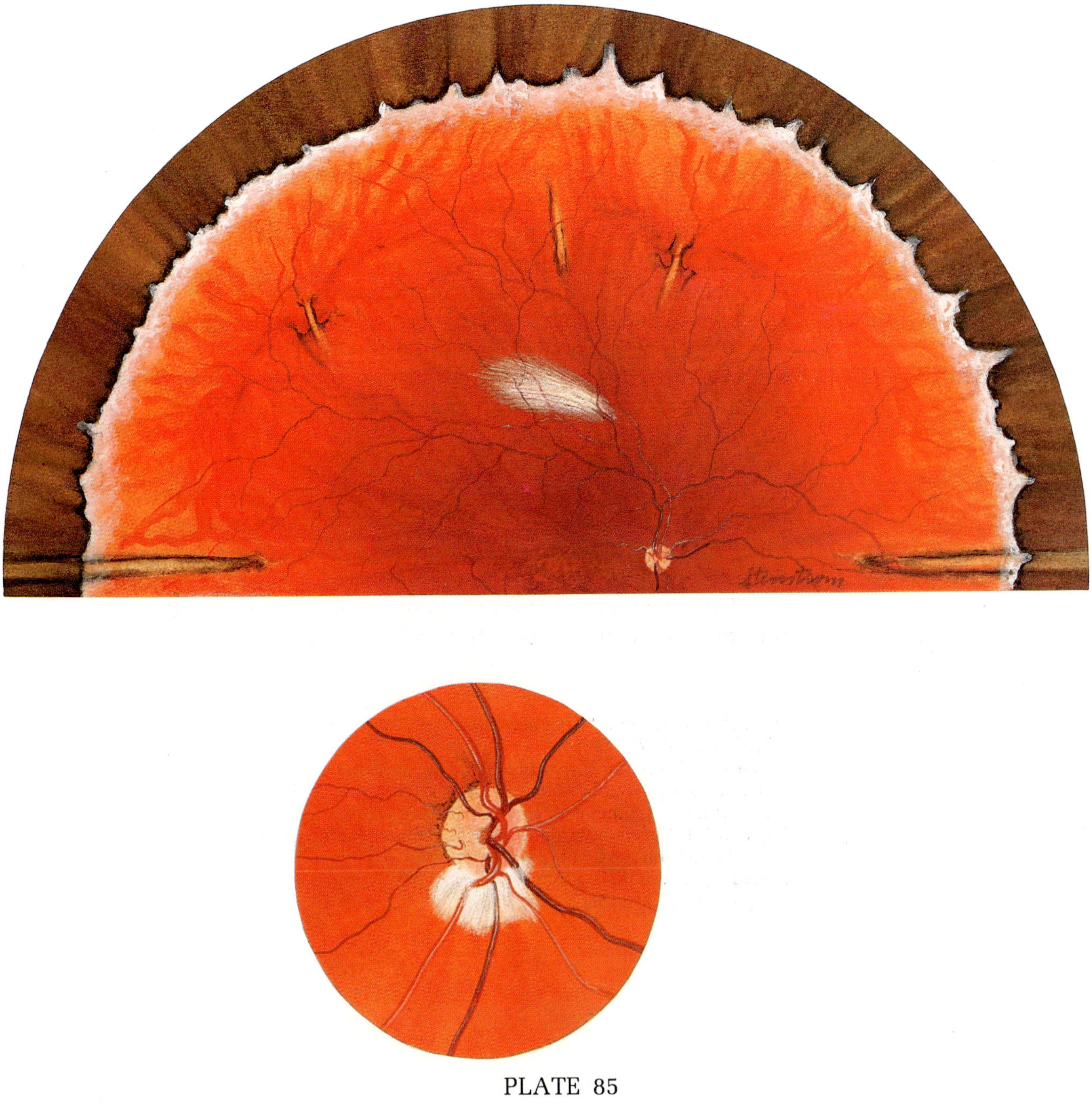

PLATE 85

CONGENITAL GROUPED PIGMENTATION (BEAR TRACKS)

Congenital grouped pigmentations appear as multiple, flat, sharply defined brown spots that typically occur in clusters, giving the subjective impression of animal tracks. These round to ovoid lesions are usually discovered in one eye of an asymptomatic patient as an incidental finding. Although these pigmentations are congenital, no hereditary pattern has been identified.

These spots may be clinically confused with nevi or old chorioretinal scars, but histologically they are quite distinct. The pigment epithelial cells show increased numbers of pigment granules, with the overlying retina normal. There is no tendency for them to develop into malignant tumors.

The distinctive pattern of these lesions has earned this entity the common name of "bear tracks."

Hoeg H: Die gruppierte Pigmentation des Augengrundes. Klin Monatsbl Augenheilkd *49*:49–77, 1911

Fursius H, Eriksson A, Nuutlia A, et al: A genetic study of three rare retinal disorders: dystrophia retinal dysacusis syndrome, x-chromosomal retinoschisis and grouped pigments of the retina. Birth Defects *7*:83–98, 1977

Legrand MJ, Hervouet F, Baron A, et al: Pigmentation groupée de la rétine. Bull Soc Ophthalmol *64*:313–315, 1964

Shields JA, Tso MO: Congenital grouped pigmentation of the retina. Arch Ophthalmol *93*:1153–1155, 1975

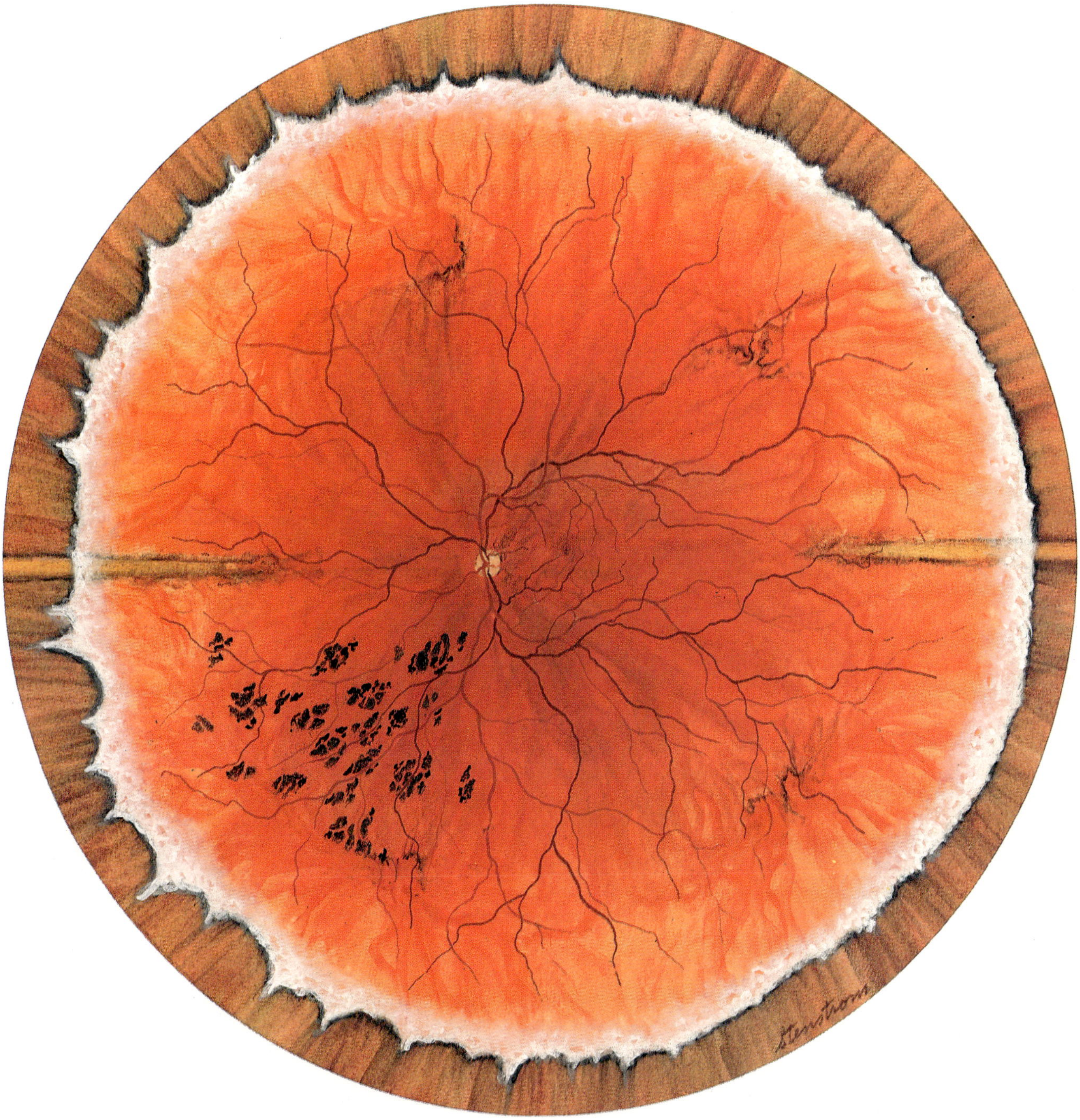

PLATE 86

COLOBOMA OF RETINA AND CHOROID

Colobomas are defects in the retina and choroid caused by failure of the embryonic fissure to fuse properly. Clinically colobomas appear as areas of absence of retina and choroid, allowing the sclera to be visualized through a very thin and transparent intercalary membrane. The intercalary membrane is a rudimentary retina, and blood vessels of various stages of development may be seen running across the coloboma. Typical colobomas are located in the inferior half of the fundus, as the embryonic fissure is located inferonasally in the developing eye. Colobomas may extend from the optic nerve to the iris, or may occupy a small area inferior to the disc, depending on the degree of nonclosure of the embryonic fissure. The margins of colobomas are rather sharply defined, with a pigmented border marking the rather abrupt transition from coloboma to normal choroid and retina.

Colobomas are congenital defects. Data on incidence, race, and sex incidence have not been accurately determined. Some colobomas are known to be transmitted genetically as an autosomal dominant trait, but autosomal recessive and sporadic cases have also been documented.

Retinal detachment may spontaneously occur in colobomatous eyes. A retinal hole is usually not visible and may lie in the intercalary membrane, where it is very difficult to visualize.

Francois J: Colobomatous malformations of the ocular globe. Int Ophthalmol Clin 8:797–816, 1968

Jesberg DO, Schepens CL: Retinal detachment associated with coloboma of the choroid. Arch Ophthalmol 65:163–173, 1961

Pagon RA; Ocular coloboma. Surv Ophthalmol 25:223–236, 1981

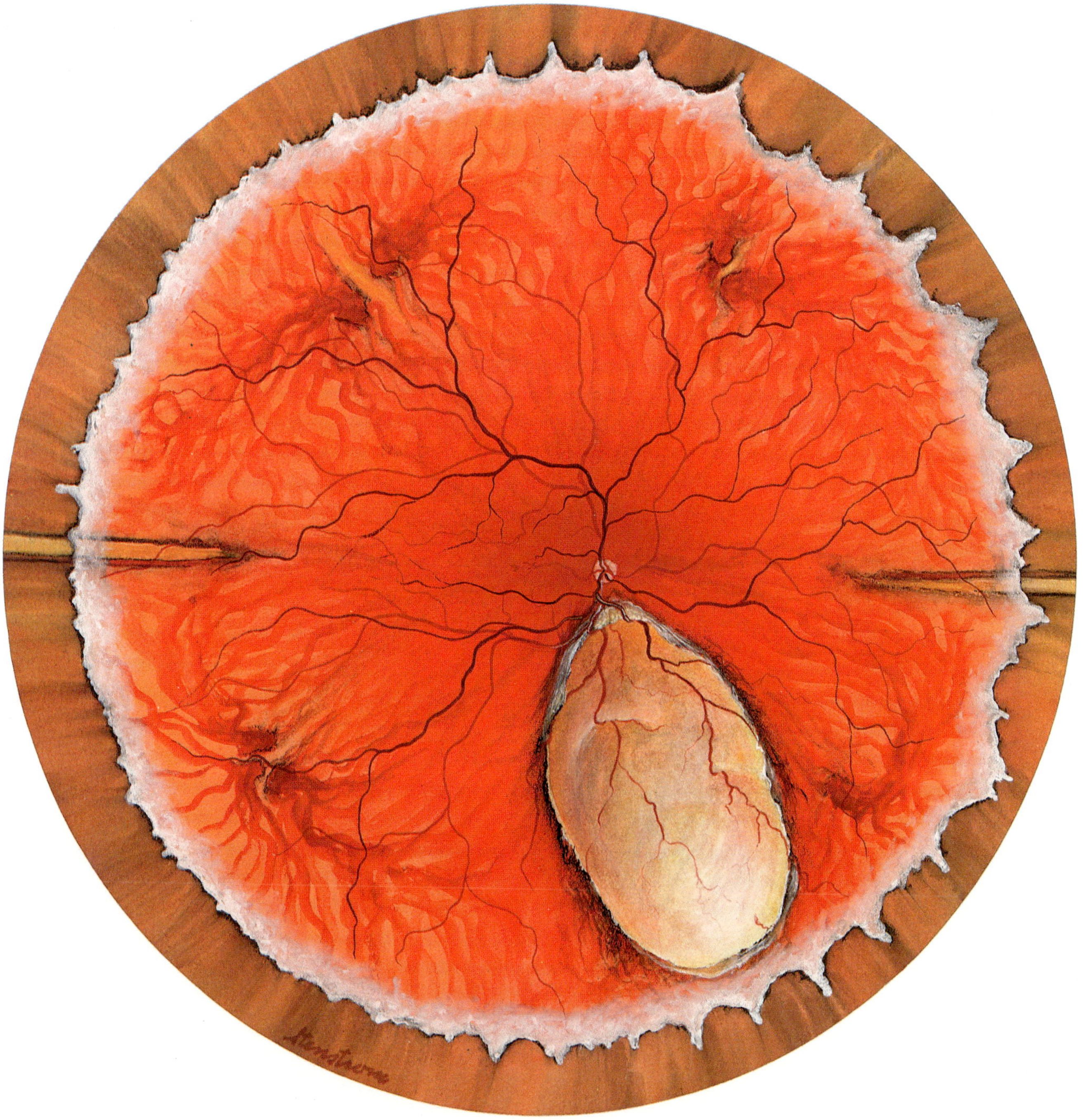

PLATE 87

PERIPHERAL DRUSEN

Drusen are discrete, small, round, white or yellow spots that represent hyaline thickenings of Bruch's membrane. Most commonly, they occur clustered in and around the macular area, and may lead to subretinal neovascularization and macular degeneration. Drusen also occur, as shown here, in the peripheral retina as relatively evenly spaced white to yellow spots, sometimes with a surrounding pigment ring. Peripheral drusen only very rarely develop subretinal neovascularization, hemorrhage, and fluid formation. The pattern of drusen in the periphery is extremely variable and may affect only one quadrant. There is usually quite striking symmetry in the two eyes. It is debatable whether drusen are a senile aging process or whether they are genetically determined. An autosomal dominant hereditary pattern has been documented in a number of families.

Drusen develop from focal hyaline thickenings of Bruch's membrane, which at first compress the pigment epithelium and ultimately erode through. The fluorescein angiogram initially shows a window defect that shows late staining but no leakage of fluorescein. Later, the drusen may calcify and become white and waxy in appearance. Peripheral retinal drusen cause very little functional disturbance of the retina. Visual fields and the electroretinogram are usually normal. Dark adapatation and the electro-oculogram are either normal or very slightly depressed.

Farkas TG, Krial AE, Sylvester VM, et al: Familial and secondary drusen: Histologic and functional correlations. Trans Am Acad Ophthalmol Otolaryngol 75:333–343, 1971

Farkas TG, Sylvester VM, Archer D, et al: The histochemistry of drusen. Am J Ophthalmol 71:1206–1215, 1971

Gass JDM: Drusen and disciform macular detachment and degeneration. Arch Ophthalmol 90:206–217, 1973

Hogan MJ: Role of the retinal pigment epithelium in macular disease. Trans Am Acad Ophthalmol Otolaryngol 76:69–80, 1972

Krill AE, Klien BA: Flecked retina syndrome. Arch Ophthalmol 4:496–508, 1965

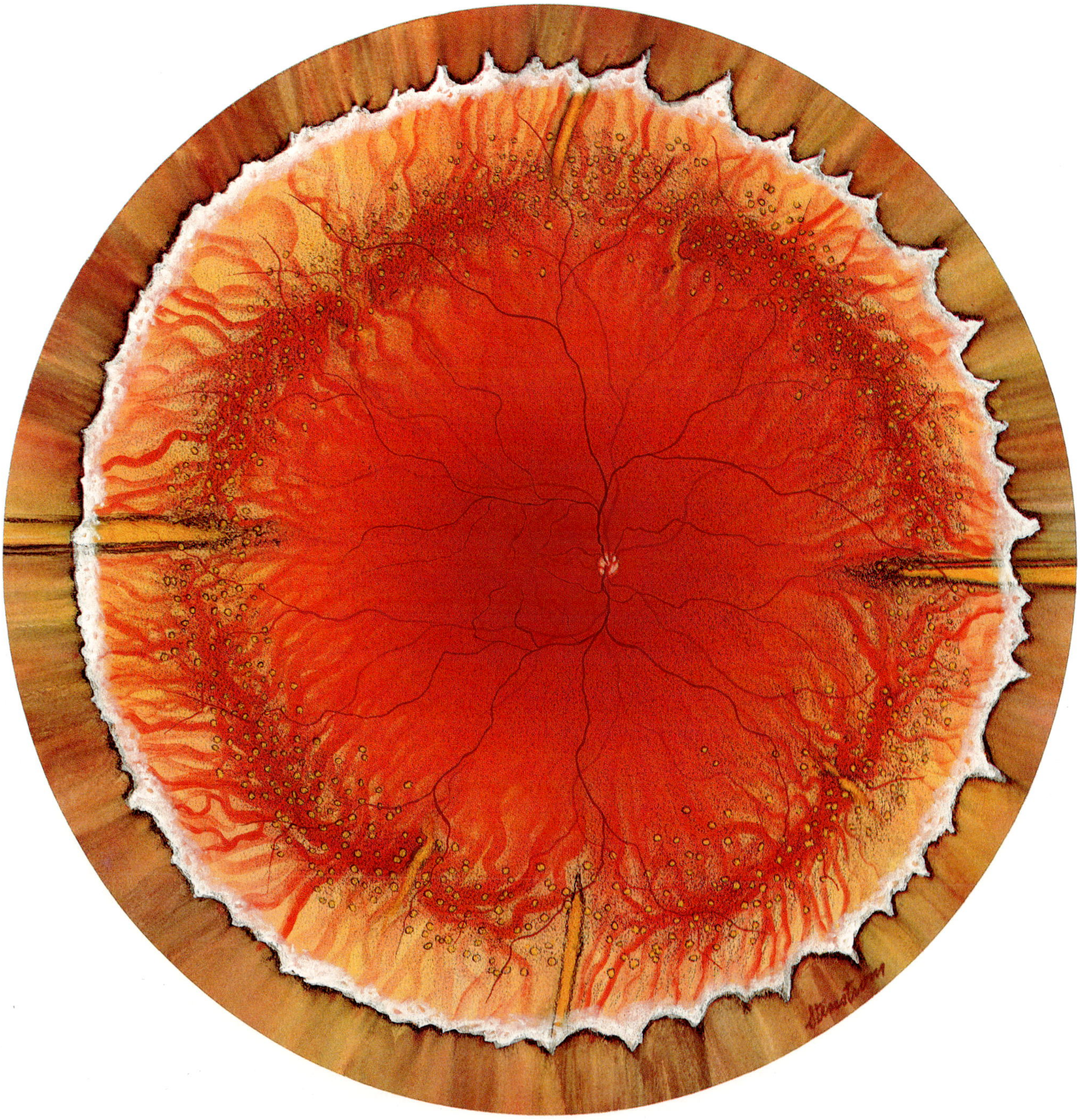

PLATE 88

FUNDUS ALBIPUNCTATUS; RETINITIS PUNCTATA ALBESCENS

Fundus albipunctatus and retinitis punctata albescens have similar funduscopic appearances yet appear to be separate entities. Both are inherited as an autosomal recessive trait and can be recognized ophthalmoscopically from youth onward. Night blindness is an early symptom of both disorders. Funduscopically, each entity appears as myriads of punctate white dots in the fundus that spare the macula and extend into the far periphery.

Fundus albipunctatus is fundamentally a stable condition with a slow rate of dark adaptation. The electroretinogram and the electro-oculogram are abnormal if tested shortly after light adaptation, but are returned to normal if tested after prolonged dark adaptation. The visual acuity, visual fields, optic nerve, and retinal vessels are all typically within normal limits.

Retinitis punctata albescens has a similar funduscopic appearance, yet it is a progressive condition with many characteristics similar to retinitis pigmentosa. The disc becomes pale and the arterioles narrow as the condition progresses. There is progressive loss of the peripheral visual field and progressive retinal and pigment epithelial atrophy. The electroretinogram and electro-oculogram both become extinguished in advanced stages.

Albert DM, Geltzer AI: Retinitis punctata albescens in a Negro child studied with fluorescein angiography. Arch Ophthalmol *81*:170–176, 1969

Carr RE: Congenital stationary night blindness. Trans Am Ophthalmol Soc *72*:449–487, 1974

Carr RE, Margolis S, Siegel IM: Fluorescein angiography and vitamin A and oxalate levels in fundus albipunctatus. Doc Ophthalmol Proc Series 4:193–204, 1974

Carr RE, Ripps H, Siegel IM: Visual pigment kinetics and adaptation in fundus albipunctatus, Doc Ophthalmol *4*:193–204, 1974

Lauber H: Die sogenannte Retinitis punctata albescens. Klin Monatsbl Augenheilkd *48*:133–148, 1910

Marmor MF: Defining fundus albipunctatus. Doc Ophthalmol Proc Series *13*:277–234, 1977

Marmor MF: Fundus albipunctatus: A clinical study of the fundus lesion, the physiologic defect and the vitamin A metabolism. Doc Ophthalmol *43*:277–302, 1977

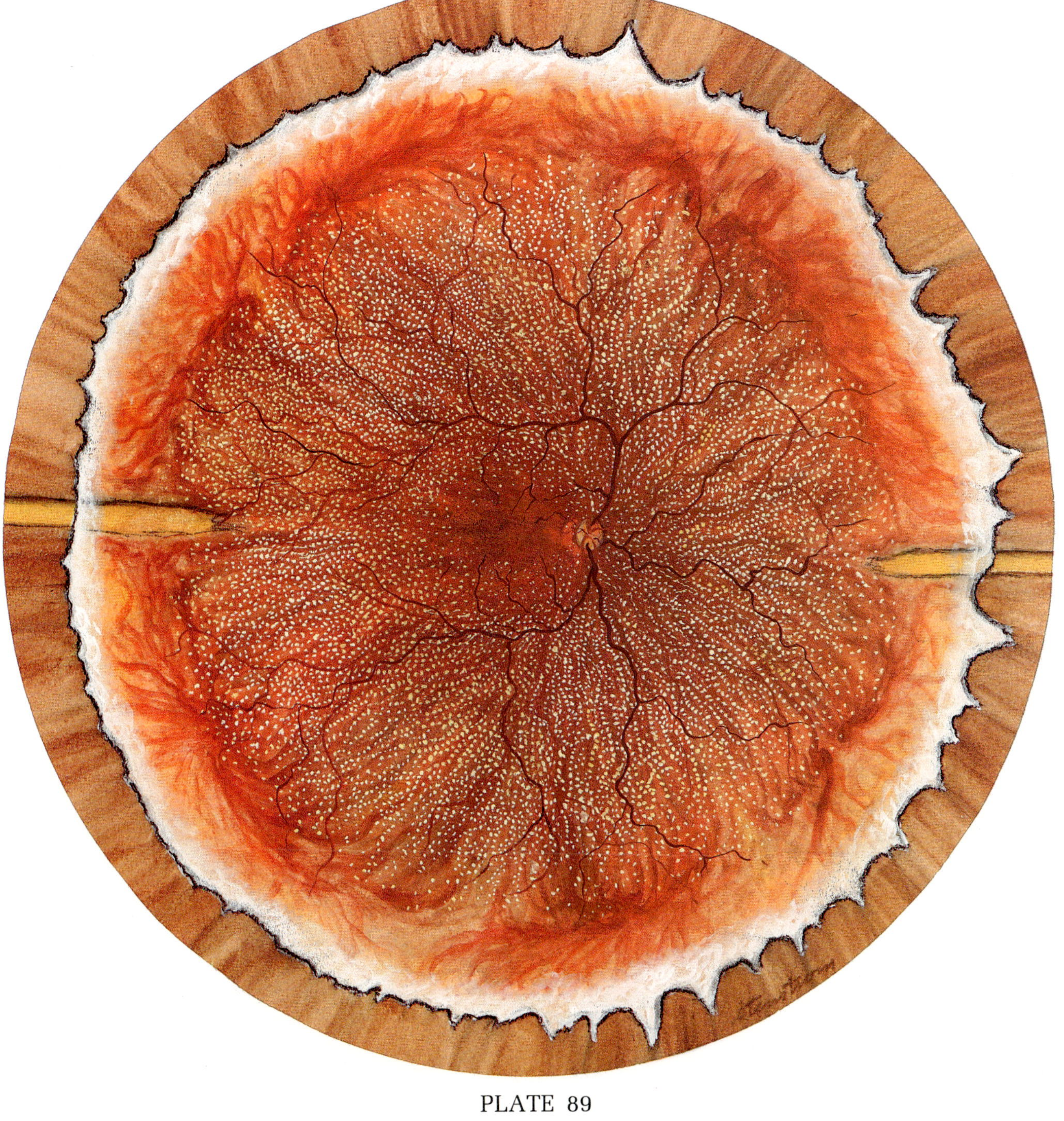

PLATE 89

LUPUS RETINOPATHY

Systemic lupus erythematosus is a chronic systemic collagen vascular disease of unknown etiology. It is characterized by systemic focal vascular changes in a pattern of exacerbation and remission. Systemic lupus erythematosus presents initially in the second to fourth decades. For unknown reasons, females are much more commonly affected than males. When the retina is involved, the appearance is usually that of white cotton wool spots of various shapes and sizes clustered around the posterior pole. These cotton wool spots represent ischemic infarcts of the nerve fiber layer caused by occlusion of the smaller retinal arterioles and capillaries. Although not present in this case, multiple dot and blot hemorrhages at the margins of cotton wool spots frequently occur. With time, the white cotton wool spots may disappear leaving large areas of capillary nonperfusion in a relatively normal-appearing retina. The retinal veins typically show slight engorgement, and may show sausage-like segmentation. The optic nerve may be normal or, in cases of severe involvement, papilledema may be present. Neovascularization of the optic nerve, which may lead to vitreous hemorrhage, has been reported. Fluorescein angiography frequently reveals numerous microaneurysms. Although not diagnostic, these retinal findings are highly suggestive of retinal involvement in systemic lupus erythematosus.

Bishko F: Retinopathy is systemic lupus erythematosus: A case report and review of the literature. Arthritis Rheum *15*:57–63, 1972

Coppeto J, Lessell S: Retinopathy in systemic lupus erythematosus. Arch Ophthalmol *95*:794–797, 1977

Gold DH, Morris DA, Henkind P: Ocular findings in systemic lupus erythematosus. Br J Ophthalmol *56*:800–804, 1972

Gold DH, Feiner L, Henkind P: Retinal arteriolar occlusive disease in systemic lupus erythematosus. Arch Ophthalmol *95*:1580–1585, 1977

Kayazawa F, Honda A: Severe retinal vascular lesions in systemic lupus erythematosus. Ann Ophthalmol *13*:1291–1294, 1981

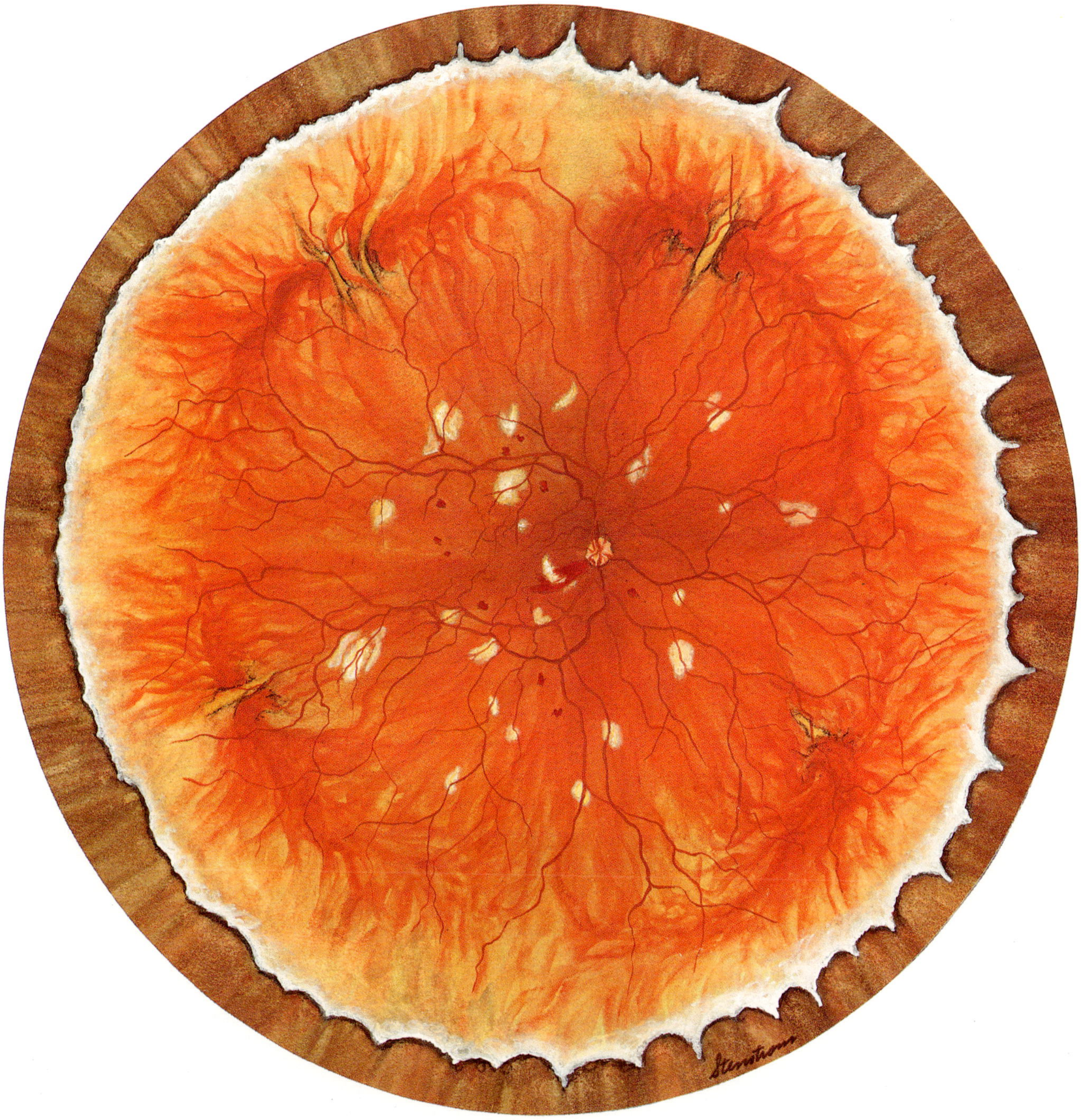

PLATE 90

SARCOIDOSIS

Sarcoidosis is a systemic disease of unknown cause that affects many organ systems. The fundamental pathological lesion is a focal granuloma consisting of nodular collections of epithelioid cells. These non-caseating granulomas can affect any ocular tissue, particularly the conjunctiva, uveal tract, and retina. An anterior granulomatous uveitis is a common manifestation of sarcoidosis. Also common is a posterior uveitis manifested by vitreous cells and retinal involvement. The classic retinal finding is a white to yellow waxy deposit appearing in or on the surface of the retina in the posterior pole. There is a tendency for these deposits, called candle wax drippings, to accumulate along the vessels, particularly retinal veins. The retinal veins may also show focal constrictions and venous sheathing. Small retinal hemorrhages may occur, but these are usually confined to the superficial retinal layers. Sarcoidosis may also involve the choroid as a diffuse subretinal grayish infiltrate that over time produces atrophy with focal pigmentation, giving the appearance of healed chorioretinitis. The optic nerve also may become involved with sarcoidosis, producing papilledema and papillitis, particularly if the central nervous system is affected. Fluorescein angiography shows late staining of areas affected by the focal granulomata of sarcoidosis.

Chumbley LC, Kearns TP: Retinopathy of sarcoidosis. Am J Ophthalmol *73*:123–131, 1972

Geeraets WJ, McNeer KW, Maxey EF, et al: Retinopathy in sarcoidosis. Acta Ophthalmol *40*:492–514, 1962.

Gould H, Kaufman HE: Sarcoid of the fundus. Arch Ophthalmol *65*:453–456, 1961

James DG, Anderson R, Langley DA, et al: Ocular sarcoidosis. Br J Ophthalmol *48*:461–470, 1964

James DG, Neville E, Langley DA: Ocular sarcoidosis. Trans Ophthalmol Soc UK *96*:133–139, 1976

Letocha CE, Shields JA, Goldberg RE: Retinal changes in sarcoidosis. Can J Ophthalmol *10*:184–192, 1975

Obenauf CD, Shaw HE, Snydor CF, et al: Sarcoidosis and its ophthalmic manifestations. Am J Ophthalmol *86*:648–655, 1978

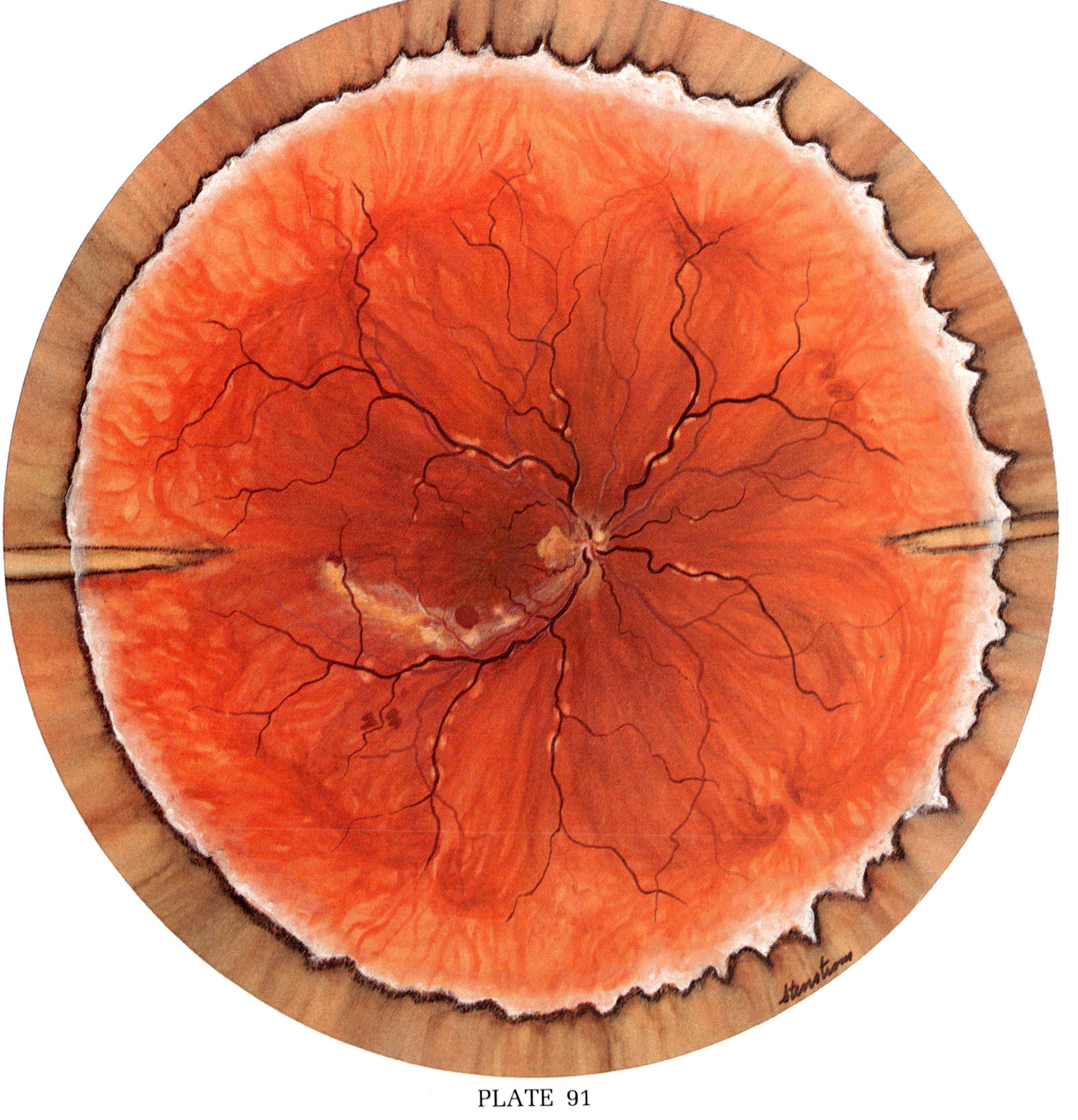

PLATE 91

CHOROIDEREMIA

Choroideremia is characterized by marked choroidal atrophy over the entire fundus, with the macular region the last to become affected. It is a genetically inherited X-linked disease, with males affected fully and females manifesting only the carrier state. Affected males first show ophthalmoscopic changes in the first decade of life consisting of atrophy of the choroid in the mid-peripheral fundus so that the white sclera becomes visible. Much of the pigment released accumulates in the retina without producing the bone spicule pattern of retinitis pigmentosa. The smaller choroidal blood vessels undergo complete atrophy, leaving only a few larger vessels present. There is mild attenuation in the size of retinal arteries, but the veins appear essentially normal. The optic nerve is normal in youth, but becomes white and atrophic with the passage of many years. Female carriers show only mild pigmentary mottling in the mid-periphery, and otherwise have entirely normal fundi and normal vision.

The presenting symptom noted is usually night blindness. Visual fields initially show multiple scotomas in the periphery, which coalesce into a ring scotoma, and eventually marked visual field constriction. As the decades pass, central vision may be obliterated. As the disease process progresses, there is secondary atrophy of the retinal pigment epithelium, and the electroretinogram eventually is extinguished.

Kurstjens JH: Choroideremia and gyrate atrophy of the choroid and retina. Docum Ophthalmol 19:1–122, 1965

McCulloch C: Choroideremia: A clinical and pathologic review. Trans Am Ophthalmol Soc 67:142–195, 1969

Rubin ML, Fishman RS, McKay RA: Choroideremia. Arch Ophthalmol 76:563–574, 1966

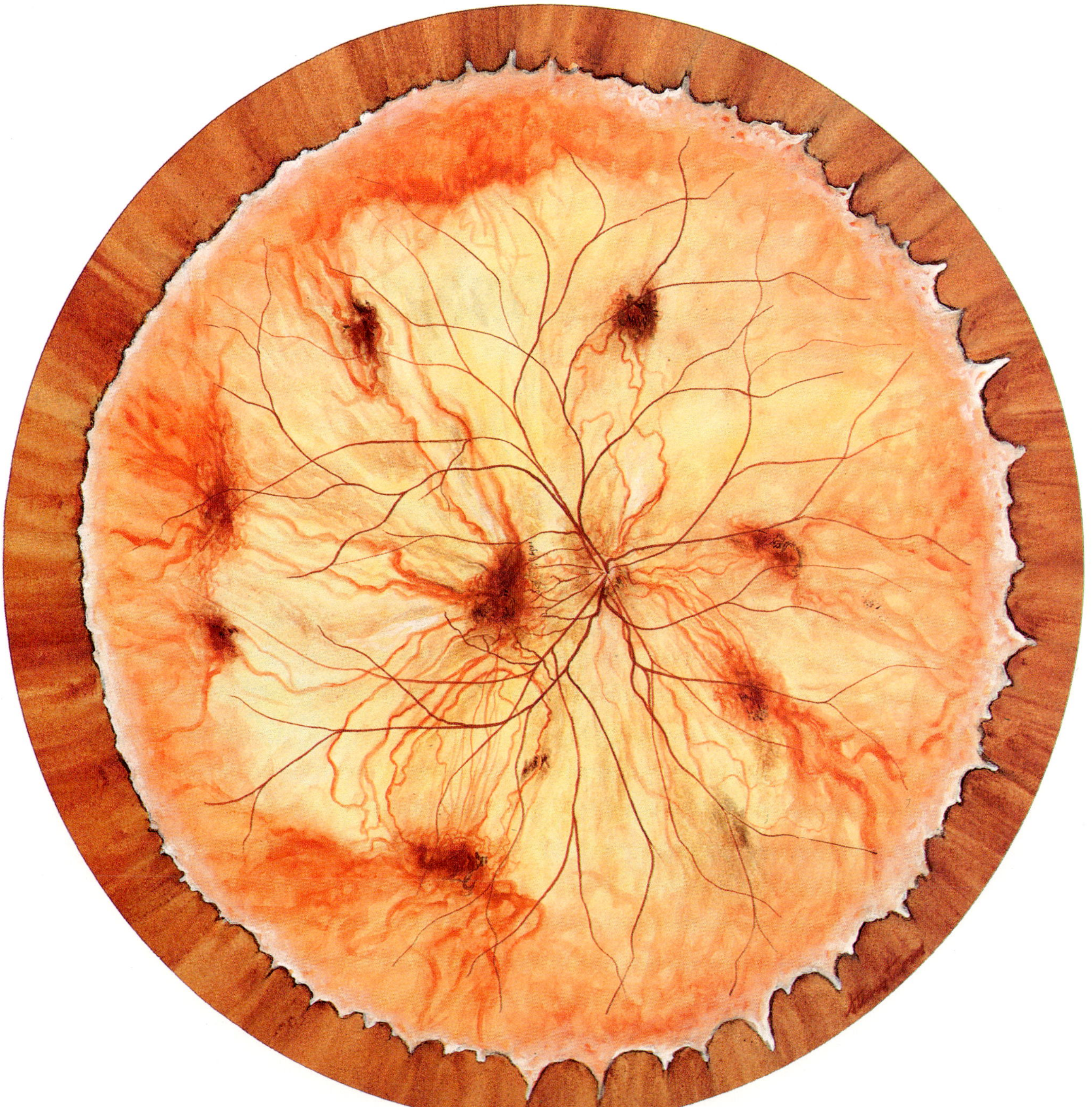

PLATE 92

FUNDUS FLAVIMACULATUS

Fundus flavimaculatus is a distinctive pattern of small yellow flecks in a variable pattern that extends from the macula into the mid-periphery. These flecks are thought to be present in the pigment epithelium, and unless there is macular involvement the flecks are asymptomatic. Fundus flavimaculatus is transmitted as an autosomal recessive condition with an occasional dominant pedigree observed. In approximately one half of the affected cases fundus flavimaculatus is associated with a macular degeneration appearing as a horizontally oval area of macular atrophy and focal pigment clumping surrounded by a characteristic beaten metal appearance. This macular degeneration is historically called Stargardt's macular degeneration, but the two conditions are now believed to be the same entity. If the macula is affected, a decrease in central vision is noted in the first or second decade that may slowly progress to legal blindness.

As observed by fluorescein angiography, the white flecks initially block the choroidal fluorescence, but more mature lesions show fluorescein staining in the later stages of the angiogram. Curiously, the pattern seen by angiography does not correspond exactly to the pattern seen ophthalmoscopically. Dark adaptation is usually normal and the electroretinogram and electro-oculogram are normal to slightly subnormal.

Franceschetti A, Francois J: Fundus flavimaculatus. Arch Ophthalmol (Paris) *25*:505–530, 1965

Hadden OB, Gass JDM: Fundus flavimaculatus and Stargardt's disease. Am J Ophthalmol *82*:527–539, 1976

Klien BA, Krill AE: Fundus flavimaculatus. Am J Ophthalmol *64*:3–23, 1967

Krill AE, Klien BA: Flecked retina syndrome. Arch Ophthalmol *74*:496–508, 1965

Newell FW, Krill AE, Farkas TG: Drusen and fundus flavimaculatus: Clinical, functional and histologic characteristics. Trans Am Acad Ophthalmol Otolaryngol *76*:80–100, 1972

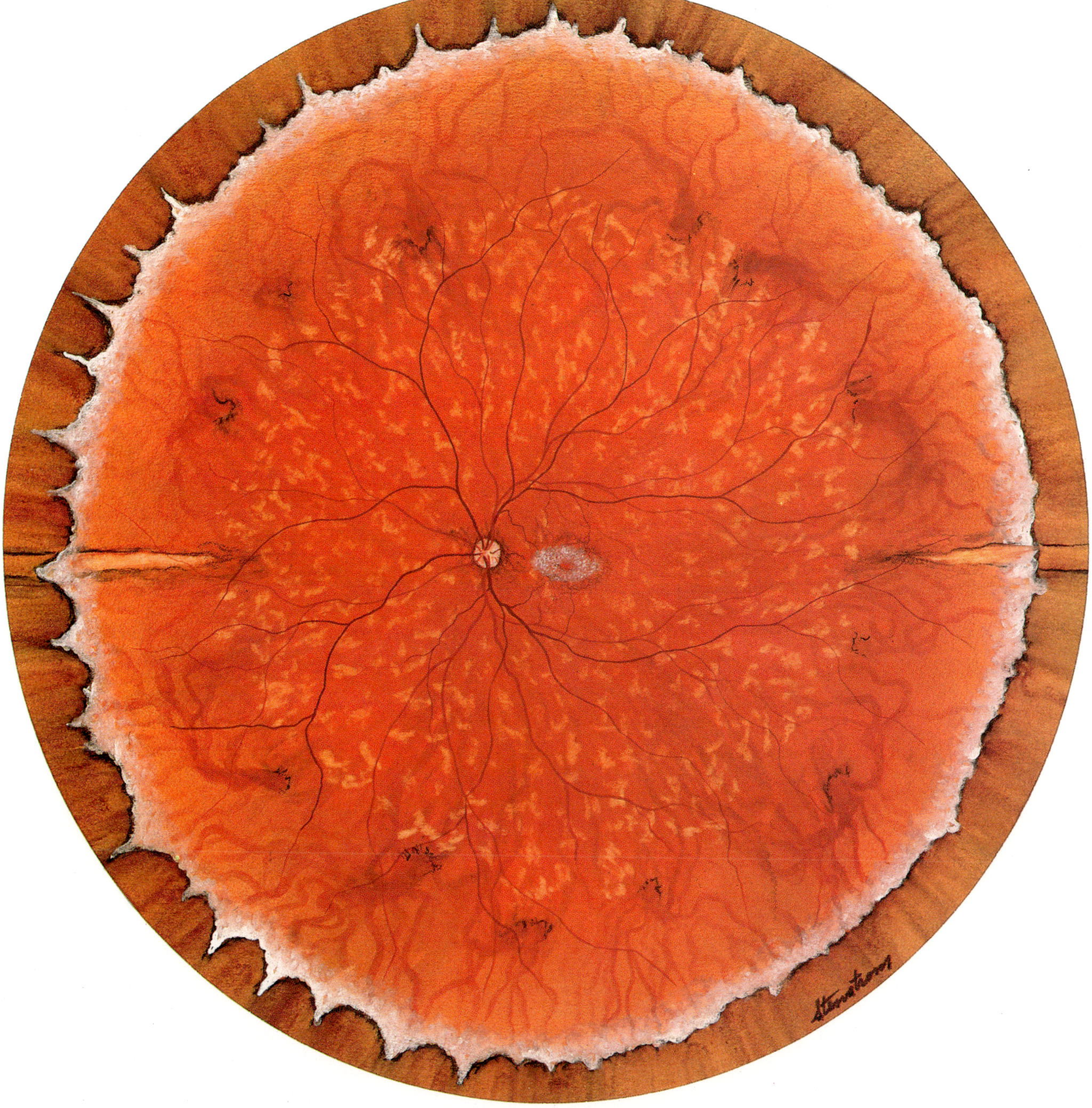

PLATE 93

THE ALBINO FUNDUS

Hereditary albinism is divided into two main types, ocular albinism, in which only the eye is involved, and oculocutaneous albinism, in which the skin, hair, and other pigmented structures are affected as well. Ocular albinism is transmitted as an X-linked trait, whereas oculocutaneous albinism is transmitted as an autosomal recessive trait. Oculocutaneous albinism is further divided into two types. In the tyrosinase-positive type there is pigment present in the normally pigmented body structures, although the amount of pigment is diminished. Affected individuals appear clinically almost normal, except for their eye findings. In the tyrosinase-negative type, individuals have white hair, pale skin, and blue irises, features immediately recognized as characteristic of albinism. All forms of albinism may have varying degrees of photophobia, nystagmus, and decreased visual acuity. In general, the less pigment present, the more pronounced these findings.

In albinism the optic nerves and retinal vessels are usually normal. The macula is abnormal with no well defined foveal reflex. Histological studies confirm that no definite fovea is present. Throughout the entire fundus, the pigment epithelium is almost transparent, so that the choroidal vascular pattern appears prominently beneath the retinal vascular system. The choroid is also devoid of pigment and the sclera is seen as a white background to the choroidal pattern. If the pigment is present in small amounts, it is usually present in the macula and becomes less prominent toward the periphery.

The several biochemical abnormalities leading to albinism occur in lower animals as well as in man. Studies of lower forms have revealed an abnormal division of neurons in the optic chiasm and there is some evidence that similar abnormalities may be present in human albinos.

Creel DJ, Witkop CJ, King RA: Asymmetric visually evoked potentials in human albinos, evidence for visual system anomalies. Invest Ophthalmol *13*:430–440, 1974

Fulton AB, Albert DM, Kraft JL: Human albinism. Light and electron microscopic study. Arch Ophthalmol *96*:305–310, 1978

Naumann GOH, Lerche W, Schroeder W: Foveola–Aplasie bei Tyrosinase-positivem oculocutanen Albinismus. Albrecht von Graefes Arch Klin Ophthalmol *200*:39–50, 1976

O'Donnell FE, Hambrick GW, Green WR, et al: X-linked ocular albinism. Arch Ophthalmol *94*:1838–1842, 1976

O'Donnell FE, King RA, Witkop CJ, et al: Autosomal recessively inherited ocular albinism: A new form of ocular albinism affecting females as severely as males. Arch Ophthalmol *96*:1621–1625, 1978

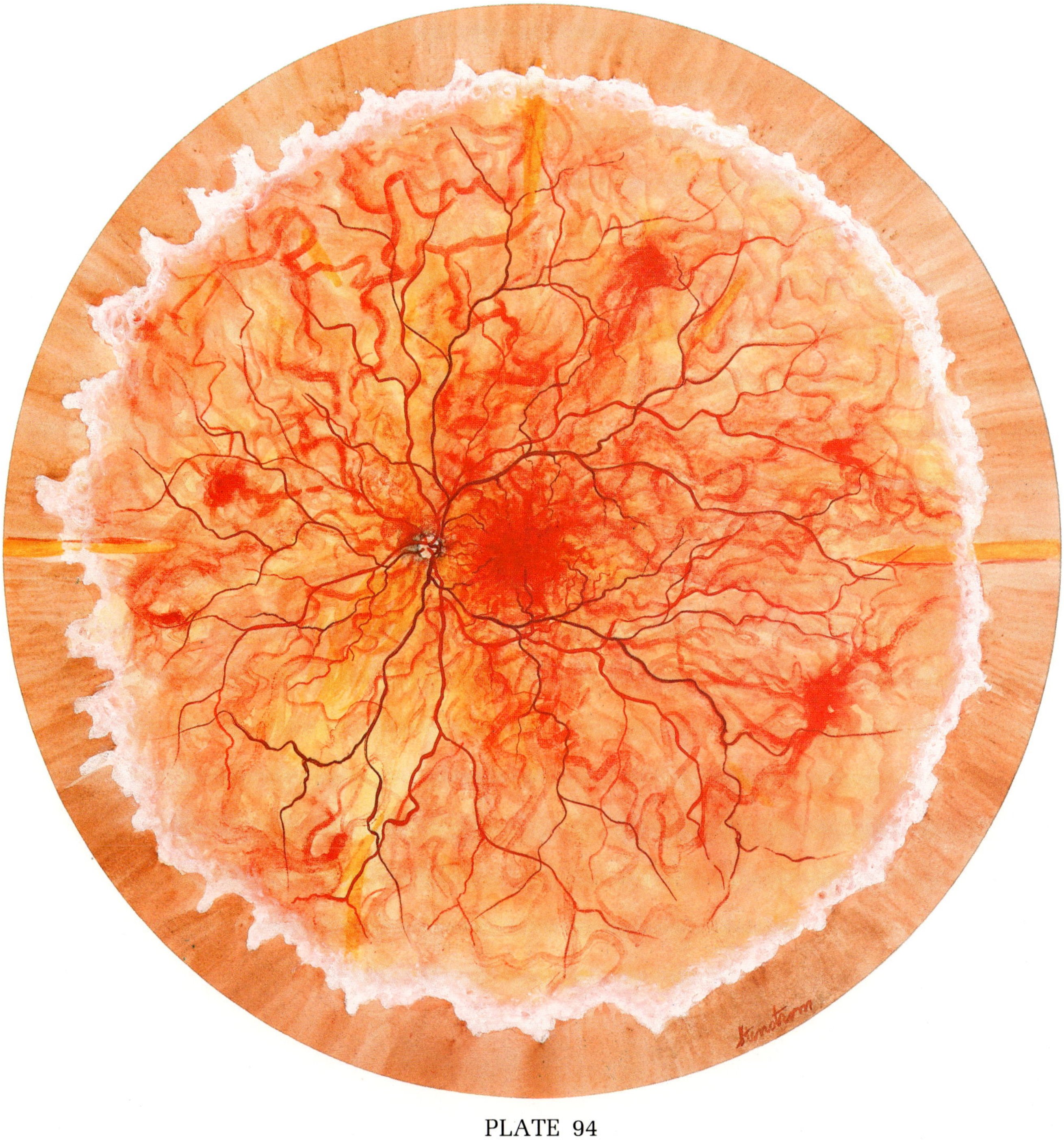

PLATE 94

GYRATE ATROPHY

Gyrate atrophy has a dramatic and specific fundus appearance that is associated with elevated levels of the amino acid ornithine in the blood. It is apparently due to the genetically inherited absence of the enzyme ornithine ketoacid aminotransferase. The fundus at birth is apparently normal, but in childhood yellow-white spots appear in the peripheral fundus and the macular reflex is diminished. By young adulthood, sharply demarcated punched-out lesions appear initially in the mid-periphery due to atrophy of the pigment epithelium within these multiple disc-sized areas. The larger choroidal vessels are visible within the punched-out areas. By adulthood, these round areas begin to form clusters and become confluent. The far periphery of the retina and choroid eventually shows severe atrophy of the choroid, pigment epithelium, and retina, while the posterior pole is the last to become involved. There is no sign of intraocular inflammation and the optical media appear quite clear. Affected patients do have night blindness and abnormal electroretinogram. Clinical recognition of gyrate atrophy is important because specific therapy is available.

Hayasaka S, Saito T, Nakajima H, et al: Gyrate atrophy with hyperornithinaemia: Different types of responsiveness to vitamin B_6. Brit J Ophthalmol 65:478–483, 1981

Kaiser-Kupfer MI, Valle D, Del Valle LA: A specific enzyme defect in gyrate atrophy. Am J Ophthalmol 85:200–204, 1978

Simell O, Takki K: Raised plasma-ornithine and gyrate atrophy of the choroid and retina. Lancet 1:1031–1033, 1973

Takki K: Gyrate atrophy of the choroid and retina associated with hyperornithinemia. Br J Ophthalmol 58:3–23, 1974

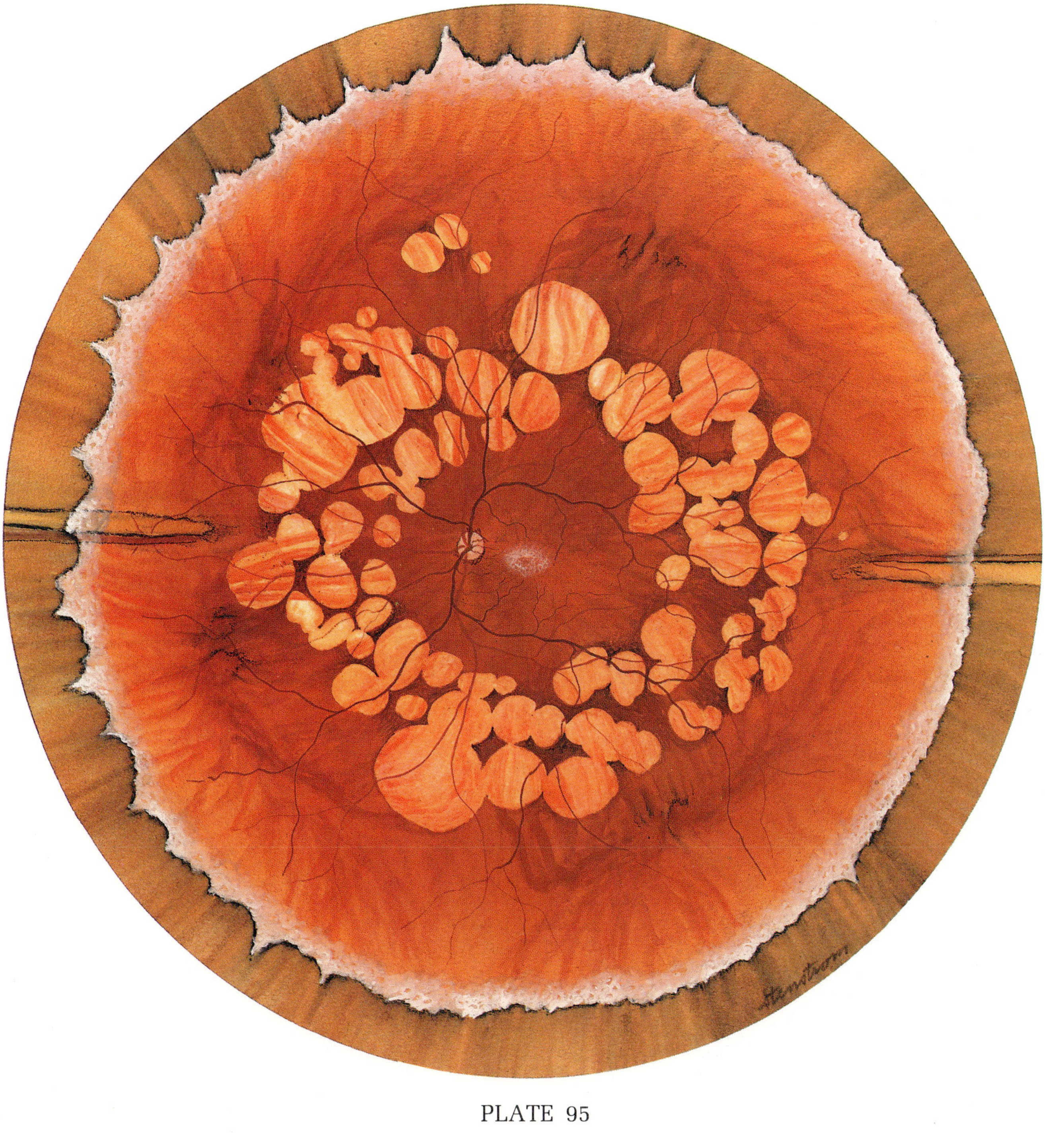

PLATE 95

ANGIOID STREAKS

Angioid streaks typically appear as relatively straight, brown or gray lines in both eyes that radiate from the optic nerve toward the mid-periphery. They may branch and give the impression of retinal vessels, but careful observation reveals that the streaks pass underneath the retinal vessels. In the posterior pole, these streaks may be several times wider than a retinal vessel, but they become thinner as they pass toward the periphery. Histologically, angioid streaks represent linear breaks in Bruch's membrane. The overlying pigment epithelium becomes thin directly over the streaks, with focal hypertrophy forming clumps of pigment. There is usually a generalized diffuse stippling of the pigment epithelium throughout the posterior pole, creating the so called "peau d' orange" appearance.

Macular degeneration is a common late complication of angioid streaks. New vessels from the choroid frequently invade the subretinal space of the macula, producing subretinal fluid and hemorrhage. Eventually, a subretinal scar of disciform macular degeneration is produced, creating decreased central vision.

Angioid streaks are associated with a large number of systemic diseases. Most commonly, angioid streaks are found in pseudoxanthoma elasticum, a degenerative disease of elastic tissue throughout the body, in which calcification and fragmentation of elastic tissue occur prematurely. Ehlers-Danlos syndrome, sickle cell disease, Paget's disease of bone, and many other diseases are also associated with angioid streaks. Angioid streaks may, in some cases, occur as an isolated ocular finding. Fluorescein angiography reveals the angioid streaks readily by demonstrating hyperfluorescence from the underlying choroid.

Archer DB, Logan WC: Bruch's membrane degenerations. II. Angioid streaks. *In*: Krill's Hereditary Retinal and Choroidal Diseases, Vol. II, Clinical Characteristics. Hagerstown Md, Harper & Row, 1977, pp 851–909

Federman JL, Shields JA, Tomer TL: Angioid streaks. II. Fluorescein angiographic features. Arch Ophthalmol *93*:951–962, 1975

Fine S: Angioid streaks. Int Ophthalmol Clin *17*:173–182, 1977

Paton D: The relationship of angioid streaks to systemic disease. Springfield, Charles C Thomas, 1972

Shields JA, Federman JL, Tomer TL, Annesley WH: Angioid streaks, I. Ophthalmoscopic variations and diagnostic problems. Br J Ophthalmol *59*:257–266, 1975

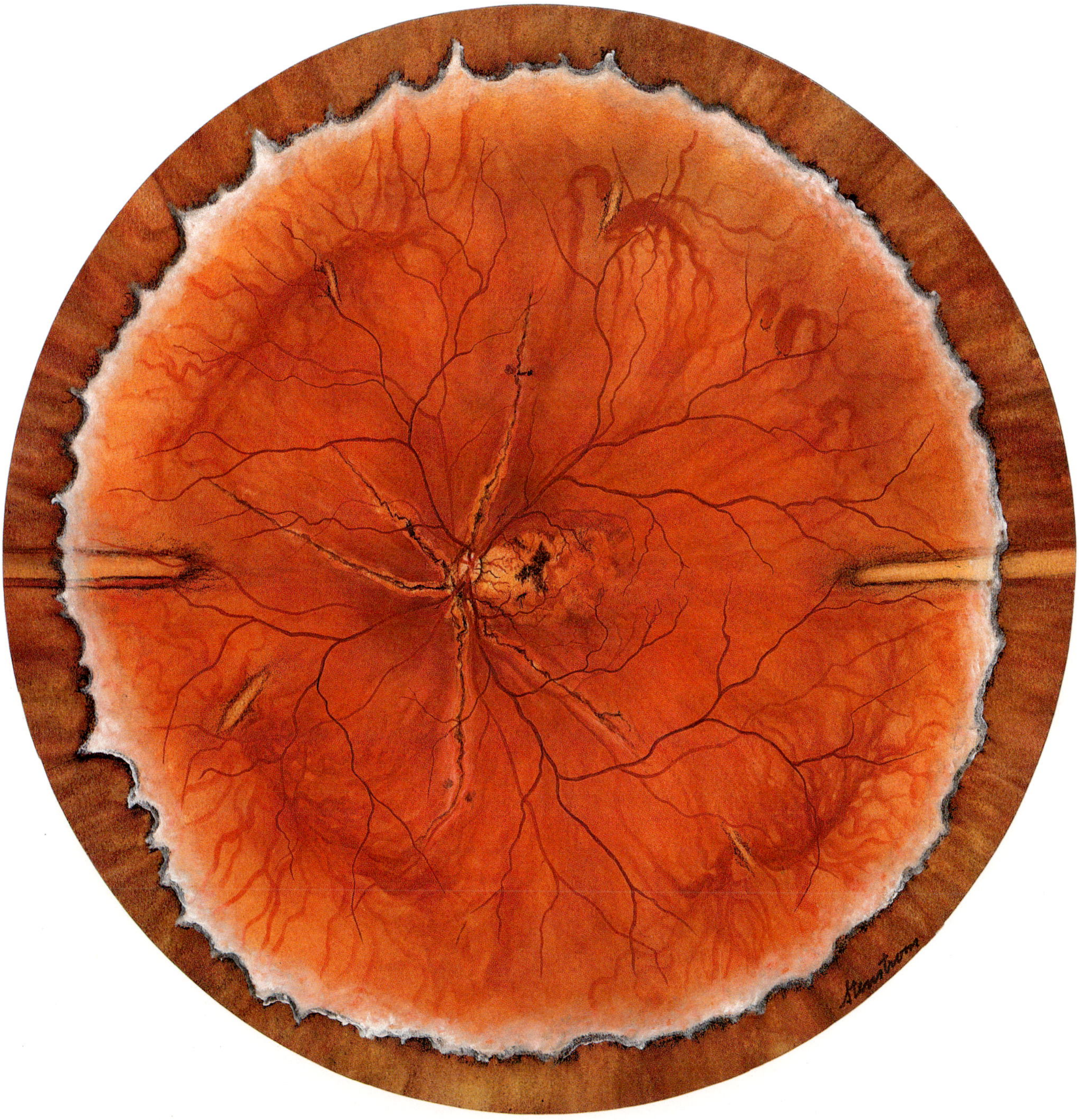

PLATE 96

ASTEROID HYALOSIS

Asteroid hyalosis consists of myriad white or yellow particles embedded in an otherwise normal vitreous. The particles range in size from dustlike to discrete, ovoid, irregular granules. Although these particles are easily seen by the observer, the patient is frequently unaware of their presence, as asteroid hyalosis infrequently causes impaired visual acuity.

Asteroid hyalosis is generally unilateral and is more common in patients of advanced age. An association with diabetes mellitus has been claimed, but most investigators have not observed a correlation with any systemic disease. When analyzed chemically, asteroid hyalosis material is found to be composed of calcium soap.

Bard LA: Asteroid Hyalitis: Relationship to diabetes and hypercholesterolemia. Am J Ophthalmol *58*:239–242, 1964

Benson AH: A case of "Monocular Asteroid Hyalitis." Trans Ophthalmol Soc UK *14*:101–104, 1894

Luxemberg M, Sime D: Relationship of asteroid hyalosis to diabetes mellitus and plasma lipid levels. Am J Ophthalmol *67*:406–413, 1969

March W, Shock D, O'Grady R: Composition of asteroid bodies. Invest Ophthalmol *13*:701–705, 1974

Rodman HI, Johnson FB, Zimmerman LE: New histopathological and histochemical observations concerning asteroid hyalitis. Arch Ophthalmol *66*:552–563, 1961

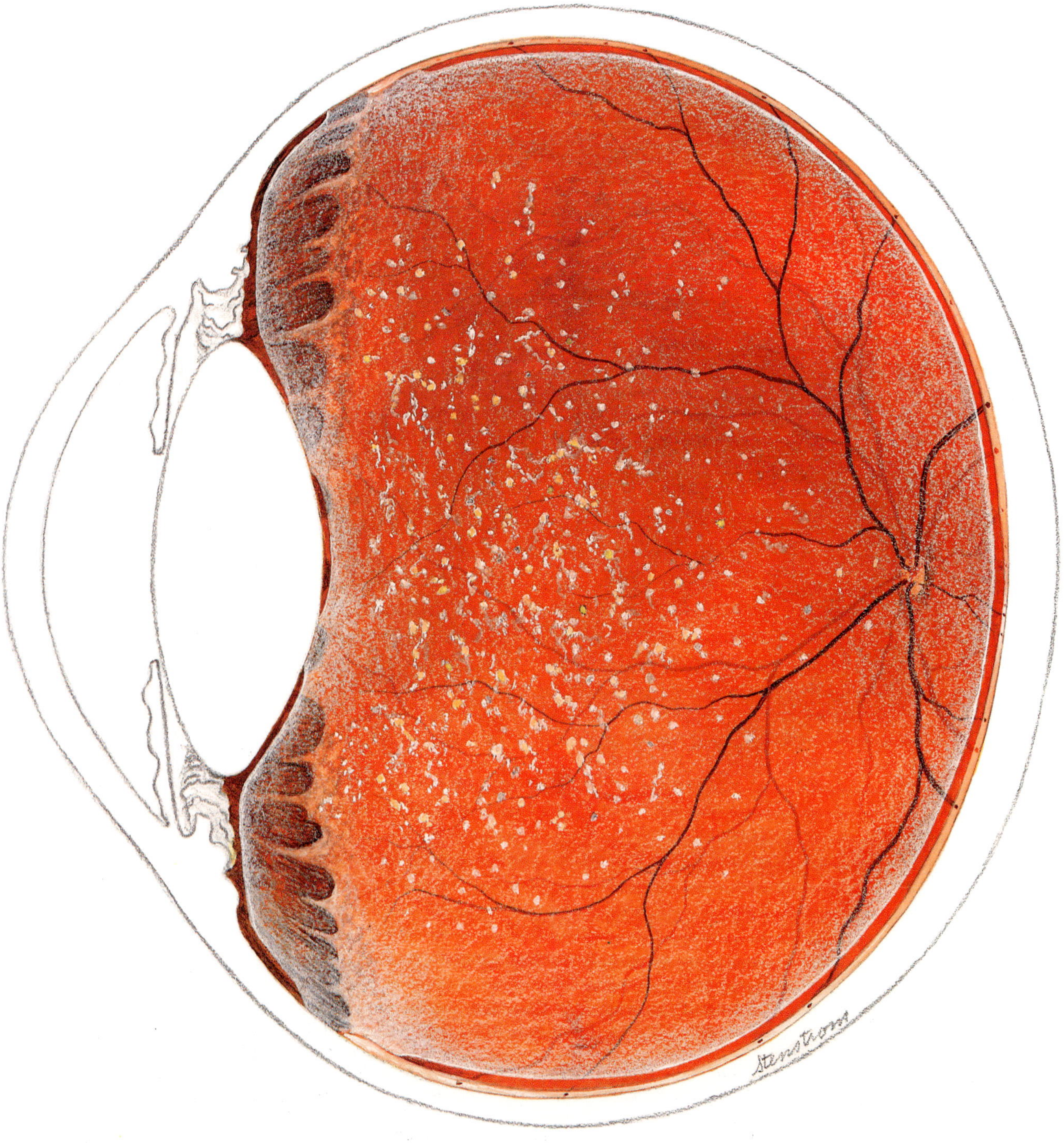

PLATE 97

JUVENILE RETINOSCHISIS

Juvenile retinoschisis is a splitting of the retina into two layers. The inner layer is very thin and consists of the retinal nerve fiber layer and the retinal vessels. The outer layer of schisis contains the remaining retinal layers and remains attached to the pigment epithelium. The area of retina affected by juvenile retinoschisis is almost always in the inferior fundus and does not extend all the way to the ora serrata. The elevated inner layer is so thin and friable that it fragments and disappears, leaving the retinal vessels suspended in the vitreous without obvious support. The retinal vessels may bleed spontaneously, producing a vitreous hemorrhage. The macula may become involved by superior extension of the schisis cavity. Even if the macula is not directly involved with the bullous elevation, some degree of foveal schisis is believed to occur in all cases. There is no well defined foveal reflex, and the surface of the macula reveals radial striae radiating in a starlike pattern from the fovea. The optic nerve is usually normal but may be atrophic if large areas of retina are affected.

Juvenile retinoschisis is inherited as an X-linked trait; hence, males are predominantly affected bilaterally. The symptoms begin in the first decade of life with minimally decreased vision in both eyes. Strabismus and spontaneous vitreous hemorrhage are common presenting signs. Typically, the course is stationary or very slowly progressive over may years.

The electroretinogram is normal or may reveal a slightly decreased b wave. The electro-oculogram is normal. Dark adaptation studies are slightly subnormal, while visual field studies reveal absolute scotomas corresponding to the areas of retinoschisis.

Brockhurst RJ: Photocoagulation in congenital retinoschisis. Arch Ophthalmol *84*:158–165, 1970

Brodrick JD, Wyatt HT: Hereditary sex-linked retinoschisis. Br J Ophthalmol *57*:551–559, 1973

Burns RP, Lovrien FW, Cibis AB: Juvenile sex-linked retinoschisis: Clinical and genetic studies. Trans Am Acad Ophthalmol Otolaryngol *75*:1011–1021, 1971

Ide CH, Wilson RJ:: Juvenile retinoschisis. Br J Ophthalmol *57*:560–562, 1973

Sabates FN: Juvenile retinoschisis. Am J Ophthalmol *62*:683–688, 1966

Sarin LK, Green WR, Daile EG: Juvenile retinoschisis. Congenital vascular veils and hereditary retinoschisis. Am J Ophthalmol *57*:793–796, 1964

Yanoff M, Rahn EK, Zimmerman LE: Histopathology of juvenile retinoschisis. Arch Ophthalmol *79*:49–53, 1968

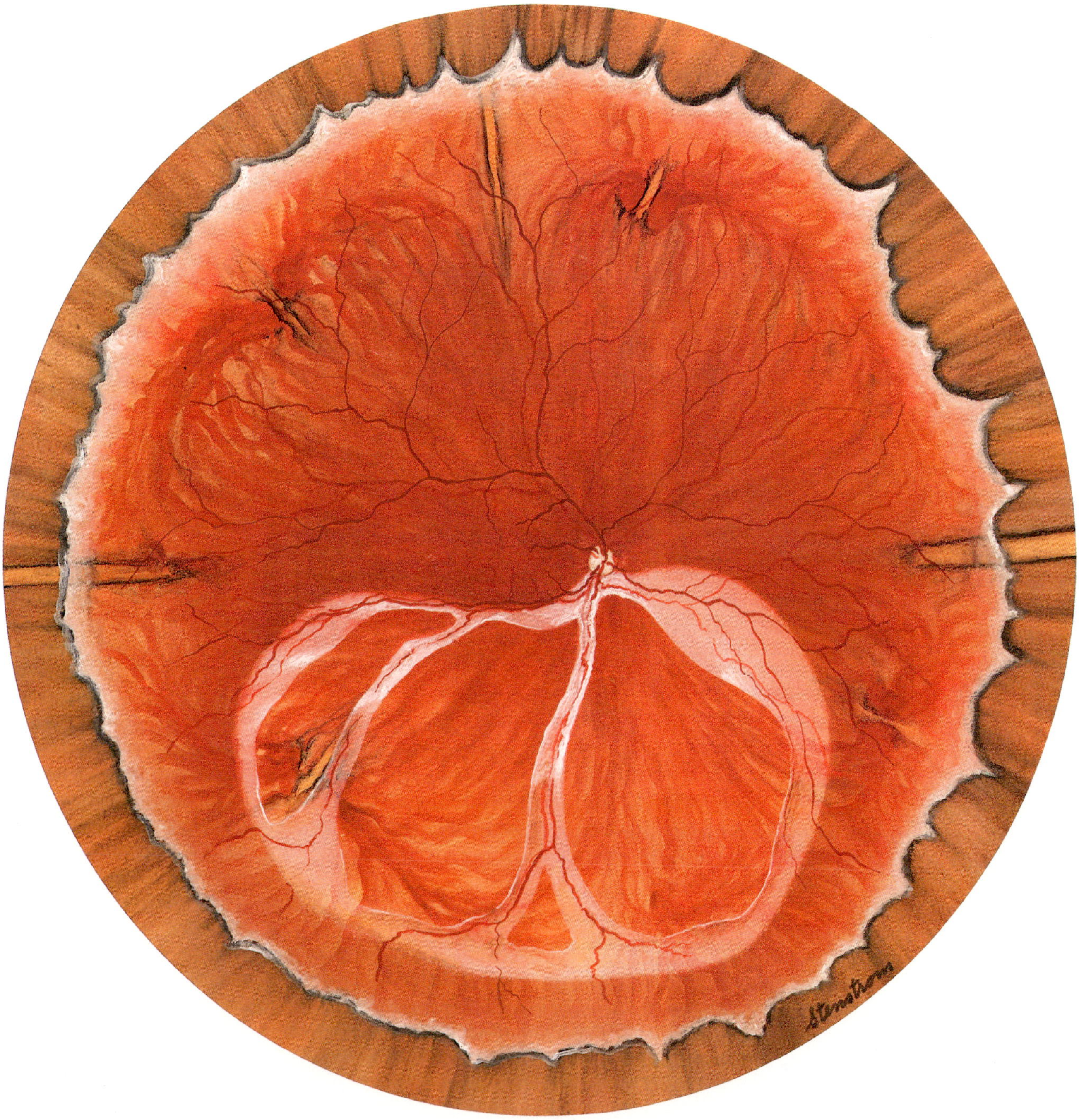

PLATE 98

SENILE RETINOSCHISIS

Retinoschisis means splitting of the retina. The adult, or senile type of degenerative retinoschisis is divided into two forms, the typical form, which is small, is minimally elevated, and rarely extends posterior to the equator, and the reticular form, which is highly elevated and frequently extends posterior to the equator. Both forms occur most commonly in the inferior temporal quadrant, with the superior temporal quadrant next most commonly affected. The peak age incidence is from 50 to 70 years and there is no marked sex predilection. Usually, there are no symptoms. Visual field testing shows an absolute scotoma in the periphery, corresponding to the affected area.

In the typical form of degenerative retinoschisis, there is a minimally elevated, smooth inner retinal layer that contains blood vessels just posterior to a row of typical cystoid degeneration. On the surface of the inner retinal layer, white flecks are usually visible. The blood vessels frequently are sheathed in white, but they are believed to remain patent.

The reticular degenerative form of retinoschisis, shown here in the inferior temporal quadrant, is much more dramatic in appearance. There is a large, highly elevated, bullous inner retinal layer containing the retinal vessels. This inner retinal layer is very smooth, convex, and transparent and appears fixed in position. It does not vary in shape or size as the eye is moved slightly. This characteristic differentiates its appearance from that of a highly elevated retinal detachment. The inner retinal layer has a characteristic watered silk or shagreen appearance, with white flecks and sheathed retinal vessels. Multiple, small, round retinal holes may occur in this inner retinal layer. The outer layer of reticular bullous retinoschisis appears much thicker than the inner layer and is generally closely applied to the pigment epithelium. There may be outer layer breaks, which are usually large, round, and may contain rolled edges. Rarely, a true retinal detachment may occur when there is a combination of inner and outer layer holes.

Beyer NE: Clinical study of senile retinoschisis. Arch Ophthalmol *79*:36–44, 1968

Foos RY: Senile retinoschisis. Relation to cystoid degeneration. Trans Am Acad Ophthalmol Otolaryngol *74*:33–51, 1970

Shea M, Schepens CL, von Pirquet SR: Retinoschisis: I, Senile type: A clinical report of 107 cases. Arch Ophthalmol *63*:1–9, 1960

Straatsma BR, Foos RY: Typical and reticular degenerative retinoschisis. Am J Ophthalmol *75*:551–560, 1973

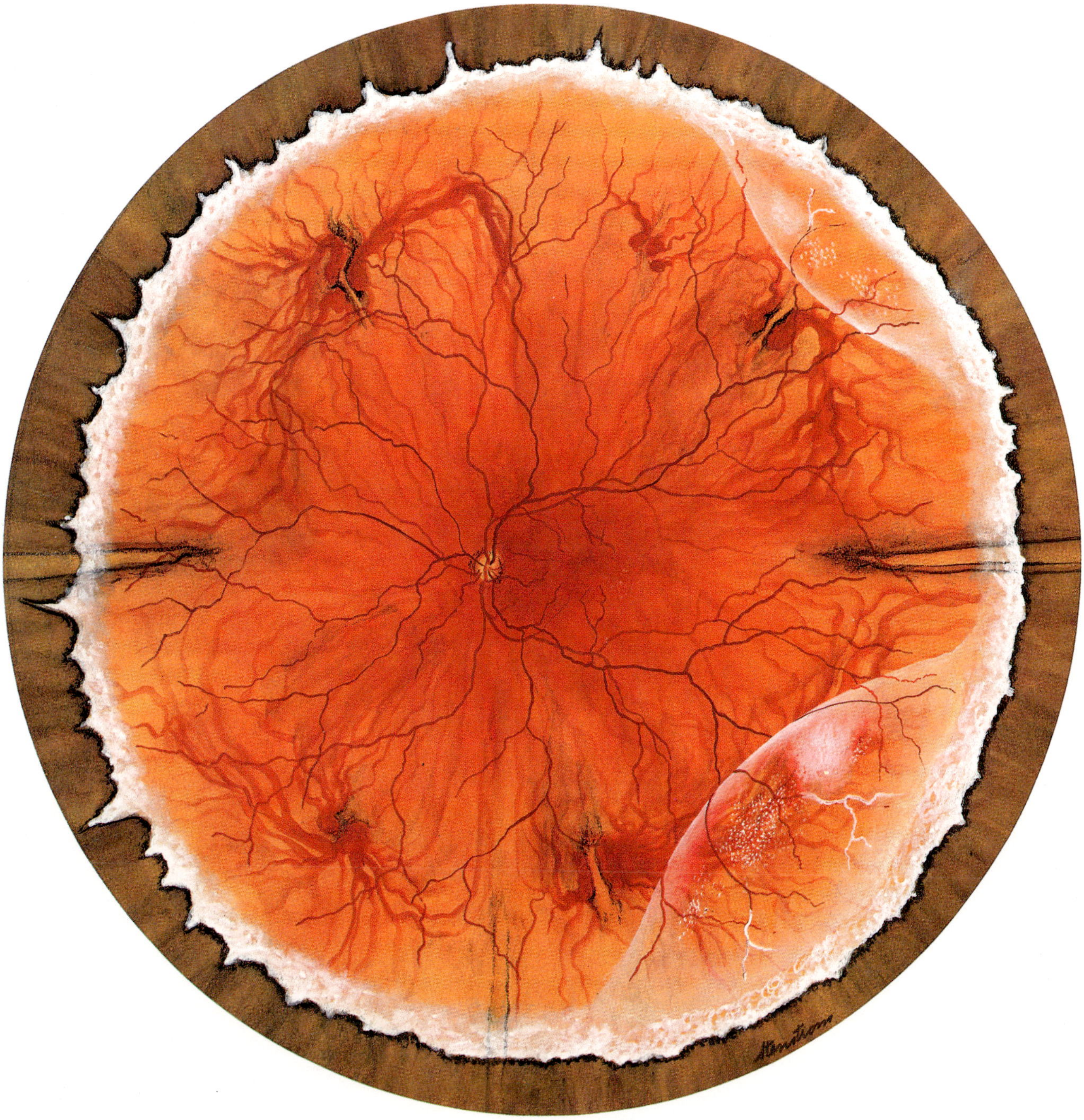

PLATE 99

GIANT CENTRAL SEROUS CHOROIDOPATHY

Central serous choroidopathy is a blister-like elevation of the retina caused by leakage of the choriocapillaris. Usually only the macular area is involved, but sometimes, as shown here, the serous elevation becomes very large and bullous and extends inferiorly toward the periphery. When the serous detachment becomes this large, the process may be confused with a rhegmatogenous retinal detachment or other causes of serous retinal detachment.

Most commonly affected are young males between the ages of 20 and 40 who are undergoing emotional stress but are otherwise in excellent health. Initial symptoms include mildly blurred vision, a central scotoma, distortion of straight lines, and objects appearing smaller than they appear with the opposite, normal eye. The visual acuity is usually near normal and can be improved with small plus lenses.

The origin of the clear fluid is a leak of the choriocapillaris through the pigment epithelium into the subretinal space. Sometimes the area of leakage can be identified as a discrete white spot in the pigment epithelium, but usually a fluorescein angiogram is required to identify the location of the leaking area. Many patterns of leakage have been described, but usually there is slow diffusion of fluorescein dye into the clear subretinal fluid. In central serous choroidopathy, there is no subretinal hemorrhage or subretinal neovascularization. Central serous choroidopathy may undergo spontaneous regression within several months and may be recurrent.

Gass JDM: Pathogenesis of disciform detachment of the neuroepithelium. II, Idiopathic central serous choroidopathy. Am J Ophthalmol 63:587–615, 1967

Gass JDM: Photocoagulation treatment of idiopathic central serous choroidopathy. Trans Am Acad Ophthalmol Otolaryngol 83:456–467, 1977

Gass JDM: Bullous retinal detachment. An unusual manifestation of idiopathic central serous choroidopathy. Am J Ophthalmol 75:810–821, 1973

Klein ML, Van Buskirk EM, Friedman E, et al: Experience with non treatment of central serous choroidopathy. Arch Ophthalmol 91:247–250, 1974

Watzke RC, Burton TC, Leaverton PE: Ruby laser photocoagulation therapy of central serous retinopathy. Trans Am Acad Ophthalmol Otolaryngol 78:205–211, 1974

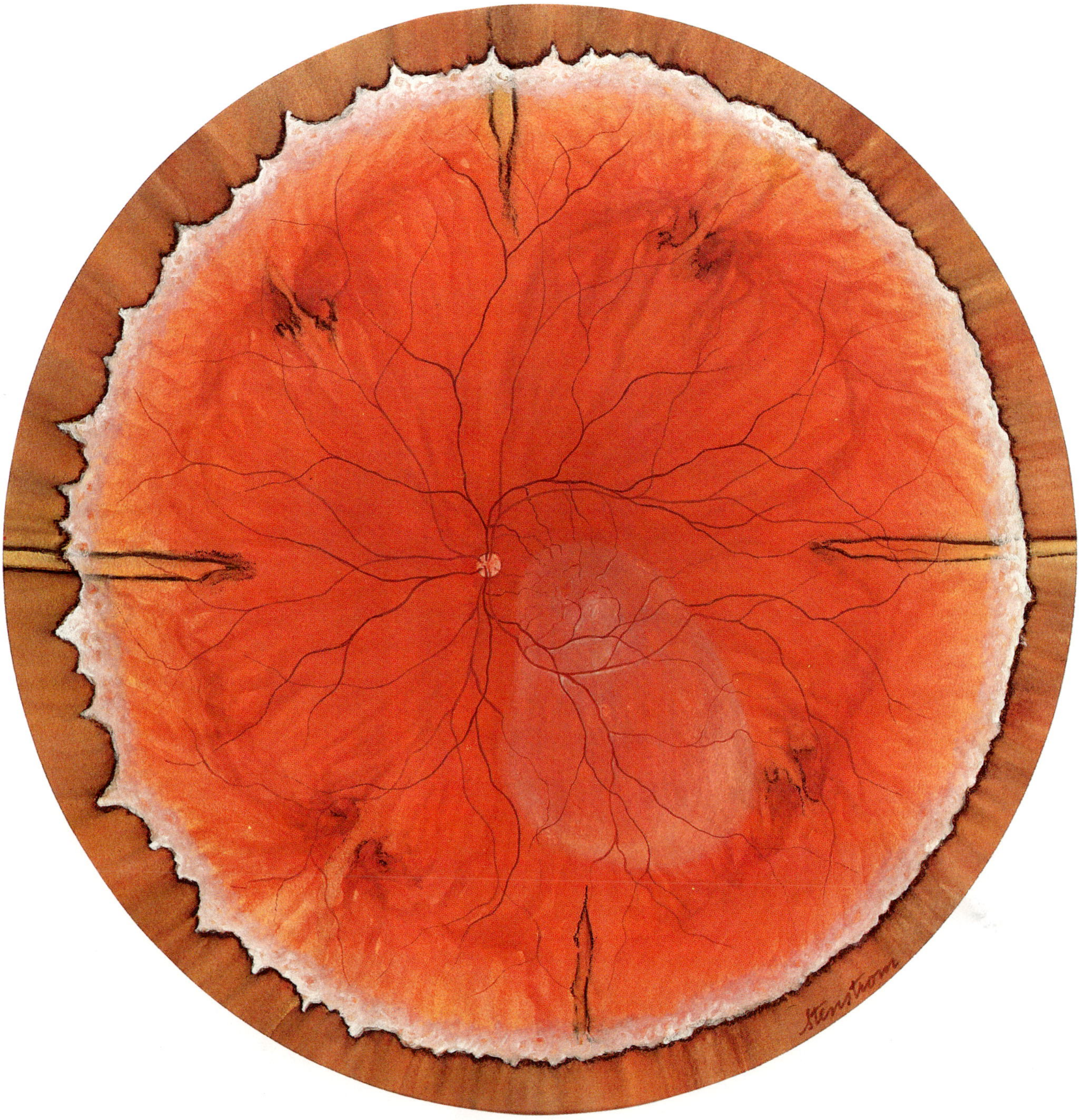

PLATE 100

VOGT-KOYANAGI-HARADA SYNDROME

The Vogt-Koyanagi-Harada syndrome is characterized by systemic manifestations and eye findings. The onset of ocular symptoms frequently follows a nonspecific viral illness with headache, stiff neck, and temporary deafness. Later in the course of the disease alopecia and poliosis may occur. The disease typically strikes young adults of the pigmented races sporadically and without warning. There is a suggested association with certain HLA histocompatibility antigens.

Symptoms include bilaterally decreased vision with pain, redness, and photophobia. Examination of the eyes reveals cells and flare in the anterior chamber, and frequently synechiae of the iris. Fundus findings include vitreous cells, retinal edema, and rarely hemorrhage. Exudative retinal detachment occurs with a profound decrease in visual acuity. The exudative retinal detachment is characterized by subretinal fluid that shifts depending on the position of the patient. The patient shown here is lying supine; therefore, the subretinal fluid collects in the posterior pole. No retinal breaks are present. As the disease runs it course, there may be spontaneous reattachment of the retina leaving focal areas of retinal depigmentation and clumps of subretinal pigment. Histological studies show a chronic, diffuse, granulomatous uveitis resembling sympathetic uveitis with involvement of the choriocapillaris.

Ohno S, Char DH, Kimura SJ, et al: Vogt-Koyanagi-Harada syndrome. Am J Ophthalmol *83*:735–740, 1977

Pattison EM: Uveomeningoencephalitic syndrome (Vogt-Koyanagi-Harada). Arch Neurol *12*:197–205, 1965

Perry HD, Font RL: Clinical and histopathologic observations in severe Vogt-Koyanagi-Harada syndrome. Am J Ophthalmol *83*:242–254, 1977

Snyder DA, Tessler HH: Vogt-Koyanagi-Harada syndrome. Am J Ophthalmol *90*:69–75, 1980

Suguira S: Vogt-Koyanagi-Harada disease. Japan J Ophthalmol *22*:9–35, 1978

Yoshioka H: Fluorescence fundus angiographic findings in early stage of Harada's syndrome. Acta Soc Ophthalmol Jap *72*:2298–2306, 1968

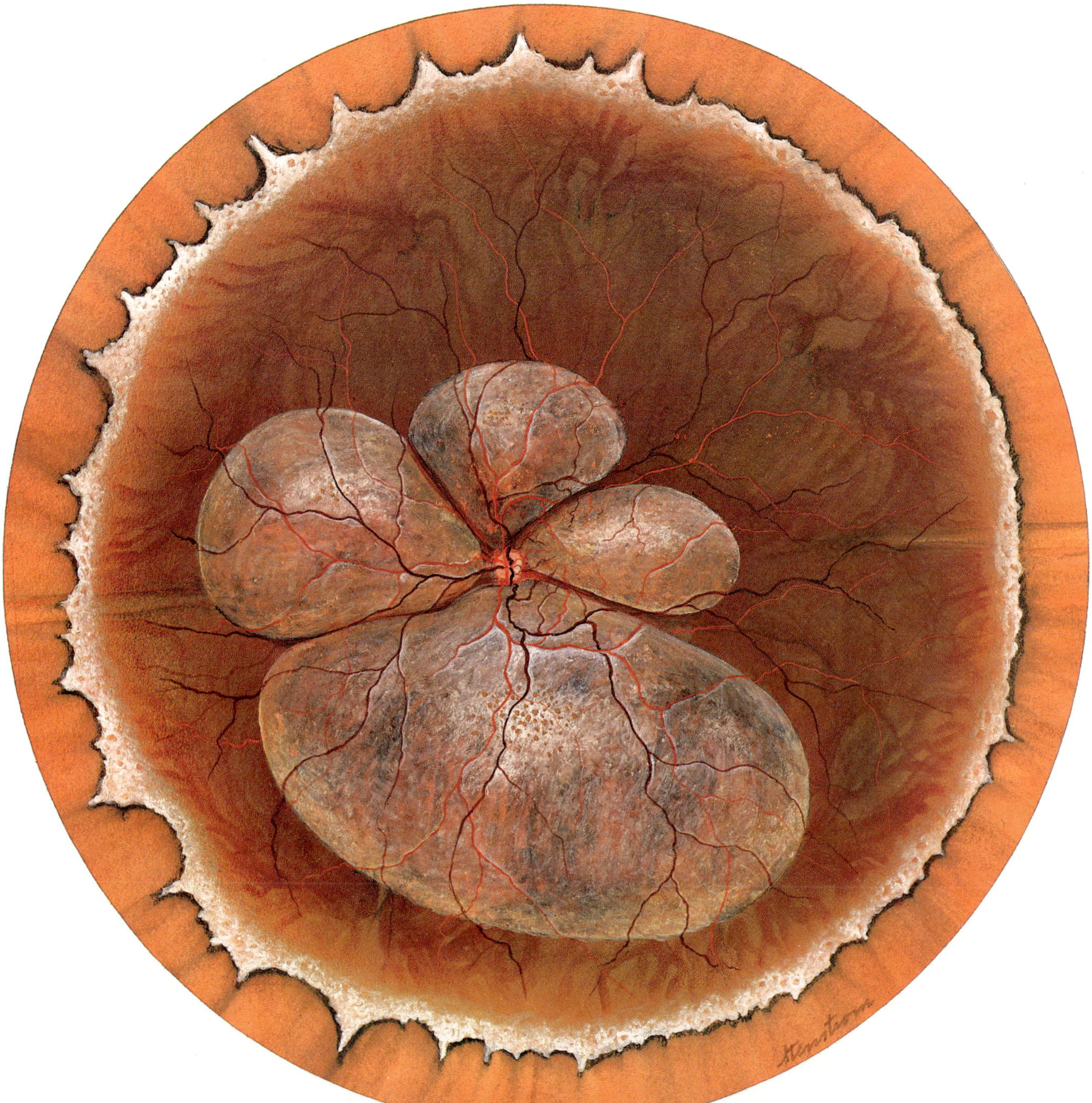

PLATE 101

INDEX

Numbers in *italics* refer to illustrations.

INDEX